Psychological Selection and Optimal Experience Across Cultures

Cross-Cultural Advancements in Positive Psychology

Volume 2

The aim of the *Cross Cultural Advancements in Positive Psychology* book series is to spread a universal and culture-fair perspective on good life promotion. The series will advance a deeper understanding of the cross-cultural differences in well-being conceptualization. A deeper understanding can affect psychological theories, interventions and social policies in various domains, from health to education, from work to leisure. Books in the series will investigate such issues as enhanced mobility of people across nations, ethnic conflicts and the challenges faced by traditional communities due to the pervasive spreading of modernization trends. New instruments and models will be proposed to identify the crucial components of well-being in the process of acculturation. This series will also explore dimensions and components of happiness that are currently overlooked because happiness research is grounded in the Western tradition, and these dimensions do not belong to the Western cultural frame of mind and values.

For further volumes:
http://www.springer.com/series/8420

Antonella Delle Fave · Fausto Massimini · Marta Bassi

Psychological Selection and Optimal Experience Across Cultures

Social Empowerment through Personal Growth

Springer

Antonella Delle Fave
Professor of Psychology
Dipartimento di Scienze Cliniche
Luigi Saccos
Università degli Studi di Milano
20157 Milano
Italy
antonella.dellefave@unimi.it

Fausto Massimini
Professor of Psychology
Dipartimento di Scienze Cliniche
Luigi Saccos
Università degli Studi di Milano
20157 Milano
Italy
fausto.massimini@unimi.it

Marta Bassi
Assistant Professor of Psychology
Dipartimento di Scienze Cliniche
Luigi Saccos
Università degli Studi di Milano
20157 Milano
Italy
marta.bassi@unimi.it

ISSN 2210-5417
e-ISSN 2210-5425
ISBN 978-90-481-9875-7
ISBN 978-90-481-9876-4 (eBook)
DOI 10.1007/978-90-481-9876-4
Springer Dordrecht Heidelberg London New York

Library of Congress Control Number: 2010938973

Printed on acid-free paper

Springer is part of Springer Science+Business Media (www.springer.com)

We gratefully dedicate this book to
Dr. Krishna Rao
Sister Ignazia
Marida and Mario

Introduction

Human history is replete with political and economic crises, environmental disasters, wars, injustice, and destruction. It is also characterized by outstanding endeavors such as impressive artistic works, technologies, acts of altruism, gratitude, and cooperation. These highly paradoxical facets are all results of mankind, a species which has evolved on the principles of biological and cultural selection in interaction with the surrounding environment.

The evolution of the brain, the emergence of the mind, and the social nature of man have contributed to the development of a third paradigm, psychological selection, which interacts with biological and cultural instructions in adapting man to his living environment. Psychological selection represents the process according to which individuals select and replicate in time information coming from their environment, both shaping their life trajectories and actively contributing to the cultural and biological trends of their species. This is the topic the present book is about: psychological selection and the active role of individuals and communities in molding their survival on earth. In developing this topic, we will resort to our lifelong commitment as psychologists to the understanding of the contradictions in human nature, trying—like all other human beings—to give sense to human actions and behaviors, and envisaging the ways in which individuals' potentials and resources can contribute to social empowerment and to the creation of a peaceful and thriving global community.

While this aim may sound like hubris, or at best utopia, it is currently being shared by a growing number of scientists in various disciplines who aim at providing a change in focus from understanding and mending the ills of human beings to comprehending and enhancing their virtues. The theoretical background we refer to is positive psychology. As illustrated in Chapter 1, positive psychology is a novel approach to studying human behavior which aims at catalyzing a change in focus from preoccupation only with repairing the worst things in life to also building positive qualities. A key interest is the analysis of happiness which has been broadly defined according to two philosophical traditions: hedonism and eudaimonism. The hedonic view equates happiness with pleasure, comfort, and enjoyment, whereas the eudaimonic view equates happiness with the human ability to pursue complex goals which are meaningful to the individual and society. Besides analyzing the antecedents, correlates, and consequences that happiness entails for human well-being at the individual and community levels, recent trends in positive psychology call for the integration of the hedonic and eudaimonic views into a global theory of human well-being, and stress the need to adopt a cross-cultural perspective on happiness which would take into account a worldwide concept of a life worth living.

It is within the broad positive psychology perspective of eudaimonia that we contextualize the three selective paradigms we presented above. Chapter 2 illustrates the processes of selection and transmission of biological and cultural information. In particular, culture is described as an emergent inheritance system that ultimately predominates on biology in shaping and directing human behavior at both the individual and the social levels. However, culture and biology interact in complex ways that impact on the relationships among human societies. Material and symbolic artifacts represent extrasomatic cultural products which substantially mediate the relationship between individuals and their environment.

Chapter 3 is devoted to the analysis of the process of psychological selection, and the role of individuals as active agents, who create, select, and replicate in time biological and cultural information according to personal meanings, goals, and experiences which are only partially constrained by biological and cultural inheritance. Flow or optimal experience is the core of psychological selection. We owe to Mihaly Csikszentmihalyi the thorough investigation of this state of consciousness back in the mid-1970s. Through the analysis of people's self-reports and descriptions of their quality of experience in various situations and contexts—for example, while performing complex and challenging tasks at work or during leisure time—he detected a particularly complex and positive state of consciousness characterized by deep involvement, absorption and enjoyment in challenging tasks in which individuals could invest matching levels of personal resources and skills.

Because of their intrinsic reward, activities associated with optimal experience tend to be cultivated in time and can lead to the lifelong construction of personal interests and goals, namely individuals' life themes. Flow can trigger the active investment of time and effort in the practice and cultivation of the associated activities, thus progressively leading to an increase in skills and competencies and to the search for higher challenges, in order to support the engagement, concentration, and involvement that characterize optimal experience in the long term.

Ever since Csikszentmihalyi's pioneering work, a great number of instruments and methodologies have been developed for the study of flow, which are presented in Chapter 4. The majority of them are based on individuals' self-reports of the content of their consciousness. Additionally, methods vary according to the level of control exerted on the flow construct: They include observation and interview techniques, psychological surveys, and experimental studies. In particular, we present some tools we have extensively applied in our research work: (a) Flow Questionnaire and Life Theme Questionnaire, which through open-ended and scaled questions allow for the specific analysis of flow, flow-associated situations, and the meaning of such experience in the psychic organization of the individual and in the construction of her life theme and (b) Experience Sampling Method (ESM), through which individuals provide online repeated descriptions of daily situations and of their states of consciousness as daily life unfolds. By means of these instruments and methods, more than three decades of research have provided extensive information on the phenomenology of optimal experience.

An overview of the findings—gathered primarily with ESM—is shown in Chapter 5. Flow is characterized by a stable cognitive core around which affective and motivational variable fluctuate according to the kind of associated activities. In light of these findings, our research team suggested that flow may not be a monolithic experience, and that there could be a family of optimal experiences related to the characteristics of associated tasks. This chapter further delves into individual and cultural features that have been found to favor individuals' retrieval of optimal experience in daily life. These include personality traits, physical conditions, personal goals, autonomy, family context, and activity characteristics, such as challenge and structure. Moreover, this chapter presents a comparison of flow with similar constructs such as peak experience and involvement and an analysis of the relationship between flow and other positive-psychology constructs.

The analysis of the features of optimal experience extends to Chapter 6. One of the crucial aspects of flow is complete absorption and focus of attention on the ongoing task. This psychological characteristic, and its chief importance within the phenomenology of flow, led us to inquire about the analogy between optimal experience and the states of meditation that are triggered by the concentration of attention on one single object. Such states have been systematically explored within the several philosophical systems and wisdom traditions developed in ancient India, which provided amazingly deep investigations of human psychological functions and consciousness processes. Chapter 6 is thus devoted to the analysis of the shared and divergent components of optimal experience and meditation, and to the contextualization of their phenomenological analysis within cultural and epistemological dimensions.

Having presented the theoretical and methodological aspects of our research, we next turn to applications. This part of the book is primarily centered on the field studies we have conducted around the world in Western and non-Western cultures, but it also includes findings obtained by international research teams. Some areas of investigation—such as work, education, or leisure—have been extensively studied, whereas others—such as cross-cultural issues, relationships, spirituality, migration, health, and maladjustment—have been largely unexplored by international flow academics, and we thus report unique novel data.

Chapter 7 introduces this book section providing an overview of psychological selection across cultures. By drawing from our databank of more than 1,000 adult and adolescent participants gathered with Flow Questionnaire and Life Theme Questionnaire, the universality of optimal experience as well as its relevance to individual and cultural functioning is presented. In addition, the importance of flow-related activities in fostering personal growth and cultural empowerment is analyzed by focusing on crucial life domains such as productive activities, leisure, interactions, and human development. Some of the issues raised in this chapter are then extensively analyzed in the following sections.

Chapter 8 centers on work as a fundamental human activity on which the bio-cultural survival and reproduction of individuals and groups are based. Work represents a privileged area for retrieving optimal experiences, in spite of the great emphasis individuals place on leisure activities. We thus present the peculiarities of the work experience compared to leisure and highlight personal, organizational, as well as cultural factors associated with optimal experience at the workplace. Attention is also paid to the role that work plays in individuals' psychological selection and well-being, by funneling psychic and material resources into pursuing professional fulfillment.

Leisure is the topic of Chapter 9. Free time includes various activities such as playing sports, practicing hobbies, idling, volunteering, interacting, watching TV, and playing videogames. These activities vary in terms of their contribution to individuals' development and well-being. From a broad perspective, they can be divided into serious and casual leisure, based on the constancy and duration of individuals' engagement. Starting from these conceptualizations, this chapter primarily focuses on sports and hobbies and media use. It illustrates the quality of associated experience and their potential as flow opportunities, as well as the individual and cultural features associated with optimal experience in leisure. The risks of free time in terms of disengagement and deviant behavior are also presented.

Considering the importance of relationships throughout human life span, we have devoted Chapter 10 to relational issues. Biological as well as cultural pressures substantially contribute to shape the features and functions of human interaction patterns within families, communities, and broader societies. Attention is paid to the role of relationships in fostering optimal experiences and in directing the process of psychological selection. Moving from core theoretical assumptions concerning the developmental implications of relationships in both individualistic and collectivistic countries, we present cross-cultural findings from family studies, focusing on parent–children interactions, sibling relations, friendship, as well as the opposite condition of solitude.

Chapter 11 explores education as the primary means of cultural transmission. A variety of educational systems and pedagogic strategies have been created in order to deal with this challenge across cultures. By promoting the association of their instructions with individuals' psychological selection, cultures can successfully survive in the long term, and at the same time support individuals' development and well-being. Given the importance of learning for both individuals and societies, flow researchers have devoted much attention to its investigation. In this chapter, we sum up major findings related to the quality of experience during formal learning activities across cultures. We identify the activities associated with optimal experience, the contextual and individual factors favoring flow in education, and we outline the short-term and long-term consequences of flow in learning. In particular, we stress the active role of the individual in perpetrating cultural information and the importance of an educational system allowing for the integration of instructions from different cultures thus sustaining plurality, complexity, and differentiation in a global society.

In Chapter 12 we investigate the role of religious practice in promoting optimal experience, as well as in shaping the process of psychological selection. Data obtained from participants belonging to different cultures and religious traditions are discussed. More specifically, we illustrate the occurrence of optimal experience during religious practice, its psychological features, and the relevance of religion among past life influences, present challenges, and future goals. Even though findings reveal that religion is not a relevant opportunity for optimal experience in daily life, they also highlight its importance in facing stressful situations and in providing individual and collective meanings and values.

The last three chapters broadly deal with adjustment and health. Chapter 13 tackles the process of migration which characterizes our times more than any other periods in history. Globalization poses a number of challenges: These range from enhanced mobility of people across nations to ethnic conflicts and to the disruption of traditional civilizations due to the dominance of the Western mono-cultural model. This phenomenon calls for the analysis of the cultural representations of happiness and well-being and of the relations between individuals and their cultural environment. Our studies on immigrants and ethnic minorities are presented in this chapter. Results show that the occurrence of optimal experiences and the features of the associated activities, as well as perceived current challenges and future goals, are primarily connected with the life opportunities offered by the hosting country, along with participants' cultural distance and length of stay. This information can be useful in designing programs to support the psychological well-being and socio-cultural adjustment of immigrants and minority members.

In Chapter 14 the relationship between psychophysical health and optimal experience is presented through the analysis of findings coming from individuals with motor and sensory disabilities, participants with eating disorders, women who underwent breast cancer surgery, and people with mental illness. Disease is not necessarily synonymous with suffering and languishing; occasions for personal growth and meaning finding can also be retrieved when physical conditions are suboptimal, or when accidents and traumas hit individuals' lives. In these occasions, people can resort to crucial personal resources, social support, and cultural and environmental factors that can promote well-being and can favor the construction of a life worth living.

Concerning people facing severe psychosocial problems and exposed to conditions of hardship and marginalization, little research has been conducted on their opportunities for optimal experience. Do they enjoy flow experiences during their daily life, and in which domains? How do their problematic conditions affect their psychological selection pattern and their potential for development, goal setting and pursuit? Chapter 15 investigates these issues in two specific categories of people living under difficult circumstances: children and adolescents exposed to neglect, abuse, and street life in different countries and drug addicts. Findings highlight a crucial aspect of psychosocial maladjustment: Opportunities for positive feelings and elation are available in daily life, but they do not provide authentic and complex flow experiences. This issue has to be taken into account in designing intervention and treatment programs, in order to make them both appealing to users and effective in their rehabilitation aims.

Even though this book certainly does not comprise all the rich knowledge researchers have gathered over the years on such complex an issue as psychological selection, we hope that the readers may find in it useful information on the advancements in this scientific domain, may encounter suggestions on practical issues aiming to improve individuals' and communities' well-being, and may be spurred to take on the challenge of pursuing the investigation of optimal experience and positive human growth.

This book is the fruit of our personal commitment to research in this field. However, we would not have been able to write it without the precious help of all those people who have supported us in this endeavor. First and foremost, we thank Mihaly Csikszentmihalyi who has inspired our work ever since our first meeting back in the mid-1970s, at a time in which mainstream research hardly recognized subjective experience as a legitimate topic in scientific psychology. His incredible insight into the phenomenology of optimal experience and his broad-minded vision of human nature have set a cornerstone in our research and have paved the way for a fruitful collaboration and a lifelong friendship. We would also like to thank all those students and colleagues who enthusiastically joined our research group over the years and bravely helped us in collecting the largest extant cross-cultural databank on optimal experience. Last but not least, we thank all the participants in our studies who shared with us the beauties in their lives, and in so doing gave meaning to ours.

Contents

Part I
Theory and Methods

Chapter 1
Hedonism and Eudaimonism in Positive Psychology

1.1 Positive Psychology: Past and Present

In 2000, Martin Seligman and Mihaly Csikszentmihalyi officially announced the birth of positive psychology in the first twenty-first century issue of the *American Psychologist*. The two authors therein proposed an in-depth reconsideration of a psychological tradition focused on human shortcomings, deficits, pathologies, and limitations, both at the individual and social levels— and brought forward the need to catalyze a change in the focus of psychology from preoccupation only with repairing the worst things in life to also building positive qualities (Seligman & Csikszentmihalyi, 2000, p. 5). Rather than representing a new formal sector or a new paradigm, positive psychology is a novel approach to studying human behavior, encompassing all areas of psychological investigation such as development, occupation, mental and physical health. As psychologists have never studied systematically the characteristics of fulfilled individuals and thriving communities, little is known about what makes for a life worth living, and how to develop personal and collective resources at optimal levels. Across a variety of research domains, positive psychology privileges the study of the constructive, creative, and generative aspects of individuals and groups. At the subjective level, it focuses on constructs such as well-being and satisfaction, hope and optimism, and flow and happiness. At the individual level, it investigates positive traits: the capacity for love and vocation, courage, interpersonal skill, aesthetic sensibility, perseverance, forgiveness, originality, future-mindedness, high talent, and wisdom. At the group level, it addresses the civic virtues and the institutions that move individuals toward better citizenship: responsibility, nurturance, altruism, civility, moderation, tolerance, and work ethic (Seligman & Csikszentmihalyi, 2000, p. 5). To achieve its aims, positive psychology has to operate at different levels: (a) to articulate a vision of the good life that is empirically sound while being understandable and attractive; (b) to show what actions lead to well-being, to positive individuals, and to flourishing communities; (c) to help document what kind of families result in the healthiest children, what work environments support the greatest satisfaction among workers, what policies result in the strongest civic commitment (Seligman & Csikszentmihalyi, 2000, p. 5).

A. Delle Fave et al., *Psychological Selection and Optimal Experience Across Cultures*, Cross-Cultural Advancements in Positive Psychology 2,
DOI 10.1007/978-90-481-9876-4_1, © Springer Science+Business Media B.V. 2011

In spite of the recent origins of positive psychology as a movement, in the past a number of researchers involved in various psychological domains had already devoted their work to the study of well-being and personal growth. Far from mainstream psychology, these researchers paved the way for the development of positive psychology. Particularly significant in the 1950s and 1960s was humanistic psychology, which heralded a third way, beside the clinical and behaviorist approaches. Within this perspective, Abraham Maslow centered his work on the analysis of human motivation and the fulfillment of basic universal needs. According to his hierarchical model of needs, human beings, once having satisfied primary requirements such as physiological ones, express high-order needs toward self-actualization, in accordance with a subjective life plan toward the full expression of one's self (Maslow, 1970). In the same vein, Carl Rogers (1963) developed the concept of full functioning as the unfolding of one's potentials, as the realization of the healthy and creative characteristics of the individual in a process of constant personal constructive growth.

These pioneer works triggered a paradigm shift, in Kuhn's terms, from a psychology aiming at the compensation of weaknesses and deficits to a psychology focused on human resources and potentials. In the following decades, a growing number of researchers started to investigate the positive side of behavior and psychological processing, formalizing and measuring constructs such as optimism, sense of coherence, self-determination, meaning-making, subjective well-being, hope, positive emotions, wisdom, resilience, and post-traumatic growth. Most of these researchers have now gathered under the positive psychology umbrella, with the aim of developing a science of well-being.

1.2 The Pursuit of Happiness: Two Philosophical Traditions

A key interest of positive psychology is the analysis of happiness: what it is, what factors favor its achievement, what consequences it entails for human well-being at the individual and community levels. The centrality of this issue is attested by the proliferation of TV shows, newspapers and magazines, scientific journals, films, essays and novels, all dealing with happiness. Common people and professionals alike are trying to make sense of a rather elusive concept which can have different interpretations and which can be achieved through different pathways.

The problem in defining happiness primarily stems from the fact that it is not a neutral term, neither at the cultural nor at the psychological levels (Delle Fave & Bassi, 2009; Delle Fave, 2004). Individuals and social groups develop a notion of what is good and desirable as function of their characteristics. Philosophical, ethical, and religious beliefs, personal and collective *Weltanschauungen*, values, meanings, expectations, and needs play a major role in this respect. In addition, there can be fluctuations and even radical changes across time in approaching happiness, as historical and economical circumstances, as well as general beliefs, are subject to change. These are some of the reasons for the historical, geographical, cultural, and subjective heterogeneity in the identification of the nature and features of happiness.

These reasons also underlie positive psychologists' search for a better understanding of the concept, in view of devising intervention strategies that can promote and spread happiness among individuals around the world.

From the theoretical perspective, two opposing philosophical traditions have been advocated by positive psychologists in the definition of happiness: hedonism and eudaimonism—both rooted in ancient Greek philosophy (Ryan & Deci, 2001). The hedonic view equates happiness with pleasure, comfort, and enjoyment. The modern definition of hedonism is commonly referred to Epicure, who in the third century B.C. claimed that people desire pleasure and seek to avoid or minimize pain. However, central to Epicure's theory was the concept of *ataraxia* (freedom from worries or anxiety). Despite great misunderstandings throughout history, the idea of happiness proposed by Epicure does not rely upon pleasure in hedonic terms. Rather it refers to the ability of the individual to maintain balance and serenity in both enjoyable and challenging times, a position which is much closer to contemporary Asian conceptualizations of well-being (see Chapter 6) than to our current understanding of hedonism.

Hobbes argued that happiness lies in the successful pursuit of human appetites, and utilitarian philosophers such as Bentham maintained that a good society is built on individuals' attempts to maximize pleasure and self-interest. It is, however, worth noticing that two utilitarian philosophers like John Stuart Mill and Bertrand Russell sustained that subjective feelings of happiness are not the ultimate target (Ryff & Singer, 2008).

In contrast, the eudaimonic view equates happiness with the human ability to pursue complex goals which are meaningful to the individual and society. This definition dates back to Aristotle who, in *Nicomachean Ethics*, formulated an ethical doctrine to provide guidelines for how to live virtuously (Ryff & Singer, 2008). Aristotle considered hedonic happiness to be a vulgar ideal making humans slaves of desires, and proposed the full realization of the true human nature, or one's daimon, through the exercise of personal virtues and potentials in pursuit of a common good.

While both philosophical perspectives share a common interest in what makes for a good life, three major polarities distinguish happiness as hedonia from happiness as eudaimonia: state versus process, feeling versus functioning, and personal fulfillment versus "integrated fulfillment" (Delle Fave & Bassi, 2007).

First of all, the two visions differ in their focus of interest: Hedonia refers to the achievement of a homeostatic balance through the fulfillment of desires and appetites; in contrast, eudaimonia refers to a process of continuous construction and growth in complexity toward the achievement of the higher good. Second, hedonia substantially endorses pleasantness, as the presence of positive affect and absence of negative affect. Hedonic happiness can take place with no effort at all, "sitting on the couch watching TV, one hand on the remote, and the other in a bag of chips" (King, Eells, & Burton, 2002, p. 37). On the opposite, eudaimonia is related to good functioning in terms of growth opportunities, effort, and commitment. In particular, happiness as feeling good can be set aside, at least temporarily, in the pursuit of important goals, such as family relations, good health, maturity, self-control.

Finally, hedonia is basically focused on personal fulfillment of individualistic needs (Veehoven, 2003). In other words, the happiness of the person takes precedence over the happiness of the community, which is seen as the social space allowing for the fulfillment of self-interest. Vice versa, the eudaimonic view supports the harmonization of individual happiness with collective well-being in a process of mutual influence in which individuals and society collaborate in the construction of a shared project of integrated fulfillment (Nussbaum, 1993).

1.2.1 Hedonia and Eudaimonia in Psychology

Happiness as conceptualized within hedonism and eudaimonism has been investigated in a variety of domains, including economy, medicine, pedagogy, anthropology, and religion. In positive psychology, emphasis has been placed on the operationalization and measurement of hedonia and eudaimonia for the development of a science of happiness (Kahneman, Diener, & Schwarz, 1999; Waterman, 1993).

1.2.1.1 The Hedonic View

The predominant view of happiness among hedonic psychologists rests on the concept of *subjective well-being* proposed by Ed Diener (1984, 2000, 2009a). It includes an emotional component, consisting in the presence of positive emotions and in the absence of negative emotions, and a cognitive component, that is a personal judgment on satisfaction with one's life as a whole, or with specific life domains such as work or relationships. These aspects are evaluated through self-report measures such as PANAS (Positive and Negative Affect Scale; Watson, Clark, & Tellegen, 1988) that assesses a person's positive and negative affect states, and SWLS (Satisfaction with Life Scale; Diener, 1994, 2009b) that evaluates the degree of satisfaction with life. From this perspective, maximizing happiness is the highest human goal (Kahneman et al., 1999). Starting from a largely bottom-up empirical approach, any way in the pursuit of pleasure is thus equally worthy, since what counts most is the attainment of a happy state.

Research has shown that individuals generally perceive themselves as rather happy and that their level of subjective well-being tends to be constant over time (Diener, Oishi, & Lucas, 2003). Such stability is partly related to personality traits: For example, extraversion and agreeableness correlate positively with subjective well-being, while neuroticism is negatively correlated with it (DeNeve & Cooper, 1998; Diener et al., 2003). Individual differences and stability in happiness levels are also predominantly related to genetic factors, as shown in studies on twins (Caprara et al., 2009; Nes, Røysamb, Tambs, Harris, & Reichborn-Kjennerud, 2006, 2008).

Happiness itself is considered as a stable individual trait. Happy individuals tend to construe the same life events and encounters more favorably than unhappy people (Lyubomirsky & Tucker, 1998). Factors such as health, income, educational level, and marital status account for just a small portion of the variance in subjective well-being measures (Diener et al., 2003). These findings can be interpreted in light of the classical study by Brickman and Campbell (1971), showing that individuals tend to adapt to life conditions very quickly. They first react strongly to good and bad events, but they then return to their original level of happiness. This underlying adaptation mechanism could also account for the general stability in subjective well-being levels in the United States and other highly developed countries, in spite of the fact that income has risen dramatically since World War II (Myers, 2000).

However, subsequent research has shown that life circumstances do have a critical influence on subjective well-being (Diener, 2000). First of all, the measurement of the ongoing experience in daily life situations allowed researchers to detect fluctuations in the individuals' cognitive, motivational, and emotional states during the course of a day, which are strongly influenced by the external context (Schimmack, 2003; Schmidt, Shernoff, & Csikszentmihalyi, 2007). Second, people do not habituate completely to all conditions, even after many years: For example, individuals with congenital disabilities report somewhat lower levels of subjective well-being than individuals without physical disabilities (Mehnert, Kraus, Nadler, & Boyd, 1990).

Research also showed that subjective well-being has both a direct and an indirect positive influence on individuals' health, being positively correlated with physical health (Okun, Stock, Haring, & Witter, 1984), satisfactory relations (Russell & Wells, 1994), management of one's health conditions (Aspinwall, 1998), and longevity (Danner, Snowdon, & Friesen, 2001). However, the relation between subjective well-being and health may be more complex than one might expect: Some people with objectively poor health report high subjective well-being, whereas some people with low well-being have no signs of somatic illness. Ryan and Deci (2001) suggest that these findings can be more fully interpreted in light of individuals' meaning-making processes, interpretative and reporting styles—constructs that have been mostly investigated by eudaimonic psychologists.

In the Broaden-and-Build Theory, the most recent and articulated framework on positive emotions, Barbara Fredrickson (2001) showed that positive emotions can facilitate the mobilization of personal resources, as well as goal planning and pursuit. Individuals experiencing positive emotions show thought schemes that are unusual, creative, integrative, open to information and effective (cognitive broadening). Broadening thought/action repertoires can have long-term benefits, in that these actions and repertoires contribute to building lasting personal resources at the physical, cognitive, and social levels. While negative emotions cause an increase in cardiovascular activity, positive emotions speed up resumption of average activation values, thus offsetting the effect of negative emotions and contributing to individuals' health (Fredrickson & Levenson, 1998).

A final relevant area of investigation in hedonist psychology is the analysis of subjective well-being across countries (Diener, 2000, 2009c; Diener et al., 2003; Veenhoven, 2009). Studies have revealed two major findings. The first one regards the differences in the mean levels of subjective well-being between nations. Observed discrepancies seem to be related to both economic and cultural factors. Wealthier nations have been found to have higher levels of subjective well-being than poorer nations (Diener & Biswas-Diener, 2002). One reason could be that wealthy nations are more likely to fulfill basic human needs for food, shelter, and health, and to score higher on human rights, equality, and democratic governance. At the cultural level, differences in subjective well-being may be due to the psychological meanings people in different nations attach to positive and negative affect. For example, among East Asians and Asian Americans negative affect seems to play a major role in the assessment of subjective well-being, whereas Europeans and European Americans tend to emphasize positive affect (Wirtz, Chiu, Diener, & Oishi, 2009). The second finding regards the levels of subjective well-being within nations. In this respect, not only have data highlighted a strong correlation between subjective well-being and wealth, they have also identified a specific trend over time (Diener et al., 2003). In poor countries, small increments in income have a substantial impact on reported well-being; by contrast, in wealthy countries, well-being levels tend to remain stable across time in spite of income increase. Again, the differential impact of wealth can be related to the idea that at low levels of income, increments are likely to be related to satisfaction of inherent human needs, whereas at high levels of income, they simply lead to the purchase of more luxury items, which do not contribute to the fulfillment of basic needs (Veenhoven, 1991, 2009).

1.2.1.2 The Eudaimonic View

While hedonic psychologists have mostly focused on happiness as subjective well-being, a variety of theories and approaches have been developed from the eudaimonic perspective.[1] All of them share the view of happiness as an ongoing process, stressing the importance of personal goals and meaning-making, rather than pleasure and enjoyment in the attainment of a good life. In addition, they argue that not all the pathways to happiness are equally good (Ryan & Deci, 2001; Veenhoven, 2003): The mere pursuit for pleasure and self-interest can have a detrimental impact on both individuals and communities, undermining personal health and enhancing depletion of resources. It is partly researchers' task to identify and analyze the virtuous ways conducive to happiness.

One essential aspect of eudaimonic happiness is meaningfulness (Baumeister & Vohs, 2002). Meaning-making represents a crucial process in organizing the individuals' experience in time (Kegan, 1994), so that daily events are integrated into unique life stories. These stories are subject to constant revision as individuals gather new information in the interaction with their environment, thus leading to the development of an increasingly complex and integrated vision of life and personal experience.

A pioneer in the study of meaning was Frankl (1959) who developed a psychotherapeutic approach centered on the importance of finding value in life, and

---

[1] In this section, we only focus on the major theories of eudaimonic happiness. For a thorough presentation of constructs and approaches, see the *Handbook on Positive Psychology* edited by Snyder and Lopez (2009). The rest of the present book is devoted to the theory of psychological selection, which also falls into the eudaimonic perspective.

on the opportunities for growth stemming from experiences of suffering and loss. Through interview methods (Davis, Nolen-Hoeksema, & Larson, 1998) or the narration of life stories (Bauer, McAdams, & Pals, 2008), researchers have shown that meaning satisfies needs for purpose, value, sense of efficacy, and self-worth (Baumeister & Vohs, 2002). Under adverse life circumstances—such as loss, bad health, or trauma—meaning-making facilitates the attribution of significance to events and their better understanding (sense-making). In addition, it can have positive effects on physical and psychological health in that a virtuous process can be triggered in which individuals frame difficult life experiences as transformative experiences, wherein they suffered deep pain but gained new insights about the self (Bauer et al., 2008).

Another contribution to eudaimonic happiness derives from the pursuit of human virtues and the mobilization of personal strengths. Seligman (2002) proposed three pathways to happiness: pleasure, engagement, and meaning. Empirical evidence showed that engagement and meaning are the most significant contributors to happiness relative to pleasure (Peterson, Park, & Seligman, 2005). In particular, analyzing the world's main philosophical and religious traditions, Peterson and Seligman (2004) identified six universal virtues, or fundamental values: wisdom, courage, humanity, justice, temperance, and transcendence. The pursuit of these virtues is favored by 24 character strengths that represent the psychological ingredients of virtues. For example, wisdom can be pursued through curiosity, love of learning, open-mindedness, creativity, and a perspective way of looking at the world. A self-reported instrument, the VIA Inventory of Strengths (VIA, IS; Peterson & Seligman, 2004), was developed to appraise character strengths. Its administration across cultures has shown that strengths require the acquisition and application of knowledge and competence, and that they can be cultivated in the long term along the pathway toward happiness achievement.

Self-determination theory by Deci and Ryan (2000, Ryan & Deci, 2001) has embraced the eudaimonic concept of happiness as process, specifying what it means to actualize the self and how that can be accomplished. Self-determination theory distinguishes different types of motivation on the basis of the perceived locus of causality and degree of autonomy in behavior regulation (Deci & Ryan, 2000). In particular, autonomous motivation—especially intrinsic motivation—represents one pole of self-determination, involving the experience of volition and choice; by contrast, controlled motivation—particularly its extreme identified with extrinsic motivation—represents the opposite pole of self-determination, involving the experience of being pressured and coerced.

Autonomous motivation favors the satisfaction of three basic psychological needs: autonomy, competence, and relatedness. The fulfillment of these needs is essential for psychological growth, the internalization and assimilation of cultural practices, psychological health, as well as the experiences of vitality and self-congruence. Starting from the analysis of basic needs, self-determination research has also distinguished the types of goals and aspirations people pursue in relation to both basic needs and well-being outcomes (Kasser & Ryan, 1996): Intrinsic aspirations comprise personal growth, affiliation and intimacy, contribution to one's community, and physical health; extrinsic aspirations include wealth and material possessions, social recognition and fame, and image or attractiveness.

Much research has been committed to the exploration of factors that facilitate versus thwart motivation and well-being in general, and in specific domains such as work, education, sport, parenting, and treatment (Deci & Ryan, 2000). Two major findings have been highlighted.

One regards the crucial effect of the environment on individuals' self-determination, in terms of both proximal family and relational context and of distal societal and cultural influences. Warm and trusting relations supporting satisfaction of basic needs facilitate natural growth processes, including intrinsically motivated behavior and integration of extrinsic motivation; whereas those environments that forestall autonomy, competence, or relatedness are associated with poorer levels of motivation, performance and well-being (Ryan, Deci, & Grolnick, 1995). While basic psychological needs are universal, research has highlighted considerable variability in the values and goals praised in different cultures. For example, within the American culture people tend to feel volitional and autonomous when they are making their own decisions, consistently with the culture's values that they have internalized. In some East Asian cultures, on the opposite, people may feel more volitional and autonomous when endorsing and enacting the values of those with whom they identify. In both types of cultures autonomy, relative to control, is crucial for intrinsic motivation and well-being, but the forms it takes can nonetheless vary in accord with what is culturally meaningful (Iyengar & Lepper, 1999).

The second crucial finding regards the relationship between wealth and happiness: Material goods and extrinsic aspirations do not satisfy per se basic psychological needs (Kasser & Ryan, 1996). Moreover, achieving money, fame, and image are often contingent on engaging in controlled activities, and can thus detract from a sense of authenticity, and result in lower well-being. The more people focus on financial and materialistic goals, the lower their well-being, both in developed countries such as the United States and Germany and in less-developed countries such as Russia and India (Ryan et al., 1999).

All these approaches point to the pathways conducive to happiness. But what *is* happiness about? From a broad perspective, Carol Ryff (1989) has addressed this question developing the concept of psychological well-being, a multidimensional construct including six substantive aspects of self-realization: self-acceptance, positive relations, personal growth, purpose in life, environmental mastery, and autonomy (Ryff & Singer, 2008). The Psychological Well-being Scale (Ryff & Keyes, 1995; Ryff, 1989) was developed to measure these aspects, Furthermore, Keyes (1998) recently developed a more exhaustive definition of well-being, adding a social component which includes five major aspects: social acceptance, social actualization, social contribution, social coherence, and social integration.

From the life span perspective, research has shown that psychological well-being varies depending on age and gender (Ryff & Keyes, 1995). In particular, autonomy and environmental mastery show incremental profiles with age, purpose in life and personal growth show sharply decremental profiles from young adulthood to old age; finally, positive relations and self-acceptance show little variation (but only for women).

As for gender, women present well-being profiles which are similar to men's, or even better. In particular, women report higher scores in positive relations and personal growth. Research has additionally shown that socioeconomic status has an impact on psychological well-being dimensions such as self-acceptance, purpose in life, environmental mastery, and personal growth (Ryff, Magee, Kling, & Wing, 1999). Finally, high levels of psychological well-being have been shown to have a protective effect on physical health (Keyes, 2007; Ryff & Singer, 2008).

1.3 Happiness: The Ongoing Debate

An increasing number of studies are showing that eudaimonic happiness and hedonic happiness are two highly correlated but separate constructs. In particular, this conclusion was reached by Linley, Maltby, Wood, Osborne, and Hurling (2009), who measured subjective well-being as satisfaction with life, presence of positive affect and absence of negative affect, and psychological well-being in its six dimensions. Similarly, Gallagher, Lopez, and Preacher (2009) identified a hierarchical structure of well-being including three components: subjective well-being, psychological well-being, and social well-being as measured by Keyes (2002) in its five dimensions. These findings attest to the importance of studying both aspects of happiness, contrary to the recent claim by Kashdan et al. (2008) that eudaimonic research may just as well be incorporated into the hedonic view. These authors claim that serious problems remain in the translation of eudaimonia from philosophy to psychology. In particular, they underline that the number of constructs and variables related to eudaimonia serve to confuse, rather than clarify, this concept. Instead of referring to qualitatively different types of happiness, it would be more precise and flexible to provide conceptual frameworks for addressing the question of why particular combinations of elements will lead to various outcomes (Biswas-Diener, Kashdan, & King, 2009, p. 209).

Eudaimonic psychologists readily acknowledge the plurality of views characterizing the eudaimonic approach, which is primarily related to the ontological complexity of the concept of happiness. Not only can happiness be understood as a transient emotion, or an experience of fulfillment and accomplishment (satisfaction with life), it can also be understood as a long-term process of meaning-making and identity development through the actualization of potentials and pursuit of subjectively relevant goals.

Happiness entails an intrinsic paradox: To get happiness forget about it (Martin, 2008). In particular, to directly pursue pleasures or success (for example, money and status) is self-defeating because the most enriching enjoyments are tied to activities and relationships valued for their own sake, and not merely for the pleasures or gains they produce. In addition, self-absorption constricts the range and depth of gratifications available in pursuing interests in other people, activities, and events. Individuals have a variety of goals and interests which they attempt to coordinate through contextual decision making and priorities in life. Some of these are tied to society and cultural values, which give them an overall meaning and do not necessarily constrain individual happiness.

1.3.1 Integrating Perspectives

Rather than dismissing the philosophical underpinnings of eudaimonic research in a premature and reductionistic attempt to homogenize the field of positive psychology (Ryan & Huta, 2009; Waterman, 2008), various researchers have recently aimed to integrate the hedonic and eudaimonic views of happiness. In particular, Martin Seligman (2002) hypothesized that the full life (being high in both eudaimonia and hedonia) leads to greater life satisfaction than pursuit of eudaimonia or hedonia alone, or than the empty life (being low in both eudaimonia and hedonia). Peterson et al. (2005) supported this claim by investigating individual differences in ways of life and priorities in the pursuit of meaning and/or pleasure.

One model integrating hedonia and eudaimonia has been proposed by Corey Keyes (2002, 2007). It is centered on the concept of mental health as a syndrome of personal well-being including symptoms of hedonia and eudaimonia, such as positive feelings (subjective well-being) and positive functioning in life (psychological and social well-being).

Keyes maintains that mental health and mental illness are not opposite ends of a single continuum, but lie on separate continua. Indeed, there is only a modest and negative correlation between them. In particular, on the mental health continuum, presence of mental health is described as flourishing and absence of mental health is characterized as languishing. To be flourishing is to be filled with positive emotions and to be functioning well psychologically and socially (high scores on at least 7 of the 13 scales measuring subjective, psychological and social well-being); to be languishing means to perceive emptiness and stagnation in life (low scores on at least 7 scales).

Research showed that the risk of mental illness onset (e.g., a major depressive episode) was six times greater among languishing individuals compared with flourishing ones (Keyes 2002). Moreover, languishing and depression—both alone and together—were associated with significant psychosocial impairment, in terms of emotional health, limitations of activities of daily living, and workdays lost or cut back. On the contrary, flourishing and absence of mental illness were associated with profiles of better psychosocial functioning and physical health, for example, in terms of cardiovascular diseases, stomach problems, and arthritis (Keyes, 2007).

Interesting results were also obtained in the analysis of those individuals who reported moderate mental health, that is individuals with either moderate levels of both hedonic and eudaimonic well-being or some combinations of each (high hedonic but low eudaimonic or low hedonic and high eudaimonic well-being). The analysis of this group of individuals allowed researcher to highlight that hedonic and eudaimonic constructs of well-being are not redundant, and have differential psychosocial consequences. In particular, individuals with moderate mental health who have high hedonic well-being do not report as good a level of functioning as flourishing individuals who also have high hedonic well-being. This finding was based on the assessment of four major mental disorders: namely, major depression, panic disorder, generalized anxiety, and alcohol dependence (Keyes & Annas, 2009).

In another attempt to integrate the hedonic and eudaimonic views of happiness, Ryan and his colleagues (2008) proposed a model based on self-determination theory. The authors maintain that major goals of eudaimonic research are to specify what living well entails and to identify the expected consequences of such living. From this perspective, living well involves (a) pursuing intrinsic goals and values for their own sake, rather than extrinsic goals and values; (b) behaving in autonomous and volitional ways rather than controlled ways; (c) being mindful and acting with as sense of awareness; and (d) behaving in ways that satisfy basic psychological needs. The consequences of living well may include hedonic satisfactions (subjective well-being), but in addition to psychological well-being, vitality, intimacy, physical health, and sense of meaning.

Indeed, positive affect and pleasure are both correlates and consequences of living well; yet their antecedents can include goals and lifestyles that are antithetical to most eudaimonic conceptions, such as living a life of shallow values, greed, or exploitation of others. The pursuit of hedonic goals cannot by itself lead to either individual or collective well-being. Research has shown that hedonic activities are consistently and positively linked with positive affect and negatively linked with negative affect (Huta & Ryan, 2009). However, eudaimonic activities on average have little relation with emotions; rather, they are strongly linked with eudaimonic outcomes, such as meaning and elevating experience.

Eudaimonia and hedonia thus have different consequences on well-being. In particular, eudaimonia gradually enhances a person's baseline level of well-being, whereas hedonia has more temporary effects. Yet, research also highlighted that individuals high in both hedonic and eudaimonic motives experience greater overall well-being than individuals who are only hedonically oriented or eudaimonically oriented, thus contributing to a full good life (Seligman, 2002).

The complex multiple nature of happiness did not only emerge in research studies guided by philosophical traditions and scientific theory, but it also emerged in the analysis of people's lay conceptions. Adopting both quantitative and qualitative techniques, Delle Fave and her colleagues (2010) investigated the content and contexts of happiness across various western countries. Results showed that individuals prominently define happiness in eudaimonic terms, as a condition of psychological balance and harmony. Moreover, findings showed that meaningfulness and experiencing positive emotions are not the same thing. In particular, they do not refer to the same life domains. Exemplary is the case of work which was quoted by participants as predominantly meaningful, but which was rarely considered as a source of positive emotions. Meaning can thus be perceived and pursued in domains which do not provide hedonic happiness per se, and can have differential effects on overall individuals' psychosocial functioning.

1.3.2 Happiness and Diversity

Acknowledging the multiplicity of pathways to happiness entails a series of crucial directions in future positive psychology research (Delle Fave & Bassi, 2009; Kashdan, Biswas-Diener, & King, 2008; Waterman, 2008). A first group of questions pertain to the measurement of happiness. More attention should be paid to the timeframe of happiness measurement. Happiness can be measured at the global level, through broad assessments across time and context; at the intermediate level, capturing mood and thoughts over durable time spans such as days, weeks, months, or meaningful life periods; and at the momentary level, evaluating immediate events and experiences as they naturally occur (Kashdan et al., 2008). Each level of analysis can provide a different complementary picture of happiness, and cross-level interactions could be explored.

A second group of questions regard the consequences of different potential sources of happiness (Waterman, 2008). The simultaneous measurement of both hedonia and eudaimonia should aim at unraveling how different people experiencing the same event, choosing the same goal or striving, or participating in the same activity may do so because they wish to derive very different things from it. Not only should researchers explore whether some event or goal or activity results in happiness, but also how strongly, and what it is about that event or goal or activity that accounts for the subjective experiences derived from it.

An even more crucial group of issues concern the exploration of the meaning of happiness across cultures (Delle Fave & Bassi, 2009; Delle Fave et al., 2010). Happiness research is primarily grounded in the western tradition, with its individualistic features shared by a minority of nations. The terms hedonia and eudaimonia themselves stem from ancient Greek philosophies. Yet, happiness has been object of investigation in most cultures. Better knowledge of cross-cultural variations in the definition, operationalization, and evaluation of happiness could help unravel its multiple meanings, and put the significance of eudaimonia and hedonia to the test.

Particularly, in this historical period, it is of paramount importance for positive psychology to contextualize the study of happiness within the broader perspective of social empowerment and cooperation across cultures (Delle Fave, Bassi, & Massimini, 2009). Taking into account the active interaction of human beings with their cultural context, individuals should be supported in the pursuit of personal growth and complexity, through the allocation of psychological resources in activities that, besides being opportunities for individual happiness, also bring about positive outcomes to their community.

The outcome of an authentic development at the psychological level is a creative and satisfied person, who is at the same time well integrated in the social environment and committed to the improvement of the cultural system she belongs to (Smith, Christopher, Delle Fave, & Bhawuk, 2002). This definition partially contradicts the present global trend toward homogenization and leveling of individual differences, and the growing emphasis on well-being as satisfaction of material and individualistic needs. Nevertheless, authentic development should be one of the aims of positive psychology, if its ultimate goals are to provide people with a life worth living, and to promote the well-being of communities and societies.

References

Aspinwall, L. G. (1998). Rethinking the role of positive affect in self-regulation. *Motivation & Emotion, 22*, 1–32.

Bauer, J. J., McAdams, D. P., & Pals, J. L. (2008). Narrative identity and eudaimonic well-being. *Journal of Happiness Studies, 9*, 81–104.

Baumeister, R. F., & Vohs, K. D. (2002). The pursuit of meaningfulness in life. In C. R. Snyder & S. J. Lopez (Eds.), *Handbook of positive psychology* (1st ed., pp. 608–617). New York: Oxford University Press.

Biswas-Diener, R., Kashdan, T. B., & King, L. A. (2009). Two traditions of happiness research, not two distinct types of happiness. *Journal of Positive Psychology, 4*, 208–211.

Brickman, P., & Campbell, D. T. (1971). Hedonic relativism and planning the good society. In M. Appley (Ed.), *Adaptation-level theory* (pp. 287–305). New York: Academic Press.

Caprara, G. V., Fagnani, C., Alessandri, G., Steca, P., Gigantesco, A., & Cavalli Sforza, L. L., et al (2009). Optimal human functioning: The genetics of positive orientation towards self, life, and the future. *Behavioral Genetics, 39*, 277–284.

Danner, D., Snowdon, D., & Friesen, W. (2001). Positive emotions in early life and longevity: Findings from the nun study. *Journal of Personality and Social Psychology, 80*, 804–813.

Davis, C. G., Nolen-Hoeksema, S., & Larson, J. (1998). Making sense of loss and benefiting from the experience: Two construals of meaning. *Journal of Personality and Social Psychology, 75*, 561–574.

DeNeve, K. M., & Cooper, H. (1998). The happy personality: A meta-analysis of 137 personality traits and subjective well-being. *Psychological Bulletin, 124*, 197–229.

Deci, E. L., & Ryan, R. M. (2000). The "what" and "why" of goal pursuits: Human needs and the self-determination of behavior. *Psychological Inquiry, 11*, 227–268.

Delle Fave, A. (2004). Positive psychology and the pursuit of complexity. Special issue on positive psychology. *Ricerche di Psicologia, 27*, 7–12.

Delle Fave, A., & Bassi, M. (2007). *Psicologia e salute. L'esperienza di utenti e operatori* [Psychology and health. The experience of patients and professionals]. Torino: UTET Università.

Delle Fave, A., & Bassi, M. (2009). The contribution of diversity to happiness research. *Journal of Positive Psychology, 4*, 205–207.

Delle Fave, A., Bassi, M., & Massimini, F. (2009). Experiencia óptima y evolución humana [optimal experience and psychological selection]. In C. Vasquez & G. Hervas (Eds.), *La ciencia del bienestar. Fundamentos de una psicología positiva* (pp. 209–230). Madrid: Alianza Editorial.

Delle Fave, A., Brdar, I., Freire, T., Vella-Brodrick, D. A., & Wissing, M. P. (2010). The investigation of eudaimonic happiness: Qualitative and quantitative findings. *Social Indicators Research*, DOI 10.1007/s11205-010-9632-5.

Diener, E. (1984). Subjective well-being. *Psychological Bulletin, 95*, 542–575.

Diener, E. (1994). Assessing subjective well-being: Progress and opportunities. *Social Indicators Research, 31*, 103–157.

Diener, E. (2000). Subjective well-being. The science of happiness and a proposal for a national index. *American Psychologist, 55*, 34–43.

Diener, E. (2009a). *The science of well-being* (Vol. 37). Dordrecht, NL: Springer.

Diener, E. (2009b). *Assessing well-being* (Vol. 39). Dordrecht, NL: Springer.

Diener, E. (2009c). *Culture and well-being* (Vol. 38). Dordrecht, NL: Springer.

Diener, E., & Biswas-Diener, R. (2002). Will money increase subjective well-being? A literature review and guide to needed research. *Social Indicators Research, 57*, 119–169.

Diener, E., Oishi, S., & Lucas, R. E. (2003). Personality, culture, and subjective well-being: Emotional and cognitive evaluations of life. *Annual Review of Psychology, 54*, 403–425.
Frankl, V. (1959). *Man's search for meaning: An introduction to logotherapy*. Boston: Beacon
Fredrickson, B. L. (2001). The role of positive emotions in positive psychology: The broaden-and-build theory of positive emotions. *American Psychologist, 56*, 218–226.
Fredrickson, B. L., & Levenson, R. W. (1998). Positive emotions speed recovery from the cardiovascular sequelae of negative emotions. *Cognition and Emotion, 12*, 191–220.
Gallagher, M. W., Lopez, S. J., & Preacher, K. J. (2009). The hierarchical structure of well-being. *Journal of Personality, 77*, 1025–1049.
Huta, V., & Ryan, R. M. (2009). Pursuing pleasure or virtue: The differential and overlapping well-being benefits of hedonic and eudaimonic motives. *Journal of Happiness Studies*, 31 October. Online first.
Iyengar, S. S., & Lepper, M. R. (1999). Rethinking the value of choice: A cultural perspective on intrinsic motivation. *Journal of Personality and Social Psychology, 76*, 349–366.
Kahneman, D., Diener, E., & Schwarz, N. (Eds.) (1999). *Well-being: The foundations of hedonic psychology*. New York: Russell Sage Foundation.
Kashdan, T. B., Biswas-Diener, R., & King, L. A. (2008). Reconsidering happiness: The costs of distinguishing between hedonics and eudaimonia. *Journal of Positive Psychology, 3*, 219–233.
Kasser, T., & Ryan, R. M. (1996). Further examining the American dream: Differential correlates of intrinsic and extrinsic goals. *Personality and Social Psychology Bulletin, 22*, 280–287.
Kegan, R. (1994). *In over our heads*. New York: Cambridge University Press
Keyes, C. L. M. (1998). Social well-being. *Social Psychology Quarterly, 61*, 121–140.
Keyes, C. (2002). The mental health continuum: From languishing to flourishing in life. *Journal of health and social research, 43*, 207–222.
Keyes, C. L. M. (2007). Promoting and protecting mental health as flourishing: A complementary strategy for improving national mental health. *American Psychologist, 62*, 95–108.
Keyes, C. L. M., & Annas, J. (2009). Feeling good and functioning well: Distinctive concepts in ancient philosophy and contemporary science. *Journal of Positive Psychology, 4*, 197–201.
King, L. A., Eells, J. E., & Burton, C. M. (2002). The good life, broadly and narrowly considered. In P. A. Linley & S. Joseph (Eds.), *Positive psychology in practice* (pp. 35–52). New York: Wiley.
Linley, P. A., Maltby, J., Wood, A. M., Osborne, G., & Hurling, R. (2009). Measuring happiness: The higher order factor structure of subjective and psychological well-being measures. *Personality and Individual Differences, 47*, 878–884.
Lyubomirsky, S., & Tucker, K. L. (1998). Implications of individual differences in subjective happiness for perceiving, interpreting, and thinking about life events. *Motivation & Emotion, 22*, 155–186.
Martin, M. W. (2008). Paradoxes of happiness. *Journal of Happiness Studies, 9*, 171–184.
Maslow, A. (1970). *Motivation and personality*. New York: Harper
Mehnert, T., Kraus, H. H., Nadler, R., & Boyd, M. (1990). Correlates of life satisfaction in those with disabling conditions. *Rehabilitation Psychology, 35*, 3–17.
Myers, D. (2000). The funds, friends, and faith of happy people. *American Psychologist, 55*, 56–67.
Nes, R. B., Czajkowski, N., Røysamb, E., Reichborn-Kjennerud, T., & Tambs, K. (2008). Well-being and ill-being: Shared environments, shared genes? *Journal of Positive Psychology, 3*, 253–265.
Nes, R. B., Røysamb, E., Tambs, K., Harris, J. R., & Reichborn-Kjennerud, T. (2006). Subjective well-being: Genetic and environmental contributions to stability and change. *Psychological Medicine, 36*, 1033–1042.
Nussbaum, M. (1993). Non relative virtues: An Aristotelian approach. In M. Nussbaum and A. Sen (Eds.), *The quality of life* (pp. 42–269). Helsinki: United Nations University and WIDER.
Okun, M. A., Stock, W. A., Haring, M. J., & Witter, R. A. (1984). The social activity/subjective well-being relation: A quantitative synthesis. *Research on Aging, 6*, 45–65.

Peterson, C., Park, N., & Seligman, M. E. P. (2005). Orientations to happiness and life satisfaction: The full life versus the empty life. *Journal of Happiness Studies, 6*, 25–41.
Peterson, C., & Seligman, M. E. P. (2004). *Character strengths and virtues: A handbook and classification*. New York: Oxford University Press
Rogers, C. (1963). The actualizing tendency in relation to "motives" and to consciousness. In M. R. Jones (Ed.), *Nebraska symposium on motivation* (pp. 1–24). Lincoln, NE: University of Nebraska Press.
Russell, R., & Wells, P. (1994). Predictors of happiness in married couples. *Personality and Individual Differences, 17*, 313–321.
Ryan, R. M., Chirkov, V. I., Little, T. D., Sheldon, K. M., Timoshina, E., & Deci, E. L. (1999). The American dream in Russia: Extrinsic aspirations in two cultures. *Personality and Social Psychology Bulletin, 25*, 1509–1524.
Ryan, R. M., & Deci, E. L. (2001). On happiness and human potentials: A review of research on hedonic and eudaimonic well-being. *Annual Review of Psychology, 52*, 141–166.
Ryan, R. M., Deci, E. L., & Grolnick, W. S. (1995). Autonomy, relatedness, and the self: Their relation to development and psychopathology. In D. Cicchetti & D. J. Cohen (Eds.), *Developmental psychopathology* (pp. 618–655). New York: Wiley.
Ryan, R. M., & Huta, V. (2009). Wellness as healthy functioning or wellness as happiness: The importance of eudaimonic thinking (response to the Kashdan et al. And waterman discussion). *Journal of Positive Psychology, 4*, 202–204.
Ryan, R. M., Huta, V., & Deci, E. L. (2008). Living well: A self-determination theory perspective on eudaimonia. *Journal of Happiness Studies, 9*, 139–170.
Ryff, C. D. (1989). Happiness is everything, or is it? Explorations on the meaning of psychological well-being. *Journal of Personality and Social Psychology, 57*, 1069–1081.
Ryff, C., & Keyes, C. (1995). The structure of psychological well-being revisited. *Journal of Personality and Social Psychology, 69*, 719–727.
Ryff, C. D., Magee, W. J., Kling, K. C., & Wing, E. H. (1999). Forging macro-micro linkages in the study of psychological well-being. In C. D. Ryff & V. W. Marshall (Eds.), *Self and society in aging processes* (pp. 247–278). New York: Springer.
Ryff, C. D., & Singer, B. H. (2008). Know thyself and become what you are: A eudaimonic approach to psychological well-being. *Journal of Happiness Studies, 9*, 13–39.
Schimmack, U. (2003). Affect measurement in experience sampling research. *Journal of Happiness Studies, 4*, 79–106.
Schmidt, J., Shernoff, D., & Csikszentmihalyi, M. (2007). Individual and situational factors related to the experience of flow in adolescence: A multilevel approach. In A. D. Ong & M. van Dulmen (Eds.), *The handbook of methods in positive psychology* (pp. 542–558). Oxford: Oxford University Press.
Seligman, M. E. P. (2002). *Authentic happiness: Using the new positive psychology to realize your potential for lasting fulfillment*. New York: Free Press
Seligman, M. E. P., & Csikszentmihalyi, M. (2000). Positive psychology: An introduction. *American Psychologist, 1*, 5–14.
Smith, K. D., Christopher, J. C., Delle Fave, A., & Bhawuk, D. P. S. (2002). Post-Newtonian metatheories in the natural sciences and in cross-cultural psychology. In P. Boski, F. J. R. van de Vijver, A. M. Chodynicka (Eds.), *New directions in cross-cultural psychology* (pp. 107–125). Warsaw, Poland: Wydawnictwo Intytutu Psychologii PAN.
Snyder, C. R., & Lopez, S. J. (2009). *Handbook of positive psychology* (2nd ed.). New York: Oxford University Press.
Veenhoven, R. (1991). Is happiness relative? *Social Indicators Research, 24*, 1–34.
Veenhoven, R. (2003). Hedonism and happiness. *Journal of Happiness Studies, 4*, 437–457.
Veenhoven, R. (2009). Trend average happiness in nations 1946–2008: How much people like the life they live. World Data Base of Happiness. Trend Report 2009-1. http://www.worlddatabaseofhappiness.eur.nl/hap_nat/findingreports/list_of_reports.htm. Accessed 8 August 2009.

Waterman, A. S. (1993). Two conception of happiness: Contrasts of personal expressiveness (eudaimonia) and hedonic enjoyment. *Journal of Personality and Social Psychology, 64*, 678–691.

Waterman, A. S. (2008). Reconsidering happiness: A eudaimonist's perspective. *Journal of Positive Psychology, 3*, 234–252.

Watson, D., Clark, L. A., & Tellegen, A. (1988). Development and validation of brief measures of positive and negative affect: The PANAS scale. *Journal of Personality and Social Psychology, 54*, 1063–1070.

Wirtz, D., Chiu, C., Diener, E., & Oishi, S. (2009). What constitutes a good life? Cultural differences in the role of positive and negative affect in subjective well-being. *Journal of Personality, 77*, 1167–1195.

Chapter 2
Biology, Culture, and Human Behavior

2.1 Genetic and Epigenetic Transmission: A New Perspective

A wide range of research studies in social sciences have focused on the deep and multifaceted relationship of individual and group behaviors with biological and cultural heritage. In particular, in the last decades culture as a dynamic system undergoing changes in time has been investigated from the evolutionary perspective first outlined by Charles Darwin (Darwin, 1859). Various approaches have been used to interpret culture's modification patterns and interaction with the biological inheritance system.

The influence of biology on human behavior has been widely proved in evolutionary studies. In particular, the frameworks of sociobiology and evolutionary psychology (Barkow, Cosmides, & Tooby, 1992; Buss, 1999; Wilson, 1975) were developed from the basic assumption that most human individual and social behaviors evolved to promote survival and reproduction in our ancestors' Environment of Evolutionary Adaptedness (EEA; Symons, 1990) during Pleistocene. The differential replication and transmission of behavioral sequences is therefore related to the enhancement of fitness, i.e., the ability to survive and to successfully reproduce in a given natural environment (Alexander, 1987; Aunger, 2000; Buss, 1999, 2000; Mace & Holden, 2005; Pagel & Mace, 2004). The concept of fitness is closely related to adaptation: Species evolve in that their members acquire new and more adaptive traits which help individuals better cope with the requirements of the ecosystem they live in. Within this framework social learning and the development of culture (including material and symbolic artifacts, social rules, moral norms, and group interaction patterns) are also explained in terms of biological adaptation (Flinn, 1997; Grinde, 1996; O'Neill & Petrinovich, 1998). From this perspective, differences in the natural environment, with its specific pressures and demands, account for most of the striking variations in survival and reproduction strategies adopted by human groups in terms of eating habits, family structure, artifacts production and use, economical and social organization (Peterson & Somit, 1978). As far as social structure is concerned, the ecological constraints also determine the labor and role division between men and women. Parenting and fertility rates evolve in response to the environmental niche pressures (Low, 1989). In a wide cross-cultural

A. Delle Fave et al., *Psychological Selection and Optimal Experience Across Cultures*, Cross-Cultural Advancements in Positive Psychology 2,
DOI 10.1007/978-90-481-9876-4_2, © Springer Science+Business Media B.V. 2011

study, Werner (1979) noticed— for example— that child rearing practices in stratified agricultural societies are based on strict authoritarian rules: This would lead to cooperative, non-self-assertive adults, well adapted to an environment requiring cooperation and interdependence in subsistence activities as means to successfully survive and reproduce.

However, the most recent acquisitions in biology and genetics have broadened the perspective, expanding previous assumptions which confined this influence to genes and to their selective transmission across generations on the basis of individuals' fitness to the pressures of the natural environment. An exhaustive overview of this expanded perspective has been provided by Jablonka and Lamb (2005, 2007). Relying on evidence obtained from a wide range of empirical studies, they showed that DNA is not the only biological source contributing to human heredity. More specifically, they highlighted the role of epigenetic variations, which can be recognized at various levels. Epigenetic variations are much more frequent than genetic mutations, and they often occur as non-random consequences of environmental pressures on the organism, thus enhancing its plasticity in adaptation.

The first kind of transmissible epigenetic information is evident at the cell level. Differences in gene expression and in cell structure, which account for the differentiation of organs in multicellular organisms, occur during mitosis and meiosis and involve RNA, chromatin marks, and feedback loops by cytoplasmic gene products acting as regulators of gene activities. Studies on the structural changes in the eye and visual cortex after exposure to environmental stimuli have specifically highlighted this pathway of transmission (Bridgeman, 2007; Hirsch & Spinelli, 1970).

Epigenetic information can also use body-to-body routes of materials' transmission. This pathway is particularly relevant in mammals, for example as the transfer of materials from the mother during pregnancy and lactation. Its consequences on the psychophysical health of the individual after birth and even in later stages of life have been extensively proved (Gluckman & Hanson, 2005; Sword, Watt, & Krueger, 2006). In addition, parents use another route of epigenetic transmission. Through their active interaction with the environmental demands they contribute to shape a developmental niche (Freedman & Gorman, 1993; Gauvain, 1995; Laland, Odling-Smee, & Feldman, 2000; Super & Harkness, 1986) which the offspring grows adapted to, and therefore tends to maintain with time and to pass on to the next generation.

Social learning is another form of transmission of epigenetic information, whose importance among nonhuman species has become increasingly evident in the studies on animal traditions (Fragaszy & Perry, 2003). It uses more complex routes than the previous ones, such as imitation and display by experienced individuals, and it can occur between genetically unrelated members of a group. Moreover, it can undergo variations by virtue of the active role of the learners, who— far from being passive recipients— can rather selectively acquire or reject parts of the information, can modify it, and can idiosyncratically integrate the new information within their set of behavior repertoire, based on their previous experiences, abilities, and patterns of interaction with the environment.

Jablonka and Lamb (2005) finally refer to an additional epigenetic pattern of information transmission: the symbolic one, which is especially typical of humans, and which represents the major drive behind the evolution of culture. A more thorough analysis of this pattern will be conducted in the following paragraphs.

In our opinion, this important systematization allows for a better understanding of the various patterns of information transmission in our species and offers an overarching model in which most of the theories on biocultural evolution that have been developed in the last 30 years can find their place and rationale. Moreover, it promotes a new and expanded interpretation of the role of biology and genetics in the evolutionary process. By emphasizing the impact of developmental components in adaptation, it accounts for the flexibility in adaptation which can be observed in most vertebrate species, as well as for the emergence of new and unique traits in humans, with their amazing consequences on the earth's ecosystem and on the evolution of our species itself.

2.2 The Emergence of Culture

At the biological level, the most remarkable emergent features that enhanced human fitness and promoted adaptation are the upright standing position, the hand structure with opposing thumb, the development of the neocortex and of the phonatory system, and neoteny, that is the biological immaturity of the newborn, which fosters attachment relations with caregivers, thus supporting parental care and the long period of education necessary to acquire adaptive behaviors within the context of human groups (Brune, 2000; Tomasello, Kruger, & Ratner, 1993). Mind also emerged as an adapted organ, a flexible learning instrument that increased the chances of human survival and reproduction during evolutionary history (Changeux & Chavaillon, 1995; Nicholson, 1997). In particular, humans evolved specific psychic processes: the awareness of external world, or subjective self-awareness; the awareness of one's own internal state, or objective self-awareness (Crook, 1980); the higher-order consciousness (Edelman, 1992), consisting in the uniquely human ability to remember, make plans, and set goals on the basis of memorization and selective retrieval of information acquired through the interaction with the environment; the ability to develop a theory of mind, recognizing the shared nature of mental processes and representations (Tomasello, 1999).

Through their direct interaction with the environment and through social learning, humans actively contributed to the construction of their own developmental niche (Laland et al., 2000). However, the prominently active role of individuals in acquiring information from the environment and from other group members, already identified in other species, was amplified in humans thanks to the above-mentioned psychic processes and features.

In particular, thanks to these features humans evolved the capacity for culture (Baumeister, 2005): They started to build artifacts, to integrate past memories and future expectations in their daily behavior, to develop language, to establish strong social ties outside kinship and proximate groups, to live in large and stable communities characterized by work and social role division, to set norms and rules, to interpret reality according to symbolic meanings (Dunbar, 1998; Jablonka & Lamb, 2005, Somit & Peterson, 1996).

Culture, therefore, can be understood as information originally produced and stored in the human brain, and transmitted through various mechanisms (Cloak, 1975; Henrich, Boyd, & Richerson, 2008). The prominent one originally was social learning; however, additional transmission systems can be detected. In particular, besides its intrasomatic localization in individuals' CNS, culture is also embedded in material and symbolic artifacts: tools, books, buildings, art works, every object which is not present in nature, but is the product of human activities. The storage in extrasomatic carriers has important implications for the survival of the cultural information developed by individuals and groups. The products of scientists, poets, painters, and philosophers outlive their biological creators. Throughout the millennia entire human communities— such as ancient Egyptians, Aztecs, and Sumerians— biologically disappeared, but their writings, buildings, art works, and utensils still resist the vagaries of time and nature.

Culture originally developed within the constraints of ecological niches; this led to remarkable differences between human communities. Specific climatic conditions, available sources of food and of raw materials gave rise to highly diversified societies. However, the differentiation of cultures played the same role that the creation of new species and subspecies plays in biology: It improved flexibility and it increased the amount of information and survival strategies which humans could adopt to cope with the environmental demands. Ultimately, cultural inheritance influenced the features and history of human communities much more than biology.

In particular, the flexibility of cultural transmission provided humans with an extremely adaptive equipment, which allowed to counterbalance biological constraints and weaknesses. Thanks to the ability to plan, to formulate abstract theories, to build mental representations of reality, and to create basic survival artifacts— such as knives, clothes, buildings, and a variety of transportation tools— humans could survive in every kind of ecological niche.

Biocultural theories (Boyd & Richerson, 1985; Durham, 1982, 1991; Ruyle, 1973) were developed in order to identify the elements and mechanisms underlying the intermingling of genetic and cultural inheritance in human behavior. A dual biocultural inheritance system was identified, in which culture originally evolved thanks to the adaptive advantages it provided to our species. Due to its increasing impact on earth's ecosystem, culture gradually became the dominant environment where humans live (Henrich et al., 2008). Cultural traditions, rules and artifacts actively shaped and created environments often very different from the original ones in which human communities had settled. As a consequence, our species needed to adapt genetically to these modified conditions, leading to the coevolution of genes and culture (Newson, Richerson, & Boyd, 2007). The phenomenon was originally defined genetic assimilation, a typical example of it being the increased frequency of the gene that allows adults to process milk sugar lactose among populations who domesticated cattle (Durham, 1991). Within the same perspective, Oyama (2000) proposed the Developmental Systems Theory, in which the genome is considered a source of potentials, flexibility, and learning opportunities, rather than a set of predetermined constraints.

2.2.1 Cultural Evolution

In the effort to delve into the mechanisms of cultural transmission and evolution, scholars approached the study of culture as an evolutionary system, which undergoes changes with time like biology (Durham, 1991; Mace & Holden, 2005; Mundinger, 1980; Richerson & Boyd, 1978). In time, cultural systems show modifications both in the set of socially transmitted intrasomatic rules and in the set of artifacts (Cloak, 1975; Massimini & Calegari, 1979). However, while the capacity for culture undoubtedly represents a biological adaptation, the role of genes and of biological epigenetic inheritance in determining the contents of culture is very limited. Cultural changes are often related to modifications of the ecological niche, but in several cases they take part in the differentiation process between human groups sharing the same natural environment. Therefore, culture can be seen as an inheritance system which evolved with increasing autonomy from biology (Richerson & Boyd, 2005). Moving from these premises, analogies and differences can be detected between the two inheritance systems. Cultural information undergoes vertical, horizontal, and oblique transmission through epigenetic routes such as social learning and imitation; in addition, it substantially relies on symbol-based transmission through language and artifacts. New cultural information can arise randomly, like genetic mutations, but more often it emerges as an intentional response to environmental pressures originating in the mind of individuals as ideas, concepts, solutions to problems. Thus, cultural changes are often intentionally directed, and actively searched for, by humans. Moreover, in most cases innovation stems out of a long preparation (Henrich et al., 2008). An efficient engine is the product of various people working together to improve a previous, less powerful one. Inventors often rely on previous findings and implement them. Similarly, a new law derives from slow, subtle changes in the cultural habits which make it necessary to modify previous behavioral rules, as happened with the provisions developed during last century to promote gender equality in most countries. Several studies have highlighted the cumulative change mechanism in the evolution of culture (Tomasello, 1999) and in particular of technological artifacts (Basalla, 1988). Cumulative cultural evolution has been also detected in laboratory experimental models (Caldwell & Millen, 2008).

Thanks to material and symbolic artifacts, cultural information can spread faster than biological information: A single individual can transmit it to several people at the same time, and across time and space. Sociological studies (Rogers, 1995) have highlighted the rapid horizontal spreading of technological innovations within a single biological generation. This has been further facilitated by industry production, which allows for the mass creation of copies of the same artifact, guaranteeing high-fidelity to the original (Blackmore, 2007). The learning mechanism underlying the acquisition of cultural information (Tomasello et al., 1993) poses virtually no limits to the amount of cultural information individuals can acquire during their life. Humans can learn something new every day; they can store in their brain networks a much larger amount of information chunks than their average life span and physiological needs allow them to do.

Richard Dawkins identified basic cultural information units, or memes (Dawkins, 1976, 1982), stored in the human CNS, as well as in material and symbolic artifacts, which compete for their own survival and transmission against other memes in the cultural system they belong to. Their selective replication and transmission across generations shapes the cultural system and its changes in time (Boyd & Richerson, 1985; Durham, 1991; Massimini & Delle Fave, 2000). However, the interpretation of memes is still controversial. The approach of memetics (Blackmore, 1999; Heyligen, Joslyn, & Turchin, 1995) assumes that memes are by-products of the evolved human capacity for imitation and social learning. They behave like parasites that "infect" minds, using humans to evolve in their turn for their own benefit, independent of individuals' intention and control, and also independent of their consequences on human biological adaptation. Memetics, therefore, foresees a cultural evolution process— lacking of intentionality like biology— based on the memes' ability to survive and reproduce in time through the natural selection of their human carrier phenotypes. The differential reproduction of memes is related to the level of their cultural fitness, i.e., their adaptiveness to the cultural environment in which they are located.

Other authors, however, argue that to consider memes as the units of cultural information, which can be replicated through human and extrasomatic vehicles, does not necessarily imply that individuals are passive carriers, or that memes only act as infectious parasites. As a matter of fact, meme competition engenders a cultural evolution trend whose outcomes can be very different from, and in some cases even opposite to the ones natural selection would produce (Boyd & Richerson, 1985). Cultural fitness can be compatible with the biological one, but not necessarily so. For example, the differential survival of memes can also imply the suppression of genes, as shown by martyrs, political dissidents, monks and nuns, who choose to give up their capacity for biological survival and genes' transmission to the benefit of memes' reproduction.

However, while the contents of culture are not necessarily adaptive (Durham, 1991; Mesoudi, Withen, & Laland, 2006), the interplay between the two systems appears to be more complex than outlined by memetics. More specifically, the cultural differentiation of human communities can interact with biological fitness in three different ways: enhancing it, decreasing it, or being neutral in respect to it. As we have previously outlined, culture originally contributed to enhance the biological fitness of human groups, and this cooperative role can be observed worldwide across different cultures and related traditions. Food and housing habits, parenting practices and healing systems, though in some cases deeply differing from one another, generally aim at enabling and improving human biological survival and reproduction.

In other cases, culture changes in time and space are neutral as concerns their impact on biology. Examples can be found in the differentiation of art forms, cuisine recipes, dressing fashions, and house furniture within societies and across human communities sharing the same natural environment.

Human history is also interspersed with cases of competition between biological and cultural fitness (Boyd & Richerson, 1985; Delle Fave & Massimini, 2000). Intraspecific violence and biological suppression of individuals and whole populations due to religious, political, and economic reasons, as well as religious celibacy, female infanticide and family size reduction are only few aspects of this phenomenon. A striking example is the highly debated habit of female infibulation and/or circumcision in several African countries (Caldwell, Orubuloye, & Caldwell, 1997; Leonard, 1996). Some scholars argue that the main reason for such a practice is a biological one: Hrdy (1981) claims that infibulation preserves wives' chastity, making males certain of their paternity. Grassivaro Gallo and Viviani (1992) suggest a relation between infibulation and women's role as shepherds: The practice reduces the production of female sexual odors, which both negatively affect herbivores and attract predators. However, this devastating mutilation of female's outer genitalia can find a more satisfying explanation in cultural norms concerning sexual stratification, women's social role and expected behavior within a patrilineal society (MacCormack & Strathern, 1980). Recurrent urinary tract infections, high-risk pregnancies, difficulties at delivery, transmission of infectious diseases to the newborn, and last but not least, impairment in sexual pleasure and orgasm are only few of the problems infibulated women have to face (Cook, 1976): These are serious constraints for biological fitness, and paternity certainty can hardly counterbalance such maladaptive outcomes.

The same general explanation can be applied to the widely spread habit to artificially modifying the sex ratio of children in favor of males. In preindustrial societies this goal is usually pursued after birth, through female infanticide or reduced care and nutrition levels (Cleland, Verrall, & Vaessen, 1983; Mealey & Mackey, 1990; Williamson, 1976). In more recent times, technology advancements made this practice possible already during pregnancy: Ultrasound scanning is often used in various urban areas of the world to carry out abortion if the fetus is female (Park & Cho, 1995). In People's Republic of China the selective suppression of females is justified in the name of the recent one-child family policy, adopted to cope with excessive population growth. These customs are mostly connected to the high costs of raising a girl in a patrilineal culture, where a dowry is needed to find a husband, and where a married daughter is of no help to her parents, because she lives with her husband's family. The artificial sex-ratio modifications mostly stem from cultural rules, but they can also influence natural selection: Within a population, an excessively low number of females can result in biological maladaptation for the survival and reproduction of the whole group.

Less striking, but more global examples of competition between cultural traditions and biological fitness are the steadily growing incidence of back pain, diabetes, and cardiovascular diseases in affluent societies, associated with unbalanced diet, prolonged sitting posture, reduced physical activity, and exposure to culturally related stressors.

Similarly, cultures can radically damage the natural environment in which they have developed, with negative consequences for both other living beings and for themselves. Whenever a human community settles down in a geographical area, it introduces changes in the ecosystem. In several circumstances, however, these changes turned to be nonadaptive for the biocultural survival of the community itself: Many cultures have become extinct because of their disruptive exploitation of the environmental resources (Diamond, 2005).

As a contemporary paradigmatic example of environmental disruption, we can take the worldwide spreading of genetically modified seeds, patented by few Western industries and sold to farmers all over the world. Their productivity and their resistance to parasites are artificially improved, and this can represent a substantial advantage, especially in developing countries facing chronic food scarcity and lack of efficacious pesticides (Finucane & Holup, 2006). However, this practice also entails negative consequences (Paarlberg, 2000). Many varieties of crops are disappearing in Asian and African countries: This homogenization trend contradicts the tendency toward differentiation, which is the basis of biological evolution. Moreover, the natural emergence of new species of parasites able to destroy the artificially obtained seeds cannot be ruled out. This could provoke dramatic famines and food shortage, which would be much more severe than before because of the reduced number of available crop varieties (Schmidt & Wei, 2006). Finally, farmers usually save some seeds for the following sowing season, but genetically modified seeds expire after some months, and farmers have to buy them every year from industries. This controversial issue is presently debated from two opposing positions, basically grounded in culturally divergent perspectives, with the prospect of reconciling the two sides seemingly still bleak (Magnus, 2009).

2.2.2 Cultural Differentiation and Inter-cultural Relations

The emergence and unfolding of different cultures generate a unique phenomenon among humans: intraspecific communication. Two individuals raised in different cultures, however belonging to the same species, can often hardly understand each other. Languages, habits, beliefs, social structures show great diversity. This progressive differentiation has two consequences on human relationships. Within cultures, it fosters cooperative behavior, trust, altruism, and the preferential information exchange with individuals showing similar cultural features (Boyd, Gintis, Bowles, & Richerson, 2003; Labov, 2001; Schaller, Simpson, & Kenrick, 2006). At the same time, it promotes cultural segregation and ingroup–outgroup discrimination (Buchan, Croson, & Dawes, 2002; Triandis, 1994; Yamagishi, Jin, & Kiyonari, 1999). Thus, when two or more human communities get into contact, the building of inter-cultural relationships can be problematic.

At the inter-cultural level, societies may fruitfully exchange and borrow memes. Though, the most frequent event in human history has been competition and imposition of cultural information by one society on another one. Wars, mostly grounded in cultural beliefs and values, are the very basic Leitmotiv of the interaction among societies (Mays, Bullock, Rosenzweig, & Wessells, 1998). This poses a key dilemma to the researcher, and to the field workers dealing with inter-cultural relationships. How can we evaluate the "superiority" of a culture, or the higher desirability of a value system, in comparison with another one? This is not an academic question. The history of mankind is characterized by cultural contacts which only rarely have been cooperative, more often resulting in conflicts and cultural competition. Some cultures survived to the detriment of others, some cultures subjected others, some cultures imposed their value system to others. Is there any matter of superiority and higher desirability in the outcomes of these conflicts?

In order to deal with this thorny issue, we have to consider what previously discussed about cultural evolution. Like in biology, within a cultural context some information is selectively transmitted across generations, while some other becomes extinct in that it proves to be unfit for survival in that environment. Like biological evolution, cultural evolution is a process of change in neutral terms: Change, per se, does not imply any ethical or evaluative judgment, rather it promotes better adaptation. One of the most investigated examples of this evolution process is the adoption of agriculture and of a sedentary lifestyle (see Diamond, 1997, for a historical review), which produced astonishing modifications in human biocultural inheritance. It gave rise to labor division, differentiation of skills, technological innovations and advancements, more articulated patterns of social organization, and a more systematic codification of social norms and behavioral rules. Thanks to these changes, some cultures became better equipped to cope with the environmental demands, in that they showed a higher flexibility, and specialized strategies and tools to face a variety of difficulties. But this is very different from saying that their memes were "more valuable" than the ones reproduced by other societies.

Given the possibility for cultural information to spread through imposition, some cultures can dominate others because of their ability to survive and reproduce in respect with other cultural variants, and not because of the absolute desirability of the values they convey (Massimini & Delle Fave, 2000). For example, during the second millennium BC patriarchal warfare societies defeated and suppressed more egalitarian and peaceful cultures settled in the Middle East, South Asia, and the Mediterranean area. These cultures were based on agricultural and trading economy, gender equality and a religious system centered on Mother Goddess and fertility rituals (Eisler, 1987; Gimbutas, 1991). They disappeared not because of the low desirability of their value system but because of their lack of artifacts and know-how related to war. In the last four centuries, cultural extinction has been repeatedly caused by means of violent colonization, wild modernization, and supremacy of technological power. This form of meme selection through imposition inhibits the differentiation process, which is a basic feature of living systems, be they species or cultures.

The dominance relationships among cultures have been traditionally rooted in the level of sophistication of the artifacts. More specifically, the development of technology was— and is nowadays— the key factor influencing the chances a culture has to win a war, to spread its values, to colonize other populations (Diamond, 1997). This process has imposed a specific evolution trend to the human communities living on earth. Technological artifacts and various techniques gradually dominated the world throughout history, until the most recent manifest spreading of modernization. In the last centuries some cultures— mainly the Western technological ones— have been prevailing because of their adaptive traits, i.e., ability to survive and successfully reproduce, and not because their memes and values are absolutely better or ethically more desirable than others. Far from being grounded in ethical principles, the real power of a country is based on the efficiency of its artifacts, be they weapons, computers, or industrial machines. This has caused the extinction of many human societies in the millennia. Today, we can sadly hear the swansong of previously numerous and complex cultures, suffocated by the relentless advance of globalized values and objects (Delle Fave & Massimini, 2002).

Globalization represents one of the most recent myths created by the human species. It is related to the idea of uniting cultures, peoples, and values in order to build a "global village" out of a world that for millennia has consisted of different and often competing human groups, a world based much more on warfare than on welfare and peace. Of course, we must acknowledge that religions, philosophical theories, and cultural movements the world over have often highlighted the universal traits of human beings and the need for positive and peaceful relations between peoples, their ethnic or cultural background notwithstanding. However, the present concept of globalization has not been formulated by mankind as a whole. Rather, it looks as a product of Western postmodern cultures. Globalization is basically conceived as a political–economical process, and substantial emphasis is placed on the potentials of a unified world market system.

Nevertheless, globalization could represent an adaptive strategy for our species, if based on the sharing of social values that could promote peaceful and cooperative inter-cultural relations. It favors spatial and social mobility of individuals and groups (Bongaarts & Watkins, 1996); it promotes circulation of cultural information in a more fast and efficient way; it fosters social and community encounters. Moreover, Western customs spread through globalization are often adapted to local practices, rather than being passively embedded in the cultural system (Hong, Wan, No, & Chiu, 2007). In its present version, however, globalization can represent a serious threat to cultural diversity. In order to foster its development as a culturally fair tool for world betterment, a greater awareness should be developed of the value of each society, regardless of its technological or economical power. Ethnicity is a basic human value, when not misused for suppressing other groups. To combine the preservation of cultural diversity with the need for inter-cultural alliance is the real challenge humans have to face nowadays. An attempt to partly investigate these issues from the point of view of psychological selection and optimal experience will be proposed in Chapter 13.

2.2.3 Social Norms and Their Analysis: The Cultural Network

As previously stated, culture evolved as an autonomous system thanks to the creation of material and symbolic artifacts, the latter comprising— among others— behavioral norms, rules, and values that do not stem from biology, but from social history. Symbolic artifacts, which represent one of the epigenetic category of inheritable information according to Jablonka and Lamb (2005), rely on two basic features of human beings: their tendency to follow rules (Harré & Secord, 1972) and their capacity for response to the "invisible reality" of meanings, ideas, values, and mental representations. Cultures shape individuals' behavior and conception of what a good and just life is, both providing a meaning-making system for daily events and interactions and fostering or limiting opportunities for goal setting, personal growth, and self-expression (Ryan & Deci, 2001; Uchida, Norasakkunkit, & Kitayama, 2004). Cultural differences in value systems substantially concern the weight and the meaning attributed to collective norms, daily activities, and social roles (Triandis, 1994, 1999). Specific activities or behaviors do not necessarily have the same meaning or function in different cultures.

The shared understanding of reality and the meaning attribution process ceaselessly performed by cultural groups throughout the millennia gave rise to rules, norms, and values formalized in laws and institutionalized normative systems (Baumeister, 2005). As any other form of cultural information, norms and values— be they institutionalized or informal— undergo a dynamic process of change with time. Their differential replication primarily depends upon criteria that are "purely cultural," autonomous from the biological fitness of the group, and substantially related to socially shared meanings, as well as to basic duties and rights grounded into a culture-specific world outlook (Leung & Morris, 2001; Miller, 2001; Nucci & Lee, 1993). Norms and values are institutionalized in normative artifacts (Calegari & Massimini, 1978; Massimini & Calegari, 1979).

In particular, constitutions— be they written or oral— represent the core of institutionalized cultural information regulating individual and group behavior, selected and stratified across generations (Pospisil, 1974). They comprise the basic social values, which can be defined as assumptions on what is desirable for the individual and for the group in a specific culture (Calegari & Massimini, 1976; Rokeach, 1974; Schwartz & Bilsky, 1987).

Constitutions can also be considered as sets of cultural instructions or attempted solutions to universal human problems. All human populations, in all times, have a fixed set of common problems to solve (Kluckhohn & Strodtbeck, 1961; Massimini, 1982). The solutions to these problems can, however, vary across human communities. Variation can occur at two different levels: The first one refers to differences in the specific cultural instructions used to solve a problem; the second one refers to differences in the hierarchical relevance attributed to a given problem in relation to the other problems that a population has to solve. Solutions therefore vary from one population to the other, even if not indefinitely; a society can give more emphasis

Table 2.1 The information units identified in constitutional texts aggregated in overarching categories

Categories	Units
Biocultural reproduction	Work
	Property
	Income
Cultural reproduction	Education
	Information exchange
	Participation
	Decision making
Prescription	Legal system
	Status
Evaluation and justification	Individual values
	Social values

to a given problem: Its solution thus becomes a priority. Different solutions and priorities are the foundations of cultural diversity.

On the basis of theoretical and empirical analyses, Calegari and Massimini (1978) have systematized universal human problems and related solutions into 11 units of information, operationalizing them as units of a cultural network (Table 2.1). Units can be grouped into overarching categories, representing more general issues each community has to deal with: biological and cultural survival, the group's social structure and organization, and the core values on which the system is built. The whole set of units has been defined "network" because its elements interact with one another and are connected by mutual influences.

The identification of the above-mentioned units was based on the analysis of single articles in constitutional texts from different Western and non-Western countries (Massimini & Calegari, 1979). Through a mathematical approach based on matrix algebra and graph theory (Mesarovic, Macko, & Takahara, 1970; Pattee, 1973; Weiss, 1971), the authors detected specific relation and hierarchical patterns among units, as well as the peculiar structure of each nation's constitution, which was characterized by the prominent role of few defined units (Calegari & Massimini, 1978). The primacy of these units determined the nature of the social and political relations selected with time by that specific country. For example, socialist democracies (such as China and the former USSR) attribute priority to the Social Values unit (in terms of social ownership of means of production), which constrains the behavioral instructions concerning Property and Work. On the contrary, in Western European democracies, Individual Values (such as freedom of choosing a job according to one's own preferences and attitudes) are prominent, and therefore primarily affect the Work unit. This cultural specificity in the reciprocal influence of units leads to the mathematical definition of cultural networks as *oriented graphs*.

Each unit deals with a major problem that society has to solve in order to survive and reproduce in time. The linguistic expression of written constitutions is usually extremely synthetic, has high informative power, and poses no particular coding difficulties.

In particular, the cultural network model allows for a systematic investigation of the core cultural information characterizing a human community (Csikszentmihalyi & Massimini, 1985). The number of problems considered and the description of the matching solutions can be analyzed and compared across societies. It is also possible to detect hierarchical links among the units, since most of them are interrelated and constrain one another's presence. For example, across cultures, opening access to formal education programs either to all citizens or to only specific groups affects individuals' status, job opportunities, and decisional power within the society.

In each culture, different specific solutions develop according to historical peculiarities. Moreover, each culture will set forth different priorities for the goals to be pursued. For example, a given population can attribute more relevance to the distribution of wealth than to formal education. In another case, the affiliation to a religious group can give to the individuals more prestige than economic status. Cultural networks have been detected in written Constitutions, as well as in orally transmitted instruction sets, like the one in use among the Papua Kapauku of Western New Guinea (Massimini, 1982).

The study of Constitutions as operationalized through the cultural network can provide fruitful insight in the structure of human societies and in their cultural selection patterns. It can help detect recurrences and divergences in the cultural pool of different societies. Within a longitudinal perspective, it can allow for investigating the process of cultural change, thanks to the fact that constitutions are written sets of instructions and norms. However, as per our knowledge, it has not been adopted in other research domains. Nevertheless, as stated by Henrich and colleagues (2008), the construction of formal cultural evolutionary models is still necessary, especially at the large-scale level of population processes, and it is exactly this level of investigation that could benefit from the study of laws and constitutions.

2.3 The Role of Individuals

As highlighted in the previous sections of this chapter, one of the major acquisition derived from the recent studies in biology is the non-random pattern of transmission which characterizes epigenetic information, and the interpretation of genome as a source of flexibility and potentials.

From the same perspective, scholars from different areas are increasingly pointing out that individuals are not simply vehicles of genetic and cultural information. As clearly emphasized by Jablonka and Lamb (2005), intentionality and direction are two crucial elements supporting the selection and evolution or culture. Decision-making forces are at work in the evolution of culture, and they prevail on random changes: Learning a skill or developing an opinion are not the result of a random and blind selection process; rather they stem from a conscious or unconscious decision of a single individual (Newson et al., 2007).

Individual cognition directs social learning and makes use of the available cultural information according to principles that deeply differ from random selection, such as biases related to the information contents, the situations in which information is exchanged, and its popularity within the group (Henrich et al., 2008). Moreover, individuals are able to introduce innovations, by inventing new cultural variants or modifying previously existing ones.

In particular, the active role of individuals emerges in the construction and transmission of cultural norms. Individuals can easily memorize a wide number of rules and prescriptions, regulating their behavior accordingly, but also retaining a certain plasticity in rule replication and interpretation. Normative artifacts, as lists of behavioral instructions aiming to regulate social interactions, are primarily interneural instructions (Cloak, 1975) that are subsequently encoded in extrasomatic carriers through processes of externalization, anonymization, institutionalization, and ritualization (Bateson & Hinde, 1976; Hinde, 1974). Humans used their ability for self-description to develop collective prescriptions, progressively moving from the micro-level of individuality and contingent interaction to the macro-level of groups and institutionalized relations (Berger & Luckman, 1966; Simon, 1969).

The individual is, therefore, not a passive carrier infected by memes (Sperber, 2000), but an active and self-organizing system, that exchanges information with the environment, attaining progressively higher levels of complexity (see Chapter 3 for more details on this aspect). Each person plays the multiple role of heir, transformer, and transmitter of biological and cultural information. In particular, individuals build their culturetype (Richerson & Boyd, 1978) by acquiring memes throughout their lives from various sources, and by actively constructing their developmental niche (Laland et al., 2000). Cultural systems thus interact with the individual in an interdependent process of circular causality (Massimini, 1982).

This approach gives to subjectivity a key role in the differential production and transmission of cultural information. The person is connected to the cultural meaningful world through idiosyncratic processes of internalization and externalization (Vaalsiner, 1998, 2007). The individual experience of the world "transforms collective-cultural meanings into a personal-cultural system of sense" (Vaalsiner, 2007, p. 62), which undergoes a personal reconstruction and can be externalized through behaviors, goals, and strivings.

Through meaning-making, humans organize their experience moment by moment (Kegan, 1994), progressively integrating new events and information into their own life history and developmental trajectory (Singer, 2004). Meaning-making is therefore a dynamic process: Throughout their lives, individuals ceaselessly revise their experiences, attribute new meanings to them, expand or narrow their own meaning system (Kunnen & Bosma, 1996, 2000). Moreover, individuals can attribute meaning to activities that are not valued or approved by the cultural context. The consistency or discrepancy between the meaning and relevance attributed to a given idea or activity by the individual and by her cultural environment is a critical issue (Delle Fave, 2009). In case of consistency, the social context will support individuals' investment of resources on that activity, encouraging its cultivation, and eventually deriving benefits from the competencies individuals develop in that activity. In case of discrepancy, a conflict can arise between the individual's meaning-making process and the social expectations, whose consequences will depend on the individual's motivation system, on the cultural evolution trend, and on the hierarchical organization of the cultural network.

This centrality of subjectivity has been also emphasized in the field of motivational studies. As described with more details in Chapter 3, approaches centered on material rewards and incentive-based models have been supplanted by theories emphasizing the active and creative role of the individual (Maslow, 1968; Ryan & Deci, 2000). Intentional goal setting and its influence on identity development have been investigated among different groups and in various life domains (Gollwitzer, 1999; Kalaloski & Nurmi, 1998; Taylor & Gollwitzer, 1995). All these studies highlight the relevance of self-selected goals and meanings in supporting development and personal growth. Moreover, they identify autonomy, creativity, and potential for innovation as structural components of humans (Simonton, 1994; Sternberg, 1988).

Finally, individuals differ from each other in experiencing the same situation. Studies on daily experience fluctuations as a whole, as well as comparative analyses of social contexts, activities, emotional and motivational patterns, can detect and track the interaction patterns between biocultural background and individual features (Csikszentmihalyi & Massimini, 1985).

On the basis of meaning attribution, motivation, and experience, day after day and throughout their life span, individuals select and reproduce a limited number of information chunks within their cultural pool (activities, interests, political, and moral beliefs). This process is especially evident within highly articulated societies, where people can specialize in a wide variety of jobs, areas of education, personal interests. The cultural system, and more specifically the constraints imposed by the relationship among units within the cultural network, can nevertheless restrict its members' opportunities for choice. For example, in theocratic societies individuals are forced to follow the dominant religious system. In rigidly stratified societies people have access to only specific jobs, according to the class or caste they belong to. In cultures characterized by gender stratification, women are usually restrained from getting involved in activities, interests, and professions which are considered males' domain. However, if we exclude the most extreme conditions, each person usually has a more or less wide range of alternative activities to be engaged in during her life.

We can thus assume that a process of selection— like in biology and in culture— takes place at the psychological level. People differentially reproduce memes in their daily life, supported by non-random elements of intentionality, goal pursuit, and meaning construction. Cross-cultural studies have been conducted in order to detect the basic criterion which guides this psychological selection (Csikszentmihalyi & Massimini, 1985; Massimini, Csikszentmihalyi, & Carli, 1987; Massimini, Csikszentmihalyi, & Delle Fave, 1988). A major role is played by the quality of experience individuals associate with the cultural information— activities, social contexts, situations— they come in contact with. This will be the core topic of the remaining chapters of this book.

References

Alexander, R. D. (1987). *The biology of moral systems*. New York: Aldine de Gruyter.

Aunger, R. A. (Ed.) (2000). *Darwinizing culture: The status of memetics as a science*. New York: Oxford University Press.

Barkow, J. H., Cosmides, L., & Tooby, J. (1992). *The adapted mind: Evolutionary psychology and the generation of culture*. New York: Oxford University Press.

Basalla, G. (1988). *The evolution of technology*. New York: Cambridge University Press.

Bateson, P. P. & Hinde, R. A. (Eds.). (1976). *Growing points in ethology*. London: Cambridge University Press.

Baumeister, R. F. (2005). *The cultural animal*. New York: Oxford University Press.

Berger, P. L., & Luckman, T. (1966). *The social construction of reality*. New York: Doubleday & Co.

Berger, P. L., & Luckman, T. (1966). *The social construction of reality*. New York: Double-day & Co.

Blackmore, S. J. (1999). *The meme machine*. New York: Oxford University Press.

Blackmore, S. (2007). Those dreaded memes: The advantage of memetics over "symbolic inheritance". *Behavioral and Brain Sciences, 30*, 365–366.

Bongaarts, J., & Watkins, S. C. (1996). Social interactions and contemporary fertility transitions. *Population and Development Review, 22*, 639–682.

Boyd, R., Gintis, H., Bowles, S., & Richerson, P. J. (2003). The evolution of altruistic punishment. *PNAS— Proceedings of the National Academy of Sciences USA, 100*, 3531–3535.

Boyd, R., & Richerson, P. J. (1985). *Culture and the evolutionary process*. Chicago: Chicago University Press.

Bridgeman, B. (2007). One-generation Lamarckism: The role of environment in genetic development. *Behavioral and Brain Sciences, 30*, 367–368.

Brune, M. (2000). Neoteny, psychiatric disorders and the social brain: Hypotheses on heterochrony and the modularity of the mind. *Anthropology & Medicine, 7*, 301–318.

Buchan, N. R., Croson, R., & Dawes, R. M. (2002). Swift neighbours and persistent strangers: A cross-cultural investigation of trust and reciprocity in social exchange. *American Journal of Sociology, 108*, 168–206.

Buss, D. M. (1999). *Evolutionary psychology: The new science of the mind*. Boston: Allyn and Bacon.

Buss, D. M. (2000). The evolution of happiness. *American Psychologist, 55*, 15–23.

Caldwell, C. A., & Millen, A. E. (2008). Experimental models for testing hypotheses about cumulative cultural evolution. *Evolution and Human Behavior, 29*, 165–171.

Caldwell, J. C., Orubuloye, I. O., & Caldwell, P. (1997). Male and female circumcision in Africa from a regional to a specific Nigerian examination. *Social Science & Medicine, 44*, 1181–1193.

Calegari, P., & Massimini, F. (1976). *Introduzione alla teoria del valori umani*. Milano: ISEDI.

Calegari, P., & Massimini, F. (1978). *Psicologia dell'artefatto normativo sociale*. Milano: Franco Angeli.

Changeux, J. P., & Chavaillon, J. (1995). *Origins of the human brain*. Oxford: Clarendon.

Cleland, J., Verrall, J., & Vaessen, M. (1983). Preference for the sex of children and their influence on reproductive behaviour. World Fertility Survey, *Comparative Studies, 27*. Voorborg: International Statistical Institute.

Cloak, F. T. (1975). Is a cultural ethology possible? *Human Ecology, 3*, 161–182.

Cook, R. (1976). *Damage to physical health from pharaonic circumcision (infibulation) of females: A review of the medical literature*, Report from regional advisor of World Health Organization to Division of Family Health. Geneva: WHO.

Crook, J. H. (1980). *The evolution of human consciousness*. Oxford: Oxford University Press.

Csikszentmihalyi, M., & Massimini, F. (1985). On the psychological selection of bio-cultural information. *New Ideas in Psychology, 3*, 115–138.

Darwin, C. (1859). *On the origin of species by means of natural selection*. London: Murray.

Dawkins, R. (1976). *The selfish gene*. Oxford: Oxford University Press.
Dawkins, R. (1982). *The extended phenotype*. Oxford: W.H. Freeman & Co.
Delle Fave, A. (2009). Optimal experience and meaning: Which relationship? *Psychological Topics. Special issue on positive psychology*, *18*, 285–302.
Delle Fave, A., & Massimini, F. (2000). Subjective experience and the building of parental roles in a bio-cultural perspective. In A. L. Comunian & U. P. Gielen (Eds.), *International perspectives on human development* (pp. 159–175). Lengerich: Pabst Science Publishers.
Delle Fave, A., & Massimini, F. (2002). Cultural change and human behaviour: Evolution or development? In A. Delle Fave & M. B. Pun (Eds.), *In pursuit of a sustainable modernisation: Culture and policies in Nepal* (pp. 13–34). Milano: Arcipelago Edizioni.
Diamond, J. (1997). *Guns, germs, and steel: The fates of human societies*. New York: W.W. Norton & Co.
Diamond, J. (2005). *Collapse: How societies choose to fail or succeed*. New York: Viking Books.
Dunbar, R. J. M. (1998). The social brain hypothesis. *Evolutionary Anthropology*, *6*, 178–190.
Durham, W. H. (1982). Interactions of genetic and cultural evolution: Models and examples. *Human Ecology*, *10*, 289–323.
Durham, W. H. (1991). *Coevolution: Genes, culture and human diversity*. Stanford, CA: Stanford University Press.
Edelman, G. M. (1992). *Bright air, brilliant fire: On the matter of the mind*. New York: Basic Books.
Eisler, R. (1987). *The chalice and the blade*. San Francisco: Harper and Row.
Finucane, M. L., & Holup, J. L. (2006). Psychosocial and cultural factors affecting the perceived risk of genetically modified food: An overview of the literature. *Social Science & Medicine*, *60*, 1603–1612.
Flinn, M. V. (1997). Culture and the evolution of social learning. *Evolution and Human Behavior*, *18*, 23–67.
Fragaszy, D. M., & Perry, S. (2003). *The biology of traditions*. New York: Cambridge University Press.
Freedman, D. G., & Gorman, J. (1993). Attachment and the transmission of culture: An evolutionary perspective. *Journal of Social and Evolutionary Systems*, *16*, 297–329.
Gauvain, M. (1995). Thinking in niches: Sociocultural influences on cognitive development. *Human Development*, *38*, 25–45.
Gimbutas, M. (1991). *The civilization of the goddess*. San Francisco: Harper.
Gluckman, P., & Hanson, M. (2005). *The foetal matrix: Evolution, development and disease*. Cambridge: Cambridge University Press.
Gollwitzer, P. M. (1999). Implementation intentions: Strong effects of simple plans. *American Psychologist*, *54*, 493–503.
Grassivaro Gallo, P., & Viviani, F. (1992). The origin of infibulation in Somalia: An ethological hypothesis. *Ethology and Sociobiology*, *13*, 253–265.
Grinde, B. (1996). Darwinian happiness: Biological advice on the quality of life. *Journal of Social and Evolutionary Systems*, *19*, 249–260.
Harré, R., & Secord, P. F. (1972). *The explanation of social behavior*. Totawa, NJ: Rowman and Littlefield.
Henrich, J., Boyd, R., & Richerson, P. J. (2008). Five misunderstandings about cultural evolution. *Human Nature*, *19*, 119–137.
Heyligen, F., Joslyn, C., & Turchin, V. (Eds.) (1995). *The quantum of evolution: Towards a theory of metasystems transition*. New York: Gordon and Breach Science Publishers.
Hinde, R. A. (1974). *Biological bases of human social behavior*. New York: McGraw Hill.
Hirsch, H. V. B., & Spinelli, D. N. (1970). Visual experience modifies distribution of horizontally and vertically oriented receptive field in cats. *Science*, *168*, 869–871.
Hong, Y., Wan, C., No, S., & Chiu, C. (2007). Multicultural identities. In S. Kitayama & D. Cohen (Eds.), *Handbook of cultural psychology* (pp. 323–345). New York: Guilford Press.
Hrdy, S. B. (1981). *The woman that never evolved*. Harvard: Harvard University Press.

Jablonka, E., & Lamb, M. J. (2005). *Evolution in four dimensions: Genetic, epigenetic, behavioural and symbolic variations in the history of life*. Cambridge, MA: MIT Press.

Jablonka, E., & Lamb, M. J. (2007). Précis of "evolution in four dimensions". *Behavioral and Brain Sciences, 30*, 353–392.

Kalaloski, V., & Nurmi, J. (1998). Identity and educational transitions: Age differences in adolescent exploration and commitment related to education, occupation, and family. *Journal of Research on Adolescence, 8*, 29–47.

Kegan, R. (1994). *In over our heads*. New York: Cambridge University Press.

Kluckhohn, F., & Strodtbeck, F. (1961). *Variants in value orientation*. New York: Row Peterson.

Kunnen, E. S., & Bosma, H. A. (1996). Adolescent conflict and the development of meaning making. In L. Verhofstadt-Denève, I. Kienhorst, & C. Braet (Eds.), *Conflict and development in adolescence* (pp. 61–74). Leiden: DSWO Press.

Kunnen, E. S., & Bosma, H. A. (2000). Development of meaning making: A dynamic systems approach. *New Ideas in Psychology, 18*, 57–82.

Labov, W. (2001). *Principles of linguistic change: Social factors* (Vol. 29). Malden, MA: Blackwell.

Laland, K. N., Odling-Smee, J., & Feldman, M. W. (2000). Niche construction, biological evolution, and cultural change. *Behavioral and Brain Sciences, 23*, 131–146.

Leonard, L. (1996). Female circumcision in southern Chad: Origins, meaning, and current practice. *Social Science & Medicine, 43*, 255–263.

Leung, K., & Morris, M. W. (2001). Justice through the lens of culture and ethnicity. In J. Sanders & V. L. Hamilton (Eds.), *Handbook of law and social sciences: Justice* (pp. 343–378). New York: Plenum.

Low, B. S. (1989). Cross-cultural patterns in the training of children: An evolutionary perspective. *Journal of Comparative Psychology, 103*, 311–319.

MacCormack, C., Strathern, M. (Eds.). (1980). *Nature, culture and gender*. Cambridge: Cambridge University Press.

Mace, R., & Holden, C. J. (2005). A phylogenetic approach to cultural evolution. *Trends in Biology and Evolution, 3*, 116–121.

Magnus, D. C. (2009). Ethical and social aspects of transgenic plants. In V. Ravitsky, A. Fiester, & A. Caplan (Eds.), *The penn center guide to bioethics* (pp. 435–446). New York: Springer Publishing Co. US.

Maslow, A. (1968). *Toward a psychology of being* (2nd ed). Princeton, NJ: Van Nostrand.

Massimini, F. (1982). Individuo, cultura, ambiente: I Papua Kapauku della Nuova Guinea Occidentale [Individual, culture, environment: The Papua Kapauku of Western New Guinea]. *Ricerche di Psicologia, 22–23*, 27–154.

Massimini, F., & Calegari, P. (1979). *Il contesto normativo sociale* [The normative social context]. Milano: Angeli.

Massimini, F., Csikszentmihalyi, M., & Carli, M. (1987). Optimal experience: A tool for psychiatric rehabilitation. *Journal of Nervous and Mental Disease, 175*, 545–549.

Massimini, F., Csikszentmihalyi, M., & Delle Fave, A. (1988). Flow and biocultural evolution. In M. Csikszentmihalyi & I. Csikszentmihalyi (Eds.), *Optimal experience: Psychological studies of flow in consciousness* (pp. 60–81). New York: Cambridge University Press.

Massimini, F., & Delle Fave, A. (2000). Individual development in a bio-cultural perspective. *American Psychologist, 55*, 24–33.

Mays, V. M., Bullock, M., Rosenzweig, M. R., & Wessells, M. (1998). Ethnic conflict: Global challenges and psychological perspectives. *American Psychologist, 53*, 737–742.

Mealey, L., & Mackey, W. (1990). Variation in offspring sex ratio in women of differing social status. *Ethology and Sociobiology, 11*, 83–95.

Mesarovic, M. D., Macko, A., & Takahara, J. (1970). *Theory of hierarchical multilevel systems*. New York: Academic Press.

Mesoudi, A., Withen, A., & Laland, K. N. (2006). Towards a unified science of cultural evolution. *Behavioral and Brain Sciences, 29*, 329–383.

Miller, J. G. (2001). Culture and moral development. In D. Matsumoto (Ed.), *The handbook of culture and psychology* (pp. 151–170). New York: Oxford University Press.
Mundinger, P. C. (1980). Animal culture and a general theory of cultural evolution. *Ethology and Sociobiology*, *1*, 183–223.
Newson, L., Richerson, P. J., & Boyd, R. (2007). Cultural evolution and the shaping of cultural diversity. In S. Kitayama & D. Cohen (Eds.), *Handbook of cultural psychology* (pp. 454–476). New York: Guilford Press.
Nicholson, N. (1997). Evolutionary psychology: Toward a new view of human nature and organizational society. *Human Relations*, *50*, 1053–1078.
Nucci, L., & Lee, J. (1993). Morality and personal autonomy. In G. Noam & T. E. Wrem (Eds.), *Studies in contemporary german social thought. The moral self* (pp. 123–148). Cambridge: MIT Press.
O'Neill, P., & Petrinovich, L. (1998). A preliminary cross-cultural study of moral intuitions. *Evolution and Human Behavior*, *19*, 349–367.
Oyama, S. (2000). *Evolution's eye: A systems view on the biology-culture divide*. Durham, NC: Duke University Press.
Paarlberg, R. (2000). Genetically modified crops in developing countries: Promise or peril? *Environment*, *42*, 19–27.
Pagel, M., & Mace, R. (2004). The cultural wealth of nations. *Nature*, *428*, 275–278.
Park, C. B., & Cho, N. (1995). Consequences of son preference in a low fertility society: Imbalance of the sex ratio at birth in Korea. *Population Development Review*, *21*, 59–84.
Pattee, H. H. (1973). *Hierarchy theory: The challenge of complex systems*. New York: Braziller.
Peterson, S. A., & Somit, A. (1978). Methodological problems associated with a biologically-oriented social science. *Journal of Social and Biological Structures*, *1*, 11–25.
Pospisil, L. (1974). *Anthropology of law*. New Haven, CT: HRAF Press.
Richerson, P. J., & Boyd, R. (1978). A dual inheritance model of human evolutionary process: Basic postulates and a simple model I. *Journal of Social and Biological Structures*, *1*, 127–154.
Richerson, P. J., & Boyd, R. (2005). *Not by genes alone: How culture transformed human evolution*. Chicago: University of Chicago Press.
Rogers, E.M. (1995). *Diffusion of innovations* (4th Ed.). New York: Free Press.
Rokeach, M. (1974). *The nature of human values*. New York: Free Press.
Ruyle, E. E. (1973). Genetic and cultural pools: Some suggestions for a unified theory of biocultural evolution. *Human Ecology*, *1*, 201–215.
Ryan, R. M., & Deci, E. L. (2000). Self-determination theory and the facilitation of intrinsic motivation, social development, and well-being. *American Psychologist*, *55*, 68–78.
Ryan, R. M., & Deci, E. L. (2001). On happiness and human potentials: A review of research on hedonic and eudaimonic well-being. *Annual Review of Psychology*, *2*, 141–166.
Schaller, M., Simpson, J., & Kenrick, D. (2006). *Evolution and social psychology*. Philadelphia: Psychology Press.
Schmidt, M. R., & Wei, W. (2006). Loss of agro-biodiversity, uncertainty, and perceived control: A comparative risk perception study in Austria and China. *Risk Analysis*, *26*, 455–470.
Schwartz, S. H., & Bilsky, W. (1987). Toward a theory of the universal structure and content of values: Extensions and cross-cultural replications. *Journal of Personality and Social Psychology*, *58*, 878–891.
Simon, H. (1969). *The sciences of artificial*. Cambridge, MA: MIT Press.
Simonton, D. (1994). *Greatness: Who makes history and why*. New York: Guilford.
Singer, J. A. (2004). Narrative identity and meaning making across the adult life span: An introduction. *Journal of Personality*, *72*, 438–459.
Somit, A., & Peterson, S. A. (1996). Indoctrinability as an evolutionary precondition for democracy. *Journal of Social and Evolutionary Systems*, *19*, 41–54.
Sperber, D. (2000). An objection to the memetic approach to culture. In R. Aunger (Ed.), *Darwinizing culture: The status of memetics as a science* (pp. 163–173). New York: Oxford University Press.

Sternberg, R. J. (Ed.) (1988). *The nature of creativity*. New York: Cambridge University Press.
Super, C. M., & Harkness, S. (1986). The developmental niche: A conceptualization at the interface of child and culture. *International Journal of Behavioral Development*, *9*, 545–569.
Sword, W., Watt, S., & Krueger, P. (2006). Postpartum health, service needs, and access to care experiences of immigrant and Canadian-born women. *Journal of Obstetric, Gynecologic & Neonatal Nursing*, *35*, 717–727.
Symons, D. (1990). Adaptiveness and adaptation. *Ethology and Sociobiology*, *11*, 427–444.
Taylor, S. E., & Gollwitzer, P. M. (1995). Effects of mindset on positive illusions. *Journal of Personality and Social Psychology*, *69*, 213–226.
Tomasello, M. (1999). *The cultural origins of human cognition*. Cambridge, MA: Harvard University Press.
Tomasello, M., Kruger, A. C., & Ratner, H. H. (1993). Cultural learning. *Behavioral and Brain Sciences*, *16*, 495–552.
Triandis, H. C. (1994). *Culture and social behavior*. New York: McGraw-Hill.
Triandis, H. C. (1999). *Individualism and collectivism*. Boulder, CO: Westview.
Uchida, Y., Norasakkunkit, V., & Kitayama, S. (2004). Cultural constructions of happiness: Theory and empirical evidence. *Journal of Happiness Studies*, *5*, 223–239.
Vaalsiner, J. (1998). *The guided mind*. Cambridge, MT: Harvard University Press.
Vaalsiner, J. (2007). Personal culture and conduct of value. *Journal of Social, Evolutionary, and Cultural Psychology*, *1*, 59–65.
Werner, E. E. (1979). *Cross-cultural Child Development: a view from the Planet Earth*. Monterey, CA: Brooks/COIe.
Weiss, P. (1971). *Hierarchical organized systems in theory and practice*. New York: Hafner.
Williamson, N. E. (1976). *Sons or daughters: A cross-cultural survey of parental preferences*. Beverly Hills and London: Sage.
Wilson, E. O. (1975). *Sociobiology: The new synthesis*. Harvard, MA: Bellknap.
Yamagishi, T., Jin, N., & Kiyonari, T. (1999). Bounded generalized reciprocity: Ingroup boasting and ingroup favoritism. *Advances in Group Processes*, *16*, 161–197.

Chapter 3
Psychological Selection and Optimal Experience

3.1 Human Beings and Complexity

As briefly outlined in Chapter 2, far from being passive vehicles of biological and cultural information, individuals play an active role both in determining their life trajectories and in influencing the long-term development of the human species. The scientific advancements of the twentieth century helped clarify this role.

In particular, crucial contributions came from physics and biology which incorporated the study of human beings within a wider living systems perspective (von Bertalanffy, 1968). As such, individuals present two relevant characteristics: They are autopoietic, self-organizing systems aiming at reproducing their specific organization pattern (Maturana & Varala, 1980; Varela, Thompson, & Rosch, 1991). They are also complex, far-from-equilibrium living entities, in constant dynamic interaction with their environment, be it natural or cultural (Prigogine & Stengers, 1984).

Chaos theory clearly describes the dynamical processes underlying energy exchanges (Vandervert, 1995), stressing that complexity in the living systems is promoted by the constant coordination and integration of their constituent parts that contribute to maintain their far-from-equilibrium state. Maintaining and increasing order in the living universe requires energy consumption that is partly transformed into work and ordered structures, and partly dissipated. If energy is not constantly provided, living systems will tend to homogenize, to lose the specialization and differentiation of their components, and to fall into disorder and entropy. In other words, they will face death, a process which is typical of living beings, for which life is synonymous with energy consumption and tendency to negative entropy, that is specialization and differentiation.

At the evolutionary level, the survival and replication of a complex living system are based on well-defined emerging properties typical of that system and promoting its adaptation (see Chapter 2). From this perspective, among the emerging features of human beings, mind and cognition play a key role, in that they promote self-regulated adaptation, that is self-transformation of structural characteristics with the aim to preserve the system's organization within the various patterns of interaction with the environment (Maturana & Varala, 1980).

A. Delle Fave et al., *Psychological Selection and Optimal Experience Across Cultures*, Cross-Cultural Advancements in Positive Psychology 2,
DOI 10.1007/978-90-481-9876-4_3,

The nervous system was selected to meet the demands of the chaotic possibilities of an ever-changing environment (Vandervert, 1995). The mind reflects the organization of the human brain. Indeed, the tendency toward complexity can be highlighted both in the brain and in the mind. Neurons are members of large ensembles that are constantly disappearing and arising through their cooperative interactions (Varela et al., 1991, p. 94). An individual neuron participates in many global patterns, in which multiple neurons resonate, and bears little significance when taken individually. Similarly, cognition is the emergence of global states in a network of simple components through local rules for changes in the connectivity among the elements (Varela et al., 1991, p. 99). Symbols—as the units of cognition—are higher-level descriptions of properties that are ultimately embedded in an underlying distributed system (Varela et al., 1991, p. 101).

3.2 Mind, Consciousness, and Human Agency

The scientific advances outlined above provide an overarching framework for understanding the active role of individuals in the interaction with their environment. In particular, the human mind plays a crucial role in directing, organizing, and monitoring the efforts toward energy exchange for survival and adaptation. The mind, like any other living system, tends toward order and complexity and presents various states, commonly referred to as experiences, which are ultimately determined by the mind's dynamic structure and organization. From the evolutionary perspective, consciousness can be understood as an outcome of dynamic energy principles; analogously, conscious experience can be described as the continuously generated entirety of a space–time template in the brain, reflecting the two fundamental conditions of organic existence—space and time—which represent the coordinates of the surrounding environment, including the individual's body. In other words, "consciousness continuously constructs a model of space–time in the brain as a comparator system by which the brain can movement-by-movement, moment-by-moment differentiate itself from, and make sense of, the constant barrage of incoming sensory information as it itself continuously reconfigures its own dimensionalities" (Vandervert, 1995, pp. 113–114).

The mind is then palpable both as patterns of sub-circuitry erected and nested in the brain and as exteriorizable (culturally sharable) mental models. It can be defined as an individual's collection of culturally sharable mental-model circuitry configurations in the brain. It began with cultural evolution and continues to evolve in both its composition and nature. The continuously iterated process of thinking has resulted in the increasing cultural exteriorization of the features of the organization of consciousness. This means that the evolution of culture proceeds in the direction of progressively more complete and efficient exteriorizations of the organization of the mind.

From the psychological perspective, there is no unified definition of consciousness. At the dawn of scientific psychology, William James (1890) identified two forms of consciousness: The first one is the sensational or *reproductive consciousness* (Shapiro, 1997), common to all mammalians and related to empirical knowledge. Through the interaction with the environmental stimuli, it promotes the acquisition of new information and behavior that are useful for survival and adaptation. The second form, relating or *productive consciousness* (Shapiro, 1997), implies the emergence of new knowledge from inside the individual, through new patterns of integration and connection between information units previously acquired. Productive consciousness generates relational knowledge about the world. It promotes world reconstruction and interpretation through new configurations of information that can be used to solve new problems, build new artifacts, and develop new ideas.

In contemporary neurosciences, at least the following distinct concepts have been identified (Koivisto, Kainulainen, & Revonsuo, 2009; Lambie & Marcel, 2002): (a) phenomenal consciousness, referring to subjective experience in its purest conceivable form (for example, the phenomenal character of various visual sensations); (b) reflective consciousness, that is subjective experience that can be conceptualized, categorized, named, reported, and voluntarily acted upon; and (c) self-awareness, a form of reflective consciousness focusing on the self. In particular, self-awareness is characterized by the presence of a conscious self as an agent of behavior. "The self is simply an epiphenomenon of conscious processes, the result of consciousness becoming aware of itself" (Csikszentmihalyi & Csikszentmihalyi, 1988, p. 20).

Besides being directed by internal drives, like hunger, or external rewards, like social approval, behavior is guided by priorities established by the needs of the self. In order to perform within the infinitely complex ecosystem to which it became adapted, the human organism established autonomy from the genetically determined instructions that had shaped its behavior and took on a mediating role between genetic instructions and cultural norms and rules. Like every other system, the main function of the self is to maintain itself and possibly to grow and to replicate. The self follows its own *teleonomy*, that is its own projects and goals, which are related to its intrinsic structure (Massimini & Calegari, 1979; Massimini, Inghilleri, & Delle Fave, 1996).

Since the cognitivistic revolution of the 1960s, an increasing number of studies in psychology have stressed the importance of conscious experience in steering human behavior, giving individuals the ability to self-regulate current actions, plan long-term goals, anticipate future rewards, and reflect upon obtained outcomes. Also intervention programs aiming to the promotion of individuals' health and well-being heavily rely on the ability to consciously and willingly regulate one's behavior (Delle Fave & Bassi, 2007). Conscious processes are processes that are accompanied by awareness of certain aspects of the process itself (for example, we are aware of our speaking while we do it) and/or awareness of relevant contents (e.g., the topic of our conversation) (Dijksterhuis & Aarts, 2010).

The sense of agency, defined as the experience of oneself as the agent of one's own actions, allows individuals to intentionally influence one's functions and the environment in order to contribute to life circumstances (Bassi, Sartori, & Delle Fave, 2010; David, Newen, & Vogely, 2008). Human agency is characterized by intentionality, forethought, self-reactiveness, and self-reflectiveness (Bandura, 2001). Intentionality is the ability to form intentions that include action plans and strategies to realize them. An intention is a representation of a future course of action to be performed; it is a proactive commitment to bring about future actions. Forethought involves a temporal extension of agency: Individuals set goals and anticipate outcomes of prospective actions to guide and motivate their efforts. Self-reactiveness includes the concept that people are not only planners and forethinkers but also self-regulators who motivate and adjust the execution of their actions according to circumstances and desired outcomes. Finally, self-reflectiveness implies people's ability to reflect on their personal efficacy, soundness of their thoughts and actions, meaning of their pursuits, and to make corrective adjustments if necessary.

3.3 Attention and the Stream of Subjective Experience

William James greatly contributed to the analysis of conscious experience as process (1890). As described by him "thinking of some sort *goes on*" (p. 44), namely it is individually reported as a stream of states of mind succeeding each other, which presents five important features: (a) each thought tends to be part of a personal consciousness, i.e., to be subjective and not directly accessible by others; (b) thought is in constant change since no state, once gone, can recur and be identical with what it was before, considering that mental reactions on every given thing are a resultant of individual experience of the whole world (internal and external) up to that date; (c) thought is sensibly continuous as the individual perceives no interruptions in it; (d) thought always appears to deal with objects independent of itself, belonging to an outer reality; (e) thought is interested in some parts of these objects to the exclusion of others, and welcomes or rejects—or chooses—from among them while it thinks.

The latter point stresses a crucial aspect of conscious experience: Its content is selected among many possible concurrent "objects" or information (sensory or previously formed mental representations) through the selective focus of attention. According to James (1890, p. 277), "the mind is at every stage a theatre of simultaneous possibilities. Consciousness consists in the comparison of these with each other, the selection of some, and the suppression of the rest by the reinforcing and inhibiting agency of attention." With another fine metaphor, James maintains that "the mind works on the data it receives very much as a sculptor works on his block of stone. In a sense the statue stood there from eternity. But there were thousand different ones beside it, and the sculptor alone is to thank for having extricated this one from the rest" (p. 277).

Research in cognitive sciences has widely investigated the selective characteristic of attention as a means to choose information. Selection is based on either bottom-up exogenous or top-down endogenous factors (Koch & Tsuchiya, 2006). Exogenous cues are object features that transiently attract attention or eye gaze and are of instinctive or learned biological importance (i.e., automatic orienting based on object saliency); whereas endogenous cues are task-dependent factors volitionally controlled by the individual (e.g., driven by personal goals). Research has further established that attention is multidimensional (Posner, Inhoff, Friedrich, & Cohen, 1987; Raz & Buhle, 2006), involving alerting, orienting, and executive processes. Alerting or vigilance is the ability to strengthen and maintain response readiness in preparation for an impending stimulus. Orienting refers to the ability to choose incoming sensory information to which to attend. Executive attention involves planning or decision making, error detection, regulation of thoughts and feelings, and overcoming of habitual actions (Raz & Buhle, 2006).

Much debate has focused on the relationship between attention and consciousness (Dijksterhuis & Aarts, 2010; Koch & Tsuchiya, 2006; Koivisto et al., 2009). While some researchers have argued that top-down attention and consciousness are inextricably interwoven (Dehaene, Changeux, Naccache, Sackur, & Sergent, 2006; Posner, 1994), increasing psychophysical and neuropsychological evidence supports researchers who maintain that they are distinct phenomena, with distinct neural mechanisms. This implies that four combinations are possible between attention and consciousness: attention with consciousness, no attention/no consciousness, attention without consciousness, and consciousness in the near absence of attention (see Koch & Tsuchiya, 2006, for a review of the empirical findings on visual perception). A great number of studies have attested to the benefits afforded by the combination of consciousness and attention in planning behavior or problem solving (e.g., working memory, verbal reportability, metacognitive skills). At the same time, complex behaviors—such as running mountain trails, climbing, playing soccer, driving home on "automatic pilot," and even goal-directed actions—can be quoted as instances of top-down attention without consciousness or consciousness with little or no top-down attention (Dijksterhuis & Aarts, 2010; Koch & Tsuchiya, 2006). These instances attest to the distinct functions of consciousness and attention in favoring individuals' adaptation to the environment: While attention plays a key role in selecting information, consciousness is involved in "summarizing all the information that pertains to the current state of the organism and its environment, and ensuring this compact summary is accessible to the planning areas of the brain, and also detecting anomalies and errors, decision making, language, inferring the internal state of other individuals, setting long-term goals, making recursive models and rational thought" (Koch & Tsuchiya, 2006, p. 17). These instances further highlight the complex relations between consciousness and attention and their differential impact on individuals' performance in given situations and tasks, confirming, for example, the long-held belief that paying attention can become counterproductive in performing tasks that require sensory-motor skills, such as playing basketball (Beilock, Carr, MacMahon, & Starkes, 2002).

3.4 Optimal Experience and Order in Consciousness

At any given moment, individuals are faced with a great number of information coming from the outer and inner worlds which greatly exceeds the limited capacity of the psychic functions devoted to its processing (Csikszentmihalyi, 1978). From the perspective of the theory of communication (Shannon & Weaver, 1963), information is "a measure of one's freedom of choice when one selects a message" (p. 9) and is commonly expressed in terms of entropy, that is in relation to the number of possible alternatives or degree of randomness in the situation: Thus, the higher the number of alternatives, the higher the number of information bits.

While this definition regards the quantitative aspects of a message, the quality and content of information is linked to (a) meaning (see Chapters 1 and 2), that is the relationship between content and individuals' life trajectories and cultural and social systems and (b) the quality of subjective experience people associate with the information content (Csikszentmihalyi & Massimini, 1985; Delle Fave, 2004).

Subjective experience is composed of cognitive, emotional, and motivational aspects and represents the conscious processing of information coming from the external environment and the inner world of a person (Csikszentmihalyi, 1982; Hilgard, 1980). Since the late 1970s, Mihaly Csikszentmihalyi has greatly contributed to the investigation of the phenomenology of subjective experience through the analysis of people's self-reports and descriptions of their quality of experience in various situations and contexts, for example, while performing complex and challenging tasks at work or during leisure time, such as surgery, art, mountain climbing, and chess playing (1975/2000, 1990, 1993). In particular, he identified *flow* or *optimal experience*, as a complex and highly structured state of deep involvement, absorption, and enjoyment. Here are some expressions individuals use to describe it (Csikszentmihalyi, 1975):

> My mind isn't wandering. I am totally involved in what I am doing and I am not thinking of anything else. My body feels good... the world seems to be cut off from me... I am less aware of myself and my problems.
>
> My concentration is like breathing... I never think of it... When I start, I really do shut out the world.
>
> I am so involved in what I am doing... I don't see myself as separate from what I am doing.

In particular, the term *flow* expresses the feeling of fluidity and continuity in concentration and action reported by most individuals in the description of this state. The term *optimal experience* refers to the pervasive positivity of cognitive, emotional, and motivational features reported in this condition.

Optimal experience is characterized by the following dimensions (Csikszentmihalyi & Csikszentmihalyi, 1988; Csikszentmihalyi, 1975, 1990; Nakamura & Csikszentmihalyi, 2009):

1. Balance between perceived high *challenges* or opportunities for action and high personal *skills*: The individuals perceive that they are facing a highly challenging activity and that they possess adequate abilities to face them. An activity need not be "active" in the physical sense, and the skills necessary to engage in it need not be physical (Csikszentmihalyi, 1990). Tasks such as reading and socializing have also been reported as *optimal activities* (or activities associated with flow).
2. Intense and focused concentration on the present moment: People report focusing attention on the task at hand, leaving no room in the mind for irrelevant information. Attention is thus undivided and focused in the present.

3. Merging of action and awareness: While being absorbed in the activity, individuals are not aware of themselves as separate from the actions they are performing. The activity becomes spontaneous, almost automatic, and is perceived as effortless even if discipline and training are required to cultivate the personal skills necessary to face the challenges.
4. Loss of reflective self-consciousness: The individual loses awareness of herself as separate from the world around her, and a feeling of union with the environment arises. Loss of self-scrutiny does not imply being unaware of what happens in one's body or mind. "What slips below the threshold of awareness is the *concept* of self, the information we use to represent to ourselves who we are. . .When not preoccupied with our selves, we actually have a chance to expand the concept of who we are" (Csikszentmihalyi, 1990, p. 64).
5. Sense of control over one's actions: Rather than the sense of *being* in control, individuals experience the sense of *exercising* control. Most importantly, they hold the knowledge that in principle they have the possibility of keeping things under control, which conveys a sense of security and power in the face of all those daily life situations in which they feel unable to influence what happens to and around them.
6. Alteration of temporal experience: Time no longer seems to pass the way it ordinarily does, and it is typically perceived to pass faster than normal (Nakamura & Csikszentmihalyi, 2009). However, in flow activities depending on clock time (e.g., running), individuals have been shown to be able to track the exact passage of time with little margin of error (Csikszentmihalyi, 1990).
7. Clear goals: Individuals must know what they want to achieve. Goals can be proximal such as winning a basketball game, or have long-term meaning such as becoming a surgeon. Without clear demands on attention, the mind becomes unfocused and begins to run toward personal problems (Jackson & Csikszentmihalyi, 1999). On the contrary, goals facilitate attention focus and commitment to meaningful activities.
8. Clear rules and positive feedback about the progress being made: It is difficult to become immersed in an activity in which one does not know what needs to be done, or how well one is doing (Csikszentmihalyi & Csikszentmihalyi, 1988). Even when the rules have to be invented, such as in creative activities, they serve to give order to individual actions; whereas, positive feedback contains the message that the performance is going well and a specific goal has been met.
9. Intrinsic motivation: Performing a flow activity is perceived as intrinsically rewarding. Flow is an *autotelic* experience in that it is an end in itself; it entails doing something for the interest in and enjoyment of it, with no expectation of external gain or reward.

The reported phenomenology was remarkably similar across settings, activities, and cultures (Massimini & Delle Fave, 2000) and will be further analyzed in the following chapters in the light of the research conducted over the last three decades.

From a historical perspective (Delle Fave, in press), Csikszentmihalyi's approach to the analysis of people's quality of experience was consistent with the prominent issues explored by the psychologists of his time, and in particular with two of them: the relationship between perceived challenges and personal skills, and intrinsic motivation.

As concerns the relationship between challenges and skills, at the beginning of the twentieth century, Yerkes and Dodson (1908) identified an inverted U-shape function between arousal and performance while studying the effects of perceived challenges on behavior. Further studies in the domain of education showed that engagement in optimally challenging situations captures attention and maximizes learning (Dewey, 1934; Piaget, 1950; Vygotsky, 1978). In the late 1950s, researchers connected the human tendency to give order and meaning to reality to the attribution of causality to events (Heider, 1958). Through the constructs of locus of causality (Weiner, 1972) and locus of control (Rotter, 1966), scholars attempted to investigate the beliefs people hold regarding the role and effectiveness of their abilities, skills, and efforts in coping with life demands and events. In the 1960s and 1970s, the relationship between perceived demands and resources was investigated moving from the assumption that environmental demands can be appraised either as challenges and opportunities for action or as threats and obstacles. The investigation of stress and coping strategies provided important contribution to this field. Particularly, according to Lazarus (1966), stress arises when individuals perceive that they cannot adequately cope with high environmental demands threatening their lives. On the other hand, Antonovsky (1979) used the term salutogenesis to describe the processes and coping strategies that promote a good quality of life in adverse situations, stressing the role of the sense of coherence (SOC) in promoting positive adaptation through a general orientation toward reality comprising comprehensibility, manageability, and meaningfulness. In the same vein, Bandura formalized the construct of self-efficacy as individuals' perceived capabilities to exercise control over their level of functioning and environmental demands. These beliefs influence cognitive, motivational, affective, and decisional processes. They further extend their influence over aspirations and strength of goal commitment, level of motivation and perseverance in the face of difficulties, causal attribution for successes and failures, perception of environmental challenges and impediments (Bandura, 1997).

In the field of motivation, researchers' attention gradually shifted from incentive-based models to models focusing on the active and creative role of the individual. Maslow (1971) introduced the concept of self-actualization, a need stemming from the person's subjective perception of her own potentials and meanings. Maslow highlighted the human capability to set goals that foster the implementation of complexity at the psychological and behavioral levels. Later on, Edward Deci (1975) formalized the concept of intrinsic motivation, namely the innate and natural tendency to pursue one's interests and exercise one's abilities (Deci & Ryan, 1985, p. 43). This aspect—which Csikszentmihalyi (1975/2000) described as characteristic of flow—was included in the framework of Self-Determination Theory (SDT, Ryan & Deci, 2000; Chapter 1).

This theoretical background provided fertile ground for the study of subjective experience and the formalization of flow. Flow presents a well-defined configuration, a precise structure, and intrinsic stability (Delle Fave, 2004). While *psychic entropy* refers to those states that produce disorder in consciousness by conflicting with individual goals—including experiences such as fear, boredom, and apathy—*psychic negentropy* is obtained when all the contents of consciousness are in harmony with each other, and with the goals that define the person's self. These include optimal experience. Therefore, in line with a "phenomenological model of consciousness based on information theory" (Csikszentmihalyi, 1990, p. 25), flow can be considered as an ordered state of consciousness, quite distant from equilibrium or entropy: Thoughts, intentions, feelings, and all the senses are focused on the same goal, and experience is in harmony.

Csikszentmihalyi further highlighted the intrinsically dynamic characteristic of optimal experience (Csikszentmihalyi, 1975; Delle Fave, Bassi, & Massimini, 2009), resting on the perceived match between high environmental challenges and adequate personal skills. "Because the tendency of the self is to reproduce itself, and because the self is most congruent with its own goal-directed structure during the episodes of optimal experience, to keep on experiencing flow becomes one of the central goals of the self" (Csikszentmihalyi & Csikszentmihalyi, 1988, p. 24). While first engaging in a new activity as beginners, people usually perceive high challenges—on the one hand—and only limited personal skills—on the other. This condition can generate a certain amount of anxiety. Nevertheless, the activity can be perceived as interesting and stimulating, the individual can derive satisfaction and enjoyment from the mobilization of personal resources, and consistency can be detected between the contents of the activity and personal goals. Under these conditions, flow is likely to be perceived, and to trigger the active investment of time and effort in the practice and cultivation of the intrinsically rewarding activity. This progressively leads to an increase in skills and competencies, and to the search for higher challenges in order to avoid a state of boredom (associated with the perception of high skills and low challenges) and to support the engagement, concentration, and involvement that characterize optimal experience in the long term.

From this dynamic perspective, flow can thus be considered as an *attractor* in consciousness (Ceja & Navarro, 2009; Delle Fave, 1996; Guastello, Johnson, & Rieke, 1999). An attractor is defined as a set of states of a dynamic physical system toward which that system tends to evolve, regardless of the starting conditions of the system. As reported by Ceja and Navarro (2009), people tend to be less predictable in positive states than in negative states. The authors build on Fredrickson's model of positive emotions (2001; see Chapter 1) which states that positive states of mind broaden momentary thought–action displays, as opposed to negative states of mind which tend to narrow those same displays. Studies have shown that flow fluctuates over time in a nonlinear dynamic fashion. Additionally, individuals organize their daily routine in a manner that maintains flow in given activities, while meeting externally imposed task and time demands (Guastello et al., 1999). Flow experience thus represents a magnetic pole that pulls the individual toward it again (Csikszentmihalyi, 1990). The dynamic process related to challenges and skills gives rise to a virtuous circle fostering individual development, through both the ceaseless acquisition of increasingly complex information and the refinement of competencies (Delle Fave, 2004; Massimini & Delle Fave, 2000).

3.5 Optimal Experience, Complexity, and Psychological Selection

In light of its positive and complex characteristics as well as its intrinsically dynamic nature, flow plays a central role in the teleonomy of the self, contributing to the self's growth in complexity (Csikszentmihalyi, 1990, 1993). Optimal experience can be considered as the "psychic compass" supporting the developmental trajectory each individual autonomously builds and follows throughout life (Delle Fave, 2007). Individuals tend to reproduce and cultivate across time those activities and situations that they associate with optimal experience. Throughout their lives, they thus build a personal *life theme* that is a set of interests and goals they uniquely cultivate and pursue (Csikszentmihalyi & Beattie, 1979).

Life theme is a core component of a broader selective process ceaselessly taking place in consciousness, defined *psychological selection* (Csikszentmihalyi & Massimini, 1985). It is rooted in the moment-by-moment interactions between the biological and the cultural information that take place within the human mind, and it unfolds in the long term as the progressive development and differentiation of each individual based on the stratified outcomes of millions of such momentary person–environment interactions (Chapter 2). Psychological selection continuously integrates and modifies the information provided by the two hereditary systems, so that each person in her lifetime becomes both the object and the subject in the selective process, both the sculptor and the block of stone described by James (1890, p. 277; Section 3.3).

Psychological selection does not only have implications for single individuals, it also plays a crucial role for the entire human species in the long term. As reported in Chapter 2, individuals are biocultural entities who grow within a developmental niche that includes the natural environment, significant others, and the broader cultural set of memes and rules regulating social interactions (Delle Fave, 2004, 2007; Massimini & Delle Fave, 2000). Through the process of psychological selection, individuals become active agents in reproducing and transmitting biological and cultural information, contributing to the differential survival and replication of their biological and cultural pools.

Being rooted in the subjective elaboration and evaluation of environmental information, psychological selection is oriented by the quality of experience individuals associate to these processes. The intentional and preferential focus of attention toward information (activities, situations, social interactions) that are associated with flow make this experience a core component of psychological selection (Csikszentmihalyi & Massimini, 1985; Massimini et al., 1996), substantially contributing to its long-term direction and orientation. This process leads to individual differentiation within the social group, emphasizing the uniqueness of each individual's developmental trend (Massimini & Delle Fave, 2000).

As the self pursues its own teleonomy, related to but in principle independent of the welfare of genes and cultures, psychological selection represents a full-fledge selective paradigm (Massimini et al., 1996). "Human evolution can thus be understood through the interaction of three interacting teleonomies:

1. Intrasomatic genetic memory which tends to reproduce itself;
2. Extrasomatic cultural memories that tend to reproduce their own kind;
3. Experiences tending to replicate themselves within the life cycle of individual consciousness" (Csikszentmihalyi & Massimini, 1985, p. 132).

In attempting to keep its internal order, consciousness differentially selects among available memes. Memes that facilitate flow experiences are preserved as they provide order in consciousness by eliminating randomness, specifying clear goals into which attention can be invested, providing adequate means for reaching them, producing relatively unambiguous feedback to the actors. For example, studying—the primary means to transmit cultural information across generations—is commonly reported as a privileged flow activity across cultures (Delle Fave & Bassi, 2000; Stokart, Cavallo, Fianco, & Lombardi, 2007; Chapter 7). The same process holds true for selecting among alternatives that will affect the genetic instructions. The choice of a mate in humans depends on a variety of considerations, among which is "compatibility"; a compatible mate is one that preserves, or increases, the order in one's consciousness (Csikszentmihalyi & Massimini, 1985). Additionally, an analysis of the quality of experience in couples expecting their first child showed that fathers and mothers invest their attention in those activities that are related to the biological event under way, and that are primarily associated with optimal experience (Delle Fave & Massimini, 2004; Chapter 10).

The teleonomy of the self is even more evident in the cultivation of activities which threaten the individual's genetic survival. A climber, for instance, puts his life at risk for the sake of reproducing optimal experience (Delle Fave, Bassi, & Massimini, 2003a; Massimini et al., 1996; Chapter 9). No sophisticated utilitarian reasoning can otherwise explain such activity, since individuals spend hours and hours to reach peaks which could be easily accessible by cable-car or helicopter.

These examples attest to the strict interconnection between the three selection paradigms, namely the relation of causal circularity existing among them (Massimini et al., 1996). They highlight the possible cooperation and competition among the paradigms through the active role of individuals in influencing their cultural and biological pools. On the one hand, individuals can take part in preserving their cultural and biological pools by selecting available information. Through genetic inheritance, direct experience, socialization, and cultural learning, individuals acquire information that can be useful in developing adaptive behaviors and engaging in meaningful goal-directed activities that reflect the values of their culture (Gauvain, 1995). On the other hand, they can promote modification and innovation in their biological and cultural pools by creating ever new information; these include new technological inventions such as PCR (Polymerase Chain Reaction), the procedure used in molecular biology to amplify or replicate a particular DNA sequence manifold, generating thousands to millions of identical copies.

Optimal experience per se implies constant differentiation: In order to replicate the state of flow, individuals need to gradually increase their skills and look for progressively more complex challenges, thus introducing new elements, new information, and observations derived from previously executing the activities. In either case, the outcomes of psychological selection can have cross-generational effects, both in influencing future generations' construction of their life themes and in contributing to guide humans toward higher levels of complexity and adaptation to their living environment.

3.6 The Neurophysiological Underpinnings of Optimal Experience

Optimal experience as the core of psychological selection and the outcome of human evolution tending toward complexity can be characterized as a "biological predisposition to enjoy" the integration of cultural and biological information in consciousness (Csikszentmihalyi & Massimini, 1985). In light of the theoretical and technological advancements in the study of brain activity and conscious experience, researchers have recently attempted to identify the neurophysiological underpinnings of optimal experience.

Two major perspectives have been proposed, both resting on the conceptualization of cognitive functions as hierarchically ordered: Under evolutionary pressures, ever more integrative neural structures developed and became able to process increasingly complex information.

Arne Dietrich (2004) focused in particular on the "effortless information processing" that is characteristic of flow. The brain presents two distinct information processing systems to acquire, memorize, and represent knowledge (Dienes & Pernes, 1999). The explicit system—which has evolved to increase cognitive and behavioral *flexibility*—is associated with the higher cognitive functions of the frontal lobe and medial temporal lobe structures. Its content can be expressed verbally and is tied to conscious awareness. On the opposite, the implicit system—which favors *efficient*, effortless information processing and performance—is associated with the skill-based knowledge supported primarily by the basal ganglia. Its content cannot be expressed verbally and it is inaccessible to conscious awareness. The two systems may work together in order to maximize the flexibility/efficiency trade-off (Dietrich, 2004). For example, when learning to drive a car, the individual follows the instructor's explicit commands, the explicit system in the prefrontal cortex forms a mental representation of the task requirements and recruits the premotor cortex and primary cortex to execute it (Jenkins, Brooks, Nixon, Frackowiak, & Passingham, 1994). With increasing practice, the implicit system—including the basal ganglia, the supplementary motor cortex, the motor thalamus, and the hippocampus—gains control over the required tasks, bypasses consciousness, and promotes performance efficiency. From this perspective, flow can be considered as a "period during which a highly practiced skill that is represented in the implicit system's knowledge base is implemented without interference from the explicit system" (Dietrich, 2004, p. 746). For flow to occur, a state of transient hypofrontality is needed which temporarily suppresses the conscious analytical capacities of the explicit system, with the notable exception of executive attention, which enables the one-pointedness of mind by selectively disengaging other higher cognitive abilities of the prefrontal cortex. However, due to the variety of activities associated with flow, we can expect differences in the neurophysiological mechanisms involved in the onset of the experience. For example, the hypofrontality hypothesis is especially convincing in relation to physical activities and manual tasks. However, it may not hold for purely intellectual activities, in which the body plays a background role (Hunter & Csikszentmihalyi, 2000) and different awareness/consciousness patterns can come into play (Dietrich 2010, personal communication).

The second attempt to identify the neurophysiological foundations of flow has come from communication research and rests on the notion of synchronization of brain activity. The idea that consciousness is related to synchronization of neural activity can be found in the work by Tononi and Edelman (1998). In their theory of integrated information, the authors describe consciousness as a process emerging from dynamic cores, that is functional clusters of neurons characterized by high levels of integration and information, quite likely related to the thalamocortical system. Just like the "quantity" of consciousness can be measured as the capacity of a system to integrate information, also the "quality" of conscious experience results from the moment-by-moment integration of specific groups of selectively interacting neurons (Tononi & Massimini, 2005).

Weber and colleagues (2009) maintain that Dietrich's explanation oversimplifies the operationalization of flow, and stress that the notion of hypofrontality stands in sharp contrast to understanding flow as a state of focused attention. In particular, studies using functional magnetic resonance (fMRI) have provided convincing evidence for increased rather than reduced activity in involved prefrontal networks during states of focused attention (Raz & Buhle, 2006). According to the authors, flow is related to the ability of the brain to bind different processes together into a single conscious experience through the mechanism of neuronal oscillatory synchronization, that is synchronization of brain waves oscillations (Buzsáki, 2006; Crick & Koch, 1990). Transitions from non-synchronous to synchronous states are abrupt or discrete, and synchronization leads to qualitatively different phenomena. As described by Haken, the brain "operates close to instabilities and achieves its activity by self-organization which leads to the emergence of new qualities" (2006, p. 110). Additionally, neural synchronization is energetically cheap: Through neural coordination an increased output can be obtained with less effort. From this perspective, "flow is a discrete, energetically optimized, and gratifying experience resulting from the synchronization of attentional and rewards networks under the condition of balance between challenge and skill" (Weber et al., 2009, p. 412). Brain areas controlling alerting and orienting could be involved, such as the frontal and parietal cortical regions, as well as the superior and inferior parietal lobe regions, the frontal eye fields, and the superior colliculus. Also pleasure and reward areas of the brain could be involved, including the dopaminergic system, the orbitofrontal cortex, the ventromedial and dorsolateral regions of the prefrontal cortex, the thalamus, and the striatum.

At present, neither of the two theoretical frameworks has received full empirical investigation. This is due to the fact that they are in their infancy and that it is quite difficult to elicit and study optimal experience in a lab: While conditions favoring flow onset have been widely investigated (see Chapter 5), flow remains a fleeting experience which is extremely difficult to bridle. Nevertheless, the two perspectives provide interesting assumptions on the neurophysiological bases of this complex state of consciousness that can go hand in hand with the results obtained from its phenomenological analysis and that can help clarify, from an evolutionary perspective, the existence of a positive and complex state of mind, shared by all human beings as a part of the normal psychological functioning, and acting as a powerful engine of development and self-actualization (Delle Fave, in press).

3.7 Optimal Experience and Positive Human Functioning: A Contribution to Eudaimonia

Psychological selection has been shown to promote complexity in consciousness through the constant integration of biocultural information and, through the preferential replication of flow experiences. At the same time, it has been shown to influence human cultural and biological selections through the differential investment of attention on available information (Massimini & Delle Fave, 2000).

From the perspective of positive psychology, flow plays a crucial role in contributing to individuals' happiness. In particular, the emphasis placed on flow as an ongoing process based on personal goals and meaning-making makes it a clearly eudaimonic construct.

Seligman (2002) has identified in optimal experience the pathway to engagement in life. Flow shapes individuals' life themes (Csikszentmihalyi & Beattie, 1979), since experiencing flow encourages a person to persist in and return to an activity because of the experiential rewards it promises, and thereby fosters growth of skills over time and search for ever-increasing challenges (Nakamura & Csikszentmihalyi, 2009). Flow brings order in consciousness, promotes mental health (Delle Fave & Massimini, 1992; see Chapter 14), and engagement in activities which are meaningful for the individual. People do not describe themselves as happy when they spend life in perfect biological homeostasis, with no change or no opportunities to express their talents and to put their knowledge and abilities to the test. On the contrary, psychological well-being is associated with search for high challenges, increment in competence, construction and cultivation of meaningful relations, development of psychological characteristics which differentiate the individual from the other members of the community and promote personal identity.

Individuals' well-being is strictly related to the flow opportunities provided by society. Inasmuch as a society, for example, overwhelms its members with excessive attention-disruptive challenges in a daily multi-task rat-race (Nakamura & Csikszentmihalyi, 2009) or provides trivial and repetitive tasks quenching creativity and personal initiative (Massimini & Delle Fave, 2000), individuals can have a hard time identifying and autonomously pursuing their pathway in life. Even material rewards do not contribute to experiencing flow in spite of the overwhelming emphasis of many social systems on accumulation and consumption of artifacts, and on economic and material goals.

When societies provide their members with scarce meaningful opportunities for action, self-expression, and individual growth, it is unlikely that their memes will spread to other groups and that individuals will flourish (Csikszentmihalyi & Massimini, 1985). In addition, not all the pathways to happiness are equally good. Despite its implications in development and in the positive quality of life, flow presents an amoral character (Csikszentmihalyi, 1990; Nakamura & Csikszentmihalyi, 2009). The replication of flow activities alone does not guarantee positive consequences for the individual or society. For example, research has shown that people can associate flow—or pseudo-optimal states, see Chapter 15—with activities damaging the self or others, such as gambling (Wanner, Ladouceur, Auclair, & Vitaro, 2006), stealing (Delle Fave, Bassi, & Massimini, 2003b), graffiti spraying (Rheinberg & Manig, 2003), addiction to internet games (Chou & Ting, 2003), drug intake (Delle Fave & Massimini, 2003), computer hacking (Voiskounsky & Smyslova, 2003), pathological online shopping (Bridges & Florsheim, 2008), and combat situations in which flow-like absorption seems to contribute to both the subjective well-being and to the efficiency of soldiers (Harari, 2008).

For this reason, other eudaimonic components come into play within psychological selection, such as meaning making (Singer, 2004) and the pursuit of self-actualization through activities that are not necessarily rewarding in the short term. Within the framework of psychological selection, and taking into account the cultural and individual dimensions of meaning (Jablonka & Lamb, 2005; Miller, 2001; Chapter 2), optimal experience can be considered as both an antecedent and an outcome. Due to the psychological rewards provided by this condition, the associated activities will be preferentially replicated and cultivated in the long term, thus affecting both the developmental trajectory of the individuals—their psychological selection—and their level of integration and participation. On the other side, through the dynamic features of the meaning-making process and the ceaseless interaction with the environment, activities previously ignored by the individual can become opportunities for optimal experience, sources of new meanings, or both (Delle Fave, 2009), and the amoral aspect of flow can be counterbalanced by individual and social resources that can intervene in steering behavior toward more constructive opportunities for action.

From this perspective, authentic development at the psychological level fosters both individuals' pursuit of psychological well-being and commitment to community improvement (Delle Fave et al., 2009; Smith, Christopher, Delle Fave, &

Bhawuk, 2002). In other words, there are virtuous ways conducive to happiness, namely those which harmonize the pursuit of optimal experiences with individual and collective meanings and goals.

As sustained by Annas in her philosophical reasoning, "virtuous activity can be thought of as an example of flow because it is an unforced expression of the person's reasoning and feelings, in harmony with the rest of her character and structured system of goals" (2008, p. 30) Becoming virtuous is a process, and virtuous activity is rewarding to the virtuous person. What the virtuous person finds enjoyable is the very exercise of virtues (such as bravery, generosity), not the risks or dangers it involves. Thus, people can actively pursue goals that they consider important and valuable, though not necessarily related to their personal well-being; they can invest their resources in activities that are valuable for the community, but that undermine their quality of life in the short term (for example, through constraints on free time or material comforts) (Massimini & Delle Fave, 2000; Sen, 1992).

Virtues can be considered as socially developed skills (Annas, 2008; Haidt & Joseph, 2004). Because they are socially constructed, they will differ across societies based on the specific cultural instructions that have been developed to solve basic human problems and on the hierarchical importance of a given problem in relation to the overall network of problems in different populations (see Chapter 2; Massimini & Calegari, 1979). However, individual psychological selection can unfold not only around personal and culture-specific challenges and goals, but also around concerns for other human beings, regardless of their biological and cultural background (Massimini & Delle Fave, 2000). Interestingly enough, recent experiments have shown that social flow, associated with group activities such as team sports, is more enjoyable than solitary flow (Walker, 2010). In particular, this seems to be due not only to the fact that social tasks require more skills and are thus inherently more challenging, but to the interdependency, cooperation, and emotional contagion existing within the group.

In principle, relation with and commitment to other human beings are the very essence of mankind as an intrinsically social animal species. From the eudaimonic perspective, it is of paramount importance that individuals be supported in the pursuit of complexity and skill development, through the allocation of psychological resources in activities that, besides being opportunities for optimal experiences, also bring about positive outcomes to their community as a whole (Massimini & Delle Fave, 2000). While globalization—primarily based on westernization—has increased cultural hostilities and inequality (Sen, 1992), emphasis should be placed on cooperation and reciprocity between social systems, for the full realization of the true human nature through the exercise of personal virtues and unique potentials for a common good.

References

Annas, J. (2008). The phenomenology of virtue. *Phenomenology and the Cognitive Sciences*, *7*, 21–34.

Antonovsky, A. (1979). *Health, stress and coping*. San Francisco: Jossey Bass.

Bandura, A. (1997). *Self-efficacy: The exercise of control*. New York: Freeman.

Bandura, A. (2001). Social cognitive theory: An agentic perspective. *Annual Review of Psychology, 52*, 1–26.

Bassi, M., Sartori, R., & Delle Fave, A. (2010). The monitoring of experience and agency in daily life: A study with Italian adolescents. In M. Balconi (Ed.), *Neuropsychology of the sense of agency: From consciousness to action* (pp. 81–105). Dordrecht, The Netherlands: Springer.

Beilock, S. L., Carr, T. H., MacMahon, C., & Starkes, J. L. (2002). When paying attention becomes counterproductive: Impact of divided versus skill-focused attention on novice and experienced performance of sensorimotor skills. *Journal of Experimental Psychology, 8*, 6–16.

Bridges, E., & Florsheim, R. (2008). Hedonic and utilitarian shopping goals: The online experience. *Journal of Business and Research, 61*, 309–314.

Buzsáki, G. (2006). *Rhythms of the brain*. New York: Oxford University Press.

Ceja, L., & Navarro, J. (2009). Dynamics of flow: A nonlinear perspective. *Journal of Happiness Studies, 10*, 665–684.

Chou, T., & Ting, C. (2003). The role of flow experience in cyber-game addiction. *Cyber Psychology, 6*, 663–675.

Crick, F., & Koch, C. (1990). Towards a neurobiological theory of consciousness. *Seminars in the Neurosciences, 2*, 263–275.

Csikszentmihalyi, M. (1975/2000). *Beyond boredom and anxiety*. San Francisco: Jossey Bass.

Csikszentmihalyi, M. (1978) Attention and the holistic approach to behavior. In K. S. Pope & J. L. Singer (Eds.), *The stream of consciousness* (pp. 335–358). New York: Plenum Press.

Csikszentmihalyi, M. (1982). Toward a psychology of optimal experience. In L. Wheeler (Ed.), *Review of personality and social psychology* (Vol. 3, pp. 13–36). Beverly Hills, CA: Sage.

Csikszentmihalyi, M. (1990). *Flow: The psychology of optimal experience*. New York: Harper & Row.

Csikszentmihalyi, M. (1993). *The evolving self*. New York: Harper Collins.

Csikszentmihalyi, M., & Beattie, O. (1979). Life themes: A theoretical and empirical exploration of their origins and effects. *Journal of Humanistic Psychology, 19*, 677–693.

Csikszentmihalyi, M., & Csikszentmihalyi, I. (Eds.). (1988). *Optimal experience: Psychological studies of flow in consciousness*. New York: Cambridge University Press.

Csikszentmihalyi, M., & Massimini, F. (1985). On the psychological selection of bio-cultural information. *New Ideas in Psychology, 3*, 115–138.

David, N., Newen, A., & Vogely, K. (2008). The "sense of agency" and its underlying cognitive and neural mechanisms. *Consciousness and Cognition, 17*, 523–534.

Deci, E. L. (1975). *Intrinsic motivation*. New York: Plenum.

Deci, E. L., & Ryan, R. M. (1985). *Intrinsic motivation and self-determination in human behaviour*. New York: Plenum.

Dehaene, S., Changeux, J. P., Naccache, L., Sackur, J., & Sergent, C. (2006). Conscious, preconscious, and subliminal processing: A testable taxonomy. *Trends in Cognitive Sciences, 10*, 204–211.

Delle Fave, A. (1996) Esperienza ottimale e sviluppo del comportamento: Evidenze sperimentali [optimal experience and behavioral development: Empirical evidence]. In F. Massimini, P. Inghilleri, & A. Delle Fave. (Eds.), *La selezione psicologica umana* (pp. 569–598). Milano: Coop. Libraria IULM.

Delle Fave, A. (2004) Lo studio della qualità dell'esperienza cosciente quotidiana: Teorie, strumenti di indagine e applicazioni [the study of quality of daily conscious experience: Theories, methods, and applications]. In D. Galati & C. Tinti (Eds.), *Prospettive sulla coscienza* (pp. 177–186). Roma: Carocci Editore.

Delle Fave, A. (2007) Theoretical foundations of ESM. In J. Hektner, J. Schmidt, & M. Csikszentmihalyi (Eds.), *Measuring the quality of everyday life: The ESM handbook* (pp. 15–28). New York: Sage.

Delle Fave, A. (2009). Optimal experience and meaning: Which relationship? *Psychological Topics. Special issue on positive psychology, 18*, 285–302.

Delle Fave, A. (in press). Past, present and future of flow. In I. Boniwell & S. David (Eds.), *Oxford Handbook of Happiness*. Oxford, UK: Oxford University Press.
Delle Fave, A., & Bassi, M. (2000). The quality of experience in adolescents' daily lives: Developmental perspectives. *Genetic, Social and General Psychology Monographs, 126*, 347–367.
Delle Fave, A., & Bassi, M. (2007). *Psicologia e salute. L'esperienza di utenti e operatori* [Psychology and health. The experience of patients and professionals]. Torino: UTET Università.
Delle Fave, A., Bassi, M., & Massimini, F. (2003a). Quality of experience and risk perception in high-altitude rock climbing. *Journal of Applied Sport Psychology, 15*, 82–99.
Delle Fave, A., Bassi, M., & Massimini, F. (2003b). Coping with boundaries: The quality of daily experience of Rom nomads in Europe. *Psychology and Developing Societies, 15*, 87–102.
Delle Fave, A., Bassi, M., & Massimini, F. (2009). Experiencia óptima y evolución humana [Optimal experience and psychological selection]. In C. Vasquez & G. Hervas (Eds.), *La ciencia del bienestar. Fundamentos de una psicología positiva* (pp. 209–230). Madrid: Alianza Editorial.
Delle Fave, A., & Massimini, F. (1992). Experience sampling method and the measurement of clinical change: A case of anxiety disorder. In M. de Vries (Ed.), *The experience of psychopathology* (pp. 280–289). New York: Cambridge University Press.
Delle Fave, A., & Massimini, F. (2003). Drug addiction: The paradox of mimetic optimal experience. In J. Henry (Ed.), *European positive psychology proceedings* (pp. 31–38). Leicester, UK: British Psychological Society.
Delle Fave, A., & Massimini, F. (2004). Parenthood and the quality of experience in daily life: A longitudinal study. *Social Indicators Research, 67*, 75–106.
Dewey, J. (1934). *Art as experience*. New York: Capricorn Books.
Dienes, Z., & Pernes, J. (1999). A theory of implicit and explicit knowledge. *Behavioral and Brain Sciences, 5*, 735–808.
Dietrich, A. (2004). Neurocognitive mechanisms underlying the experience of flow. *Consciousness and Cognition, 13*, 746–761.
Dijksterhuis, A., & Aarts, H. (2010). Goals, attention, and (un)consciousness. *Annual Review of Psychology, 61*, 467–490.
Fredrickson, B. L. (2001). The role of positive emotions in positive psychology: The broaden-and-build theory of positive emotions. *American Psychologist, 56*, 218–226.
Gauvain, M. (1995). Thinking in niches: Sociocultural influences on cognitive development. *Human Development, 38*, 25–45.
Guastello, S. J., Johnson, E. A., & Rieke, M. L. (1999). Nonlinear dynamics of motivational flow. *Nonlinear Dynamics, Psychology, and Life Sciences, 3*, 259–273.
Haidt, J., & Joseph, C. (2004). Intuitive ethics: How innately prepared intuitions generate culturally variable virtues. *Daedalus, 133*, 55–66.
Haken, H. (2006). Synergetics of brain function. *International Journal of Psychophysiology, 60*, 110–124.
Harari, Y. N. (2008). Combat flow: Military, political, and ethical dimensions of subjective well-being in war. *Review of General Psychology, 12*, 253–264.
Heider, F. (1958). *The psychology of interpersonal relations*. New York: Wiley.
Hilgard, E. (1980). The trilogy of mind: Cognition, affectation, and conation. *Journal of the History of the Behavioral Sciences, 16*, 107–117.
Hunter, J., & Csikszentmihalyi, M. (2000). The phenomenology of body-mind: The contrasting cases of flow in sports and contemplation. *Anthropology of Consciousness, 11*, 5–24.
Jablonka, E., & Lamb, M. J. (2005). *Evolution in four dimensions: Genetic, epigenetic, behavioural and symbolic variations in the history of life*. Cambridge, MA: MIT Press.
Jackson, S. A., & Csikszentmihalyi, M. (1999). *Flow in sports: The keys to optimal experiences and performances*. Champaign, IL: Human Kinetics.

James, W. (1890). *The principles of psychology*. New York: Holt.

Jenkins, I. H., Brooks, D. J., Nixon, P. D., Frackowiak, R. S. J., & Passingham, R. E. (1994). Motor sequence learning: A study with positron emission tomography. *Journal of Neuroscience, 14*, 3775–3790.

Koch, C., & Tsuchiya, N. (2006). Attention and consciousness: Two distinct brain processes. *Trends in Cognitive Sciences, 11*, 16–21.

Koivisto, M., Kainulainen, P., & Revonsuo, A. (2009). The relationship between awareness and attention: Evidence from ERP responses. *Neuropsychologia, 47*, 2891–2899.

Lambie, J. A., & Marcel, A. J. (2002). Consciousness and the varieties of emotional experience: A theoretical framework. *Psychological Review, 109*, 219–259.

Lazarus, R. (1966). *Psychological stress and the coping process*. New York: McGraw-Hill.

Maslow, A. (1971). *The farther reaches of human nature*. New York: Viking Press.

Massimini, F., & Calegari, C. (1979). *Il contesto normative sociale: Teoria e metodo di analisi* [The social normative context: Theory and method of analysis]. Milano: Franco Angeli.

Massimini, F., & Delle Fave, A. (2000). Individual development in a bio-cultural perspective. *American Psychologist, 55*, 24–33.

Massimini, F., Inghilleri, P., & Delle Fave, A. (Eds.). (1996). *La selezione psicologica umana* [Human psychological selection]. Milano: Coop. Libraria IULM.

Maturana, H., & Varala, F. (1980). *Autopoiesis and cognition: The realization of the living*. Dordrecht: Reidel Pbl. Company.

Miller, J. G. (2001). Culture and moral development. In D. Matsumoto (Ed.), *The handbook of culture and psychology* (pp. 151–170). New York: Oxford University Press.

Nakamura, J., & Csikszentmihalyi, M. (2009) Flow theory and research. In S. J. Lopez & C. R. Snyder (Eds.), *Handbook of positive psychology* (pp. 195–206). New York: Oxford University Press.

Piaget, J. (1950). *Introduction à l'epistémologie génétique* [Introduction to genetic epistemology]. Paris: P.U.F.

Posner, M. I. (1994). Attention: The mechanisms of consciousness. *Procedures of the National Academy of Sciences, 91*, 7398–7403.

Posner, M. I., Inhoff, A. W., Friedrich, F. J., & Cohen, A. (1987). Isolating attentional systems: A cognitive-anatomical analysis. *Psychobiology, 15*, 107–121.

Prigogine, I., & Stengers, I. (1984). *Order Out Of chaos*. New York: Bantam.

Raz, A., & Buhle, J. (2006). Typologies of attentional networks. *Nature Reviews Neuroscience, 7*, 367–379.

Rheinberg, F., & Manig, Y. (2003). Was macht spaß am graffiti-sprayen? Eine induktive anreizanalyse [What's entertaining about graffiti spraying? An inductive analysis on incentives]. *Report Psychologie, 28*, 222–234.

Rotter, J. B. (1966). Generalized expectancies for internal versus external control of reinforcement. *Psychological Monographs, 80*, 1–28.

Ryan, R. M., & Deci, E. L. (2000). Self-determination theory and the facilitation of intrinsic motivation, social development, and well-being. *American Psychologist, 55*, 68–78.

Seligman, M. E. P. (2002). *Authentic happiness: Using the new positive psychology to realize your potential for lasting fulfillment*. New York: Free Press.

Sen, A. (1992). *Inequality reexamined*. Oxford: Oxford University Press.

Shannon, C. E., & Weaver, W. (1963). *The mathematical theory of communication*. Chicago: University of Illinois Press.

Shapiro, Y. (1997). Consciousness according to James. *Theory and Psychology, 7*, 457–481.

Singer, J. A. (2004). Narrative identity and meaning making across the adult life span: An introduction. *Journal of Personality, 72*, 438–459.

Smith, K. D., Christopher, J. C., Delle Fave, A., & Bhawuk, D. P. S. (2002). Post-Newtonian metatheories in the natural sciences and in cross-cultural psychology. In P. Boski, F. J. R. van de Vijver, & A. M. Chodynicka (Eds.), *New directions in cross-cultural psychology* (pp. 107–125). Warsaw, Poland: Wydawnictwo Intytutu Psychologii PAN.

Stokart, Z., Cavallo, M., Fianco, A., & Lombardi, M. (2007). Esperienza ottimale e identità femminile: Uno studio transculturale su tre gruppi di adolescenti [Optimal experience and female identity: A cross-cultural study with three groups of adolescents]. In A. Delle Fave (Ed.), *La condivisione del benessere. Il contributo della psicologia positiva* (pp. 325–344). Milano: Franco Angeli.

Tononi, G., & Edelman, G. M. (1998). Consciousness and complexity. *Science*, *282*, 1846–1851.

Tononi, G., & Massimini, M. (2005) Coscienza [consciousness]. In F. Conti (Ed.), *Fisiologia medica* (pp. 631–642). Firenze: Edi-Ermes.

Vandervert, L. R. (1995). Chaos theory and the evolution of consciousness and mind: A thermodynamic-holographic resolution to the mind-body problem. *New Ideas in Psychology*, *13*, 107–127.

Varela, F., Thompson, E., & Rosch, E. (1991). *The embodied mind: Cognitive science and human experience*. Cambridge, MA: MIT Press.

Voiskounsky, A. E., & Smyslova, O. V. (2003). Flow-based model of computer hackers' motivation. *Cyber Psychology*, *6*, 171–180.

von Bertalanffy, L. (1968). *General systems theory*. New York: Braziller.

Vygotsky, L. (1978). *Mind in society*. Cambridge, MA: Harvard University Press.

Walker, C. J. (2010). Experiencing flow: Is doing it together better than doing it alone? *Journal of Positive Psychology*, *5*, 3–11.

Wanner, B., Ladouceur, R., Auclair, A. V., & Vitaro, F. (2006). Flow and dissociation: Examination of mean levels, cross-links, and links to emotional well-being across sports and recreational and pathological gambling. *Journal of Gambling Studies*, *22*, 289–304.

Weber, R., Tamborini, R., Westcott-Baker, A., & Kantor, B. (2009). Theorizing flow and media enjoyment as cognitive synchronization of attentional and reward networks. *Communication Theory*, *19*, 397–422.

Weiner, B. (1972). *Theories of motivation*. Chicago: Markham.

Yerkes, R., & Dodson, J. (1908). The relation of strength of stimulus to rapidity of habit formation. *Journal of Comparative and Neurological Psychology*, *18*, 459–482.

Chapter 4
Instruments and Methods in Flow Research

4.1 The Assessment of Optimal Experience

There are many ways to measure optimal experience (Nakamura & Csikszentmihalyi, 2009), the majority of which focus on individuals' self-reports of their experiential state and of their surrounding environment. As stated by Harré and Secord (1972), these are considered as authentic descriptions based on the human abilities to observe and describe one self. Additionally, methods in flow investigation vary according to the level of control exerted by the researcher on the flow construct: These methods comprise observation and interview techniques, the administration of questionnaires in psychological surveys, the conduction of experimental studies. Methods further vary in temporal focus: Some instruments require respondents to provide a retrospective evaluation of optimal experience, others investigate flow in real time, as daily events and situations take place. The following paragraphs will present the most widespread methods and instruments, with their pros and cons. Some models of analysis will also be illustrated.

4.2 Interviews and Direct Observation

Csikszentmihalyi (1975/2000) first identified optimal experience through semi-structured interviews to people involved in highly engaging and challenging tasks, such as climbing mountains, playing chess, or dancing, in the domain of leisure, and surgery in the domain of work. Through broad descriptions on how they felt when the activity was going well, these individuals provided qualitative accounts enabling researchers to pinpoint the phenomenological characteristics of flow (see Section 4.3.4). In spite of the great amount of fine-grained qualitative information that can be gathered through interviews, this method was barely applied in flow research ever since Csikszentmihalyi's pioneering work. This may be related to the great emphasis placed on the development and use of psychometrically sound quantitative instruments in subsequent research. This may also be related to the effort and energy invested by both participants and researchers in holding an interview, coding and analyzing data. Nonetheless, today we witness to a resurge of interest

A. Delle Fave et al., *Psychological Selection and Optimal Experience Across Cultures*, Cross-Cultural Advancements in Positive Psychology 2,
DOI 10.1007/978-90-481-9876-4_4, © Springer Science+Business Media B.V. 2011

in this methodology (Hurlburt & Akhter, 2006) which can allow researchers to further explore the semantics of optimal experience—i.e., its relation to individuals' meaning-making processes—in addition to quantitative methods.

Interviews can play an important role in exploring optimal experience at the cross-cultural level. Even though flow was identified as a pan-human feature (see Chapters 3 and 7), interviews can be of help in highlighting possible culture-specific peculiarities, for example meanings attributed to flow characteristics such as challenges, intrinsic motivation, and autonomy (Delle Fave & Massimini, 2004a). Interviews can also help explore flow dimensions in specific domains, such as web-related activities (Pace, 2004), or in specific populations, such as young children, who would find it difficult to fill out questionnaires (Inal & Cagiltay, 2007). They can also help participants focus, expand, and reflect on particular moments in their lives associated with optimal experience, for example in the therapeutic setting, and thus represent a useful tool in promoting well-being among patients (Delle Fave & Massinimi, 1992; Delle Fave, 2009).

The observation technique has been applied in combination with quantitative methods. For example, in a study aiming to promote positive learning experiences among medical students (Beylefeld & Struwig, 2007), participants were engaged in a quiz-type board game as a tool to increase technical skills and knowledge base in medical microbiology. Optimal experience during the game was captured both by means of self-rating scales and through direct observation by research staff. Staff members informally observed the game and evaluated players on the basis of criteria such as participation, competition, conflict, small group communication, enjoyment, and instructiveness. The observation technique was also used in association with interviews in an ethnographic study on intrinsic motivation and flow in skateboarding (Seifert & Hedderson, 2010). In the natural setting of a state-of-the-art park, the authors repeatedly observed skateboarders spontaneously performing their activities, and took notes on participants' challenges in the situation, quality of experience while performing tricks, sense of freedom and autonomy, sense of accomplishment, and persistence in the face of failure. These topics were later tackled in semi-structured and open-ended interviews with the participants, in order to complement the authors' observations and to draw a personal picture of single participants, as well as to highlight flow experience in skateboarding. These examples suggest that, just like interviews, observation can be a viable tool in flow research, particularly for exploratory purposes, in contexts and activities that may not be captured through standard rating scales or online measurement.

4.3 Single-Administration Questionnaires

Among the available self-report instruments, the majority are single-administration questionnaires measuring flow either as a general construct or in particular life domains and life stages (sport and work, childhood and adolescence).

4.3.1 Flow Questionnaire and the Measurement of Psychological Selection

The *Flow Questionnaire* (FQ) is the first una-tantum measure of optimal experience developed by Csikszentmihalyi on the basis of the results of his early interviews (1975/2000; Csikszentmihalyi & Csikszentmihalyi, 1988). His original version was expanded (Delle Fave & Massimini, 1988), and implemented by our research group in various countries in the following years, giving rise to the largest cross-cultural databank on optimal experience. The questionnaire is currently available in English, Italian, Spanish, Portuguese, and French. It consists of both scaled items and open-ended questions, and it is divided in three parts. In the first section, participants are asked to read quotations describing optimal experience (see Section 4.3.4), to report whether they have ever had such experiences and, if so, to list the associated activities. They are subsequently asked to select, from their list, the activity associated with the most intense and pervasive optimal experiences, and to rate on twelve 0–8 Likert-type scales (ranging from "very little" to "very much") the level of cognitive, affective and motivational variables, as well as the levels of challenges and skills perceived in the situation: Sample items are "I am involved", "I enjoy doing this and using my skills", "I wish I could do something else" (reverse scored). The translation of the item "challenge" in other languages posed some problems. Changes in the item wording had to be introduced due to the reference to competition and performance embedded in the term "challenge." A thorough analysis of this issue will be provided in Section 4.5. Through the same scales, participants are also invited to rate the average experience associated with other main daily domains such as work, being with family, being alone, and religious activities.

Participants are then asked to provide a brief description of the features and meaning of the selected optimal activities and the daily ones previously rated on the scales. Four additional open-ended questions investigate the conditions facilitating flow onset and flow continuation in time. The second part of FQ includes 10 general open-ended questions pertaining to individuals' psychological selection: They investigate the thoughts commonly occupying participants' mind when they have nothing else to do, the thoughts they wish to concentrate on, the activities they wish to do and those they prefer to do, as well as the situations and conditions that disturb or interfere with thought and action. The last section of FQ investigates, with two open-ended questions, the so-called *anti-flow experience*, that is, the experiential state, opposite to flow, characterized by lack of concentration and psychic disruption (Delle Fave & Massinimi, 1992). In particular, participants are asked to report the activities, if any, they associate with the anti-flow experience, and to describe how they feel.

FQ is commonly administered along with two other questionnaires: the *Life Theme Questionnaire* (LT) and the *Order/Disorder Questionnaire* (OD) (Csikszentmihalyi & Beattie, 1979; Delle Fave & Massimini, 1988; Delle Fave, 2004). Together, they contribute to the investigation of participants' psychological selection. More specifically, LT explores positive and negative life influences, current challenges, future goals, major life accomplishments, positive and meaningful experiences during childhood and adolescence, personality characteristics, and the participants' evaluation of the positive and negative aspects of their productive life (be it work or school tasks, depending on the type of participants). OD investigates participants' concepts of order and disorder, both in the external environment and in the inner world, so as to assess order in consciousness and its manifestations in the external setting.

Concerning data analysis, manuals were created to qualitatively investigate the contents of the participants' answers to the open-ended questions in the three questionnaires. Answers are coded and grouped into broader functional categories according to the question typology. In the case of questions referring to activities and thoughts, answer categories correspond to daily life domains (such as work, study, leisure, social relations, family, introspection; Csikszentmihalyi, 1997a). In the case of questions referring to psychological evaluations, such as the descriptions of the four aspects of flow phenomenology, answer categories correspond to features of the experience (such as concentration, skills, motivation). This coding strategy allows researchers to identify idiographic as well as nomothetic trends in participants' and groups' answers, and to calculate standard descriptive statistics and non-parametric inferential tests. The features of optimal experience assessed with Likert-type scales can be analyzed with traditional statistical tests.

4.3.2 The Flow Short Scale

Another general measure of flow is the *Flow Short Scale* (Flow-Kurz-Skala; FKS) developed by Rheinberg and colleagues in Germany (2003). Individuals are asked to report the activity they are currently performing and to evaluate its psychological features in relation to optimal experience (see Section 4.3.4) on ten 7-point scales, ranging from "not at all" to "very much". Sample items are: "My thoughts/activities run fluidly and smoothly", "My mind is completely clear", "I have no difficulty concentrating". The instrument contains six additional items, three of them measuring the perceived importance of the activity, and the other three assessing the experienced difficulty of the task, perceived competence and current demands on 9-point scales.

FKS has been validated and primarily used in German-speaking countries (Engeser & Rheinberg, 2008; Rheinberg et al., 2003; Schüler, 2007). Factor analysis identified a two-factor solution for the flow items and the importance items. The participants' level of optimal experience is commonly calculated as mean value of flow items.

4.3.3 The Flow State Scale and the Dispositional Flow Scale

In the late 1990s, Jackson and Marsh (1996) developed a specific questionnaire to measure optimal experience in the sport and physical activity setting: the *Flow State Scale* (FSS). Participants are asked to describe the experience associated with the event that they have just completed by circling the score that best matches it on thirty-six 5-point items ranging from "strongly disagree" to "strongly agree". Each of the nine psychological dimensions of flow (as reported in Section 4.3.4) is tapped by four FSS items. The scale validity and reliability were primarily tested in the United States and Australia, on a large number of athletes, practicing different sports and physical activities (e.g., basketball, field hockey, aerobics, jogging). Subsequently, Jackson and colleagues (1998) developed the Disposition Flow Scale (DFS) with the aim to capture the dispositional tendency to experience flow in physical activity. DFS also comprises thirty-six 5-point items tapping into the nine flow dimensions, with instructions focusing on the frequency with which participants usually experience each characteristic in a target activity.

Factor analysis confirmed a satisfactory fit of both a model with nine first-order factors and one higher-order model with a global flow factor. However, while data analyses indicated that the scales performed reasonably well on the whole, they also highlighted high variability among items. This led the authors to replace problematic items with psychometrically sounder ones (Jackson & Eklund, 2002; Jackson, Martin, & Eklund, 2008). The new scales are called *Flow State Scale-2* (FSS-2) and *Dispositional Flow Scale-2* (DFS-2), respectively. Sample items of FSS-2 are: "It is really clear to me how my performance is going", "My attention was focused entirely on what I was doing", "I found the experience extremely rewarding". Sample items of DFS-2 are: "I am not concerned with how others may be evaluating me", "I lose my normal awareness of time", "I have a sense of control over what I am doing". FFS-2 was successfully translated and validated in Spanish (Calvo, Catuera, Ruano, Vaillo, & Gimeno, 2008), Japanese (Kawabata, Mallett, & Jackson, 2008), and French (Fournier et al., 2007).

Besides the sport setting, these scales can be fruitfully applied in other areas, such as education or work. For these purposes, Martin and Jackson (2008) recently developed two brief flow scales based on FSS-2 and DFS-2 items, and on semi-structured interviews with athletes. The first one, called *Short Flow*, comprises nine 7-point items ranging from "strongly disagree" to "strongly agree". This scale reflects an aggregate or global flow assessment based on the long multi-item multi-factor scales. The second scale, called *Core Flow*, includes ten 5-point items ranging from "strongly disagree" to "strongly agree": It taps into the phenomenology of flow experience drawing from qualitative research on what it feels like to be in flow during a target activity. Both measures demonstrated acceptable model fit and reliability (Jackson et al., 2008; Martin & Jackson, 2008); they also showed that short and core flow are not the same construct, and they can provide different perspectives under particular circumstances.

4.3.4 The WOrk-reLated Flow Inventory

In the Netherlands, Bakker (2008) developed a scale to measure flow at work, which he called the *WOrk-reLated Flow inventory* (WOLF). Flow is operationalized with a set of 13 items, four of which measure absorption (e.g., "I am totally immersed in my work"), four work enjoyment (e.g., "I feel happy during my work"), and five intrinsic work motivation ("I would still do this work, even if I received less pay"). Respondents are asked to indicate how often they experienced these elements of flow at work during the last 2 weeks on 7-point scales, ranging from "never" to "always". Data gathered among different categories of workers confirmed the three-factor structure of the inventory, as well as its validity and internal consistency. Scores of absorption, work enjoyment, and intrinsic work motivation can be analyzed separately, or can be combined into one overall flow score (Bakker, 2005; Salanova, Bakker, & Llorens, 2006).

4.3.5 Optimal Experience Survey

In Argentina, Mesurado (2008) developed the *Optimal Experience Survey* (Cuestionario de Experiencia Óptima; CEO), aiming at investigating flow among children and early teenagers (ranging from 9 to 15 years of age). Based on the nine dimensions of flow (Section 4.3.4), the ESM form (Section 5.4), and the Flow Questionnaire, CEO includes 32 scaled and open-ended questions divided into four parts. Given its similarities with extant flow measures, CEO can be considered as their Spanish adaptation in youths populations.

Like in FQ, in part 1 participants are asked to read quotations describing optimal experience, to report whether they have ever had such experiences and to indicate the associated activities. They are then asked to select the activity associated with the most intense and pervasive optimal experiences and to report the content of their thoughts while performing it. The subsequent parts of CEO focus on the selected activity. In part 2, respondents are asked about the reasons why they perform such activity; in part 3, fourteen 7-point semantic differential items and thirteen 5-point Likert-type scales ranging from "very much" to "not at all" investigate the quality of associated experience in its emotional, cognitive, and motivational components. Sample items are: "How did you feel while performing this activity? happy vs sad", "Are you concentrated while performing this activity?", "Do you wish doing something else?". The last section investigates the social context (i.e., whom participants are with) during activity performance.

CEO proved to be able to discriminate between individuals reporting high versus low scores of optimal experience. In addition, structural equation modeling of scaled items allowed the author to identify a four-factor structure consisting of affect (afecto), cognition (cognición), achievement (logro), and skills (habilidad) (Mesurado, 2009). Analyses further identified two second-order factors, one including positive affect and cognitive activation, and another one including perception of achievement and ability.

4.3.6 Choosing Between Questionnaires

All the questionnaires reported above have proven valuable in the investigation of optimal experience. Choosing which questionnaire to use ultimately depends on the researcher's comparative judgment of the questionnaires' psychometric properties as well as on his/her research aims; nonetheless, the following remarks may be of help in making one's way among the various instruments.

The first and most important remark regards the conceptualization of optimal experience. Flow Questionnaire (FQ; Delle Fave & Massimini, 1988) and Optimal Experience Survey (CEO; Mesurado, 2008) conceptualize flow as an all-or-nothing phenomenon—qualitatively distinct from other experiential profiles—by relying on individuals' ability to identify it through the quotations, and to associate with it specific activities. Variations in intensity of flow experiences can be detected through the rating scales assessing the level of flow characteristics. As first reported by Csikszentmihalyi (1975/2000), optimal experience can be associated with both "deep-flow" activities (macro flow)—i.e., structured tasks such as games, artistic performances, agonistic sports, and work activities—that require high levels of concentration, absorption, and energy investment—and daily tasks (micro flow) that may be associated with lower levels of flow characteristics. By contrast, all the other questionnaires—Flow Short Scale (FKS; Rheinberg et al., 2003), Flow State Scale-2 and Dispositional Flow Scale-2 (FSS-2 and DFS-2; Jackson & Eklund, 2002), and WOrk-reLated Flow inventory (WOLF; Bakker, 2008)—focus on continuous flow variables. Because externally validated criteria for cut-off scores on each flow dimension do not exist (Bakker, 2005), we wonder whether researchers using these instruments may tap into experiences different from flow, especially when low levels of the experiential variables are reported. One possible solution was proposed by Bakker (2005): Using WOLF, he tackled the cut-off problem by acknowledging flow among individuals who scored higher than or equal to the 75th percentile of each of the three flow dimensions in the scale.

Another comparative remark across available questionnaires regards the number of items measuring flow dimensions. Psychometric research has shown that multiple items provide a more valid and reliable assessment of the target construct (Marsh, Martin, & Hau, 2006). From this perspective, FSS-2, DFS-2, and WOLF provide better psychometric benefits than the other scales. However, FQ and CEO reduce this problem by first asking participants to focus on flow descriptions and, in FQ, by posing additional open-ended questions about individuals' psychological selection. Furthermore, as stated by Martin and Jackson (2008), brief forms may be necessary in some cases, such as in large-scale projects that include many measures.

Choice of questionnaire may also depend on the domain of application. While FQ and FKS have been applied in various domains, ranging from learning to sport, all the other scales were initially created to investigate a specific area: sport (FSS-2 and DFS-2), work (WOLF), and education (CEO). However, boundaries of the domain-specific questionnaires have not been so strict. An adapted version of WOLF, for example, was used to measure flow among music students (Bakker, 2005); also FSS-2 was used among music students (Blom & Ullén, 2008; de Manzano, Theorell, Harmat, & Ullén, 2010), and the Short Flow (Martin & Jackson, 2008) derived from FSS-2 was applied in the work, sport, and school domains.

A final remark worth mentioning in this section regards once again the conceptualization of optimal experience. All questionnaires but WOLF measure the nine flow dimensions (Section 4.3.4). Bakker (2008) included in WOLF only three dimensions (absorption, enjoyment, and intrinsic motivation), maintaining that the other ones are possible causes rather than phenomenological components of optimal experience. Distinguishing between antecedents, experiential characteristics, and consequences of flow is a crucial area of investigation that will be thoroughly treated in the following sections and chapters, in light of the results stemming from experimental and longitudinal studies, as well as from online repeated measurements. In choosing what questionnaire to use in flow assessment, however, measures investigating all nine flow dimensions intuitively provide a more exhaustive evaluation of the construct.

4.4 Experimental Studies

Flow has been investigated in experimental designs in which key experiential conditions were manipulated by researchers. In most studies the variable being manipulated was task difficulty, which was assumed to reflect the levels of challenges vis-à-vis personal skills. In a research on learning in a web environment, Pearce, Ainley, and Howard (2005) presented physics exercises, varying in difficulty, to students differing in level of physics knowledge. The authors further manipulated the degree of control in executing the exercise by allowing participants to either freely operate on the computer simulations or to simply watch them. In other studies (Eckblad, 1981; Engeser & Rheinberg, 2008; Keller & Bless, 2008; Keller & Blomann, 2008; Rheinberg & Vollmeyer, 2003), participants were presented a computer game, in which all parameters of the game and of the situation were kept constant except for the game difficulty level. In particular, Keller and Bless (2008) and Keller and Blomann (2008) adapted the computer game Tetris to allow for a dynamic and automatic increase or decrease in task difficulty depending on participants' individual performance. After carrying out exercises or games for a given time, flow as dependent variable was measured through self-reports assessing perceived challenges and skills as well as cognitive, affective, and motivational variables. Achievement, performance in the game, and personality characteristics were also assessed.

A recent study by Walker (2010) experimentally investigated the hypothesis that flow perceived in social conditions can be more enjoyable than flow perceived alone (Section 3.7). For this purpose, the social context was manipulated by selecting sports that could be practiced alone, with a partner, or with a team (tympanic paddleball and pickleball), while keeping challenges and skills constant across conditions. The dependent flow variable was measured after practicing for 10 min by assessing participants' level of enjoyment, perceived challenges and skills, and the frequency of flow, among other states.

Compared to interviews, observations, and surveys, experimental studies allow researchers to control and manipulate crucial flow dimensions, as well as possible confounding variables. For these reasons, they can provide valuable insight into the dynamics of optimal experience. However, a crucial point must be underlined. The majority of the studies required participants to perform a given activity for a fixed amount of time (8–10 min on average) and to subsequently fill out self-reported flow measures. As emerged during interviews, flow is a fleeting experience which cannot be switched on and off at will. Additionally, the performed activity must be interesting and meaningful for the individual; while some people may perceive interest and meaningfulness in computer games, others may not, depending on whether these activities are related to psychological selection. Moreover, laboratory conditions could be missing the spontaneity and complexity of real life situations, and individuals may require some time to adjust to the new conditions. For all these reasons, it could be possible that participants do not experience flow during the manipulated task. Therefore, when setting up an experiment, researchers should have special care in choosing the target task and time length vis-à-vis participants' perceived skills and meaningful challenges, and subsequently administer a self-report questionnaire which could discern whether participants have been in flow or not.

4.5 Experience Sampling Method

In order to investigate flow in everyday life, Experience Sampling Method (ESM) was developed by Csikszentmihalyi and his collaborators in the 1970s. The aim was to overcome the limitations of interviews and questionnaires which heavily rely on retrospective recall to gather flow reports, and to obtain online—i.e., real-time—data on the stream of conscious experience as daily events and situations unfold. ESM is thus an ecologically valid method of data collection in which participants' experience is repeatedly assessed at random moments over the course of time and in natural settings.

Much literature is available on ESM psychometric properties and technical characteristics (Conner Christensen, Feldman Barrett, Bliss-Moreau, Lebo, & Kaschub, 2003; Conner, Tennen, Fleeson, & Feldman Barrett, 2009; Csikszentmihalyi, Larson, & Prescott, 1977; deVries, 1992; Hektner, Schmidt, & Csikszentmihalyi, 2007; Napa Scollon, Kim-Prieto, & Diener, 2003; Tennen, Suls, & Affleck, 1991). Participants are usually provided with an electronic device—a wrist watch alarm, an electronic agenda, a palmtop computer, a mobile phone—which sends random acoustic signals (beeps) during waking hours. Type of device, length of study, number of beeps and beep schedule all depend on the investigator's aims. In general, studies have shown that sending 6–8 random signals a day for 1 week is enough to gather a representative sample of individuals' daily experiences and activities (deVries, 1992; Hektner et al., 2007). However, ESM has also been used during longer periods of time, for example, for over 1 month in a study with climbers in the Himalayan region (Delle Fave, Bassi, & Massimini, 2003; Chapter 9), and with repeated weekly sessions over 1 year in studies on twinship, friendship, and parenthood (Bassi & Delle Fave, 2009; Delle Fave & Massimini, 2004b; Chapter 10).

When the individual is signaled, she is asked to fill in one questionnaire sheet, called Experience Sampling Form (ESF), contained in a booklet or presented electronically, like a recent digital version created by transferring an HTML file over the Internet (Chen, 2006). Each form presents an identical series of open-ended and Likert-type questions investigating the ongoing participant's time-budget (activity, social context, location) and the associated quality of experience in its motivational, affective, and cognitive components. The ESF was first developed by Csikszentmihalyi et al. (1977), and subsequently translated into different languages, including Chinese (Moneta, 2004), Dutch (deVries, 1992), German (Hormuth, 1986), Japanese (Asakawa & Csikszentmihalyi, 1998), and Spanish (Ceja & Navarro, 2009). The structure of the Italian version, reported in the Appendix to this chapter, was also used as template for the Portuguese ESF (Freire, 2006). Compared to the English original form (see Hektner et al., 2007, pp. 294–297), the Italian ESF presents two major differences, one at the measurement level and one at the conceptual/semantic level. First of all, the semantic-differential scales measuring affect were substituted with Likert-type scales, in the wake of the empirical evidence that pleasant affects and unpleasant affects are distinct feeling qualities, and that it is thus not possible to describe them along a single bipolar dimension (Cacioppo & Berntson, 1994; Russell & Carroll, 1999). Second, the variables "challenges in the activity" was replaced by the item "Was the activity you were doing an occasion for self-expression and action?" This change was necessary after performing a pilot study among Italian respondents using both ESM and FQ: The literal translation of challenge—*sfida*—entails strong reference to competition and physical contest, and was thus mostly identified in agonistic sport activities. The same problem was faced by other romance-language speaking colleagues in Spain (personal communication from Lucìa Ceja). The Spanish word for challenge—*reto*—has the same reference to competition as the Italian *sfida* and was thus replaced by *desafio* which better captures the concept of challenge as opportunity for self-expression (Ceja & Navarro, 2009). *Desafio* was also the wording used by Mesurado (2008) in the CEO, with specification "Intending *desafio* in a positive meaning as overcoming an obstacle" (Entendiendo el desafio en un sentido positivo como superación de un obstáculo). In a study with Flow Questionnaire conducted with English-speaking Indian participants the same problem arose (Swarup & Delle Fave, 1999; Chapter 13). Therefore, in a subsequent study with Nepalese adolescents conducted with the English ESF, the expressions "challenges in the activity" and "Was the activity you were doing an occasion for self-expression and action?" were both inserted in the ESF (Delle Fave & Massimini, 2005). Findings showed that the longer expression managed to capture a wider variety of optimal activities than the shorter one. Finally, the same problem with the word "challenge" was found in particular domains—such as Web use—also among English-speaking individuals (Chen, Wigand, & Nilan, 1999; Pace, 2004): Challenges and skills are operationalizations that "are unlikely to be understood by subjects in all but the most mundane activities (e.g., playing a physical sport), thereby generating unreliable definitions" (Chen et al., 1999; p. 592). Since the Web should be considered as a "multi-activity medium", the two concepts should be operationalized in terms of specific Web activities (e.g., creating Web pages, retrieving information, chatting, playing games).

ESM has been widely used across cultures, in both cross-sectional and longitudinal investigations, with clinical and non-clinical samples (Conner et al., 2009; deVries, 1992; Hektner et al., 2007; Massimini, Inghilleri, & Delle Fave, 1996; Trull & Ebner-Priemer, 2009). Several methodological studies investigated its reliability and validity, as well as participants' compliance. Reliability was analyzed with test–retest split-half procedures (Csikszentmihalyi & Larson, 1987; Hektner et al., 2007). Concerning validity, several studies correlated ESM data on the internal states with individual physical conditions. For example, Hoover (1983) obtained high correlations between physiological indices (cardiac and motor frequency) and the ESM variables "active" and "awake".

Finally, participants' compliance was investigated over the last decades (Csikszentmihalyi & Larson, 1987; Hektner et al., 2007). The ESM procedure can be successfully used with different typologies of participants, ranging in age between 10 and 85 years, and widely varying in their socio-demographic features. The rate of compliance shows some variations according to sample characteristics: Over a 1-week ESM session, Csikszentmihalyi and Larson (1987) reported a signal response rate of 73% among blue-collar workers, 83% in a group of white-collar workers, and 92% among managers. Among Italian students the rate amounted to 68.8% (Bassi, Sartori, & Delle Fave, 2010), and 83.3% among climbers (Bassi and Delle Fave, 2010).

4.5.1 ESM Data Coding and Analysis

ESM provides an incredibly rich amount of information, both quantitatively and qualitatively. Researchers handling these data may be baffled by their richness: Larson and Delespaul appropriately entitled their 1992 paper on data analysis "Analyzing Experience Sampling data: a guidebook for the perplexed." Today, researchers can consult the book by Hektner et al. (2007) on ESM procedure.

In the preliminary phase of data cleaning, answers given more than 15 or 20 min after signal receipt are discarded from analysis. These response windows are arbitrary cut-offs used to avoid distortions associated with retrospective recall (Hektner et al., 2007; Napa Scollon et al., 2003). In paper ESFs (see Appendix), it is possible to ascertain the time elapsed between signal receipt and form filling-out because participants are asked to indicate the time when they were beeped, and the time when they started to fill out the sheet. In electronic ESFs, the software can be programmed to remove "late" answers automatically.

Once data have been cleaned, responses to the ESF questions must be assigned a numeric value so that the information can be entered in a database and analyzed statistically. Answers to open-ended questions (regarding, for example, activities, location, or social context) are coded using extant manuals (Hektner et al., 2007), and then are grouped into broad content categories according to functional criteria. Each researcher, however, can create her own coding system. As suggested by Csikszentmihalyi (1997a), the first step in grouping answers is to choose the level of magnification at which to look at people's typical daily life. Concerning activities, for example, three main broad classes can be detected: productive activities, maintenance, and free time. Each of them can be broken down into fine-grained categories, because every activity quoted by the participants is labeled with a numeric code. For instance, productive activities can be divided into work and study; study can be further broken down into study at home and study at school; study at school can be divided into listening to classes, taking tests, group activities, and so forth.

Concerning scaled items, *z*-scores are usually obtained for each individual based on their global mean for each item. Standardization offers the advantage of controlling for individual differences in item response. Ratings can be further aggregated using two different approaches (Hektner et al., 2007; Larson & Delespaul, 1992): the beep level and the subject level.

In the *beep-level* analysis, the unit of data organization is the self-report filled out when the participant receives a beep. *Z*-scores are created by subtracting the participant's mean for the item from the raw score, and then dividing the result by the participant's standard deviation. For each respondent, at the end of the transformation, each variable will have as many *z*-scores as are the self-reports (except possible missing values). At this point, a researcher may want to know how happy participants are while performing leisure activities. A mean score is calculated by averaging the *z*-scores obtained for that variable during leisure. Given the big number of serial self-reports each participant fills out, the most important criticism of beep-level analysis regards the possible interrelationship between adjacent reports (autocorrelations). In this respect, Larson and Delespaul (1992) acknowledged that in certain circumstances, violating the assumption of independence is almost unavoidable and may represent the best possible presentation of the data. In addition, the random way in which self-reports are gathered weakens the dependence among serial data.

In the *subject-level* analysis, the participant is the unit of data organization. The ratings of each variable are standardized for each individual, and then aggregated scores (mean *z*-scores) are obtained. In this case, in the calculation of the mean score, *N* is no longer the number of self-reports but the number of participants. This kind of analysis is more conservative in that the assumption of independence is not violated, as it is in the beep-level analysis. However, aggregating data in this way squanders repeated measurements, increasing the probability of Type II errors (Larson & Delespaul, 1992).

Choosing the most suitable approach in data organization ultimately depends on the researchers' aims. Their choice will also influence the kind of statistical analysis that can be performed (Conner et al., 2009; Hektner et al., 2007). Traditional OLS (ordinary least squares) strategies such as ANOVA or OLS regression basically require a subject-level organization of data, for the reasons reported above. Nowadays, however, the level of analysis has become irrelevant with the introduction of the multilevel approach that handles beeps and persons simultaneously (Bryk & Raudenbush, 1992; Goldstein, 1987). Multilevel modeling can successfully handle ESM nested data, with unequal numbers of observations across individuals and unequally spaced time intervals between observations. It additionally provides a way to obtain estimates of intra-individual and inter-individual variability, thus taking into account autocorrelations in data analysis.

4.5.2 The Advantages and Disadvantages of Online Measurement

Compared to single-administration questionnaires, ESM presents a series of advantages in the analysis of subjective experience (Hektner et al., 2007; Napa Scollon et al., 2003). From the methodological point of view, it combines the ecological validity of naturalistic observation with the descriptive nature of diaries and the precision of scaled questionnaires. ESM allows researchers to gather information on individuals' behavior (Napa Scollon et al., 2003) and to relate them to external contingencies (situations and contexts) as well as to subjective experience.

By far, the major advantage of ESM regards the real-time assessment of experience. Retrospective reports are subject to memory biases. For instance, individuals are more likely to recall or report experiences that seem more personally relevant (personal heuristics effect), that occurred more recently (recency effect), that stand out as significant or unusual (salience or novelty effect), or that are consistent with their current mood state (mood-congruent memory effect) (Trull & Ebner-Priemer, 2009). Studies have revealed only partial overlapping between retrospective ratings of mood and behaviors and real-time assessments (Feldman Barrett, 1997; Schimmack, 2003). Because of the short time lag between signal and response, ESM ratings validly reflect internal experiences and not individual's response styles (Schimmack, 2003) or social desirability (Hektner et al., 2007).

A final advantage of ESM consists in repeated measurement over time. This allows researchers to focus on both general psychological processes (nomothetic investigation), such as individual personality differences in experiencing emotions, and on intrapersonal processes (idiographic investigation) centering, for instance, on the individual experience fluctuation over the week (Hektner et al., 2007). The individual's week average score of a variable can represent the reference point to which to compare daily moment-by-moment scores for that variable, thus providing the within-person cut-off point that single-administration questionnaires do not have (Section 4.3.5). The same is possible at the inter-individual level, by standardizing individuals' experience ratings (z-scores) and thus providing a common metric to compare experience across participants.

ESM also presents a set of disadvantages that researchers must take into consideration. Some of them pertain to participants, and others to situation issues (see Napa Scollon et al., 2003 for a detailed description). Concerning participants, self-selection bias and attrition—which are potential problems in all studies—are especially relevant in ESM research due to time length of studies and to the onerous task of randomly filling in ESFs during the day. Additionally, ESM may not be suitable to study specific groups, such as illiterate individuals or people performing activities that cannot be easily interrupted (e.g., truck drivers or professional basketball players). In these cases, single-administration questionnaires or interviews may be advisable. Situation issues regard the declining quality of data reporting after 2–4 weeks of data collection (Stone, Kessler, & Haythornwaite, 1991), and the possibility that individuals may not want to or could not respond to one or more signals (e.g., during rituals and religious ceremonies, or while playing soccer). Further, the ESM procedure itself could alter the course of daily events, first and foremost by disrupting individuals while performing a crucial activity (e.g., athletes), by interrupting flow while it occurs, and/or by leading people to pay unusual attention to their internal states and behaviors. However, studies have shown that 80–90% of US participants reported having a "normal" week and that ESM captured their week well (Csikszentmihalyi & Larson, 1987). In a German study, only 14% of participants reported that the signal bothered them in public, and only 22% complained about disruption of their daily routine (Hormuth, 1986). Possible solutions and recommendations to address participant and situation issues can be found in Hektner et al., 2007.

4.6 The Experience Fluctuation Model

Since the early days of flow research, Csikszentmihalyi (1975/2000; Csikszentmihalyi & Csikszentmihalyi, 1988) maintained that *flow* is experienced when people perceive that opportunities for action (challenges) are evenly matched by their capabilities (skills). By contrast, when perceived skills are greater than challenges, *boredom* will follow, and when perceived challenges exceed skills, *anxiety* will arise. Later attempts to empirically test these theoretical assumptions using ESM, however, did not fully confirm these predictions. In particular, when challenges and skills were in balance individuals did not necessarily feel better than in other conditions. The major problem was that a state of flow depends on one's subjective perception of the challenges and skills associated with a given activity, and not on their objective appraisal. Massimini and his team at the University of Milano solved this problem by setting an individual's cut-off point against which perceived challenges and skills are evaluated (Massimini & Carli, 1988). Using the ESM procedure, they proposed that optimal experience should arise only when challenges and skills are in balance above a certain level. By standardizing challenges and skills ratings, the zero, which corresponds to the individual's mean for challenges and skills over the tested period, becomes the starting point above which optimal experience is likely to be reported. When both challenges and skills are balanced, but both score below the person's average (that is, below zero), a person may report a different experience.

Consequently, a model was built based on the subjective perception of challenges and skills (Carli, 1986; Massimini & Carli, 1988; Massimini, Csikszentmihalyi, & Carli, 1987). In the so-called *Experience Fluctuation Model* (EFM), the Cartesian plane is divided into eight sectors of 45°, named *channels*, using a trigonometric function. Each channel represents a specific ratio interval of skills on the x-axis, and challenges on the y-axis (Fig. 4.1). After standardizing challenges and skills, the

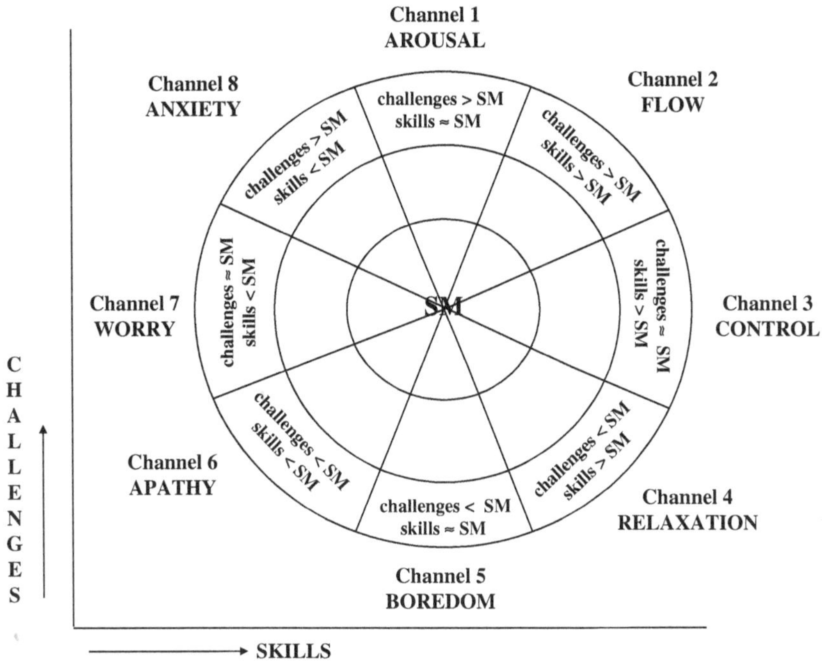

Fig. 4.1 Experience fluctuation model—the three concentric circles represent the rings (SM = subjective mean)

center of the model—zero, the *subjective mean*—corresponds to individuals' mean value of the two variables, as well as to the mean of all participants' means.

The model allowed to identify specific experiential profiles for each of the channels (Clarke & Haworth, 1994; Csikszentmihalyi, 1990, 1997b; Delle Fave & Bassi, 2000, 2003; Delle Fave & Massimini, 2005). In particular, channel 2, characterized by the balance of challenge and skill values above subjective mean, corresponds to optimal experience. Channel 4, in which skills are higher and challenges are lower than subjective mean, identifies a state of relaxation. Channel 6, where both challenges and skills values fall below the mean, is characterized by an experience of apathy. Channel 8, with challenges higher and skills lower than subjective mean, features a state of anxiety. The remaining challenges/skills ratios are called *transition channels* (Csikszentmihalyi, 1997b; Delle Fave, 1996) as they are associated with the experiential states of arousal (channel 1), control (channel 3), boredom (channel 5), and worry (channel 7).

For exemplification purposes, Fig. 4.2 depicts the experience fluctuation of a sample of 199 Italian adolescents across the channels (*N* self-reports = 7,616). The following variables have been analyzed: concentration, ease of concentration, control, involvement, wish to do the activity, happy, time perception and goals. These findings will be extensively discussed in Chapter 5, along with the great amount of additional data obtained from ESM research.

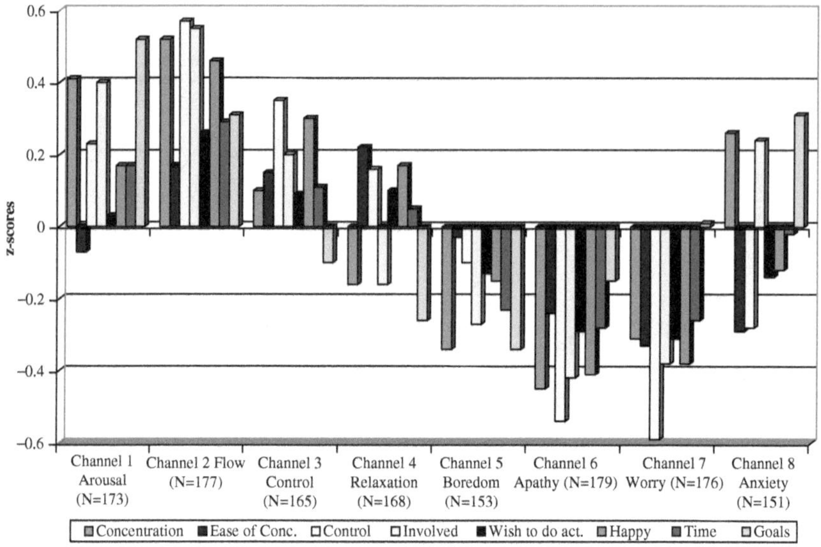

Fig. 4.2 Quality of experience in the EFM channels (N = number of participants)

Results confirm that *optimal experience* (channel 2) is a state of high and effortless concentration, involvement, control of the situation, clear goals, intrinsic reward and positive affect (Csikszentmihalyi 1975/2000; Csikszentmihalyi & Csikszentmihalyi, 1988). *Relaxation* (channel 4) is characterized by positive mood and intrinsic motivation, as well as low cognitive investment; it is primarily connected with energy restoration and low-challenging tasks, such as maintenance activities and TV watching (Delle Fave & Bassi, 2000). The experience of *apathy* (channel 6) is characterized by psychic disorganization, with low values of the cognitive, emotional, and motivational components of experience. High percentages of apathy in one's daily life can lead to potentially pathological outcomes: As shown in clinical studies, the predominance of apathy hampers mental health and personal growth (Delle Fave & Massinimi, 1992). During *anxiety* (channel 8), individuals do not feel able to cope with the situation, and they report high cognitive investment, negative affect, and often low intrinsic motivation.

The remaining experiences have not been as extensively studied as the four major channels. Indeed, some studies simplified the EFM by dividing the Cartesian plane into four quadrants corresponding to optimal experience, relaxation, apathy, and anxiety (Nakamura & Csikszentmihalyi, 2009). However, findings show consistent experiential patterns in the transition channels across samples. *Arousal* (channel 1) and *control* (channel 3) present the best experiential profiles after optimal experience: The former is characterized by high cognitive investment, involvement, and goals in the face of a discrepancy between above-average challenges and around-average skills; by contrast, the latter corresponds to a pervasive experience of control and happiness in the face of around-average challenges and above-average skills. Channels 5 and 7 are associated with *boredom* and *worry*, respectively. In both cases—when challenges are below and skills are around average (channel 5), and when challenges are around and skills are below average (channel 7), substantially negative experiences are reported. In particular, boredom is characterized by low levels of cognitive investment and lack of goals, and worry by low levels of control of the situation.

The dynamic nature of flow—related to the precarious balance between challenges and skills (Section 4.3.4)—can be fruitfully investigated by using EFM. Not only does the model allow researchers to trace how experience qualitatively fluctuates across the channels and to identify possible individual fluctuation patterns (Fig. 4.2); it can also consent researchers to analyze subjective experience from a quantitative perspective, highlighting how its characteristics can vary over time according to the reduction or increase in the levels of challenges and skills within a given channel. For this purpose, as shown in Fig. 4.1, each channel is further divided into 3 areas, called *rings*, which identify the distance of the values of challenges and skills from the center of the model (Delle Fave & Bassi, 2000; Delle Fave, 1996). Ring 1 ranges from 0 to 0.90 standard deviations from the center, ring 2 from 0.90 to 1.8, and ring 3 from 1.8 to 2.7. A fourth ring over 2.7 standard deviations has also been found; being quite rare, however, it has not been subject to systematic analysis. Table 4.1 illustrates the experience fluctuation in the rings of the EFM channels.

As expected, moving from ring 1 to ring 3—i.e., as the challenge and skill values increases, either above average or below average—the experiential profile associated with each channel tends to become more definite, or intense. For instance, in channel 2 (optimal experience), the higher the opportunities for action and the abilities in facing them, the more positive and complex the associated experience. On the contrary, in channel 6 (apathy), experience gets worse and worse when challenges and skills plunge below the average. Also in channels 4 and 8, respectively associated with relaxation and anxiety, quantitative changes in challenges and skills levels are associated with more intense experiential profiles, with higher positive mood and lower cognitive investment for relaxation, and higher cognitive investment and lower positive mood for anxiety.

4.7 Challenges and Skills in the Flow Construct

Many strategies have been proposed to evaluate the flow condition "balance between high perceived challenges and skills" by combining the values of challenges and skills assessed through ESM (Hektner et al., 2007, p. 93). In the circular EFM (Section 4.6), ratings are standardized and the flow condition is identified as the perception of a balance between above average levels of both challenges and skills (channel 2 in Fig. 4.1).

Other researchers have used different calculations based on challenges and skills raw scores. Moneta (1990) and Ellis, Voelk, and Morris (1994) multiplied challenges and skills to create an interaction term. Hektner (1996) computed the geometric mean, i.e., the square root of the product of challenges and skills, to create a continuous variable. Moneta and Csikszentmihalyi (1996) expressed the balance/imbalance of challenges and skills by calculating their absolute difference. Through multilevel models of analysis, the last two authors measured the effect of the relationship between challenges and skills on individuals' values of

Table 4.1 Experience fluctuation in the rings of the EFM channels

	Arousal			Optimal experience			Control			Relaxation		
Ring	1	2	3	1	2	3	1	2	3	1	2	3
Concentration	0.12	0.42***	0.79***	0.16**	0.45***	0.84***	−0.05	0.15	0.22	−0.11	−0.22***	−0.19
Ease of concentration	0.05	−0.13*	−0.13	0.10	0.16**	0.31***	−0.00	0.23**	0.23*	0.15*	0.27***	0.32
Control	−0.04	0.18***	0.43***	0.19***	0.48***	0.94***	0.18**	0.46***	0.52***	0.03	0.19**	0.37**
Involved	0.26***	0.33***	0.71***	0.13*	0.44***	0.99***	0.13	0.20*	0.29*	−0.16**	−0.13*	−0.15
Wish to do activity	0.05	0.04	−0.01	0.13*	0.26***	0.36***	−0.17	0.15*	0.21	−0.11	0.11	0.24*
Happy	−0.10	0.14*	0.53***	0.18**	0.32***	0.71***	0.07	0.40***	0.41**	0.07	0.21***	0.22
Time	0.03	0.12	0.36**	0.15*	0.22***	0.47***	−0.12	0.20*	0.35**	−0.05	0.04	0.13
Goals	−0.01	0.53***	1.13***	−0.05	0.20***	0.66***	−0.07	−0.12	−0.18*	−0.17**	−0.21***	−0.54***
N participants	83	129	79	78	137	117	70	96	51	80	115	45

Table 4.1 (continued)

	Boredom			Apathy			Worry			Anxiety		
Ring	1	2	3	1	2	3	1	2	3	1	2	3
Concentration	−0.16*	−0.41***	−0.65***	−0.19*	−0.47***	−0.73***	−0.09	−0.34***	−0.44***	0.10	0.25**	0.42***
Ease of concentration	−0.12	0.07	−0.07	−0.12	−0.24**	−0.37**	−0.14	−0.41***	−0.50***	−0.13	−0.28**	−0.55**
Control	0.05	−0.18*	−0.25*	−0.30***	−0.53***	−0.88***	−0.25***	−0.056***	−0.92***	−0.15*	−0.20*	−0.60***
Involved	−0.20*	−0.36***	−0.28*	−0.21**	−0.40***	−0.77***	−0.34***	−0.027***	−0.44***	0.16	0.15	0.32*
Wish to do activity	−0.14	−0.09	−0.47**	−0.09	−0.34***	−0.50***	−0.00	−0.046***	−0.57***	−0.15	−0.09	−0.19
Happy	−0.13	−0.19*	−0.33**	−0.20***	−0.45***	−0.59***	−0.16	−0.40***	−0.52***	−0.07	−0.11	−0.44**
Time	−0.13	−0.28***	−0.38*	−0.10	−0.30***	−0.58***	−0.17*	−0.25**	−0.42***	−0.05	−0.12	0.24
Goals	−0.19**	−0.35***	−0.41***	−0.12	−0.09	−0.27***	−0.05	0.06	0.04	0.12	0.44***	0.67***
N participants	82	101	36	85	127	94	77	108	113	80	87	58

Note. *T*–tests were performed to identify scores that were different from the mean (corresponding to zero). Significance levels are reported: $^{*}p < 0.05$; $^{**}p < 0.01$; $^{***}p < 0.001$. Ring 1 ranges between 0 and 0.90 standard deviations from the center; Ring 2 ranges between 0.90 and 1.8; Ring 3 ranges between 1.8 and 2.7.

concentration by comparing three different formalizations: (a) the crossproduct (b) the absolute difference, and (c) the quadratic effects of challenges and skills following a rotation of the predictor axes (the operationalization on which the EFM is essentially based). All formalizations fitted reasonably well, accounting for nearly half of the variance. With reference to goodness of fit criteria, both the rotated and the absolute difference models, however, were to be preferred (Moneta & Csikszentmihalyi, 1999)

Much debate has been spurred by the use of perceived challenges and skills as the crucial variables in identifying flow. Two intertwined issues have been raised in this debate: (a) the ability of challenges and skills balance to capture flow experience, and (b) the operationalization of flow. This debate is still going on and is bringing about useful insight into the phenomenology of optimal experience (see Chapter 5)

Concerning the first issue, the majority of studies measuring challenges and skills through ESM or manipulating them in experimental designs have substantiated that challenges–skills balance has a positive and independent effect on the quality of experience (Chen et al., 1999; Delle Fave & Massimini, 2005; Guo & Poole, 2009; Keller & Bless, 2008; Massimini et al., 1996; Mesurado, 2009; Moneta & Csikszentmihalyi, 1996; Pearce et al., 2005; Sherry, 2004). Nevertheless, some contrasting evidence has been reported, depending on the challenges and skills operationalization that was applied (Ellis et al., 1994; Engeser & Rheinberg, 2008; Moneta, 2004; Moneta & Csikszentmihalyi,1996). In particular, the conceptualization of challenges–skills balance as a continuous variable as shown above (Hektner 1996) has been related to deviations from theoretical expectations. For instance, Hektner et al. (2007) maintained that it is occasionally possible of a person to be anxious or bored in the high challenges/high skills condition. Such results, however, were not reported using z-scores in the EFM, suggesting that the operationalization of challenges–skills balance as a continuous variable may fail to tap fine-grained qualitative differences across experiences, which can instead be detected by the EFM. Highly complex mathematical and statistical issues, as well as concept operationalization (e.g., the definition of challenges as opportunities for self-expression and action; Section 4.6), are connected with ESM data analysis and modeling. These issues need to be addressed in future studies in order to make sense of conflicting results.

Taking into account the attempts to evaluate the relationship between challenges and skills as a continuous variable, the second issue deals with the operationalization of optimal experience. Some researchers have opted for a global score of optimal experience stemming from the repeated administration of flow scales (Rheinberg, Manig, Kliegl, Engeser, & Vollmeyer, 2007) or of the quotations describing flow (Love Collins, Sarkisian, & Winner, 2009), thus overcoming or bypassing the challenges/skills "problem." Schmidt, Shernoff, and Csikszentmihalyi (2007) maintain that the condition of high challenges and high skills is "a proxy for flow—telling us only that, statistically speaking, flow may be more likely to occur" (p. 545). In addition, they state that "to further our understanding of flow, it is necessary to consider multiple elements of the flow experience simultaneously in order to verify that the experiences we examine truly are flow experiences as defined descriptively" (p. 545). Starting from this rationale, a continuous flow variable was created as a composite score of ESM repeated ratings of concentration, enjoyment, and interest (Shernoff, Csikszentmihalyi, Schneider, & Shernoff, 2003), or concentration, enjoyment, interest, involvement, and control (Schmidt et al., 2007)—very much like in WOLF (Bakker, 2008; Section 5.3.4). In a study using multilevel modeling, this composite score was treated as dependent variable and challenges/skills relationship (measured through the geometric mean computation) as independent variable, along with other personality (e.g., self-esteem) and contextual variables (e.g., activity type). Findings showed that the challenges/skills relationship represented a significant predictor of the flow variable, as well as the personality and contextual variables.

This is certainly the first attempt to construct a single measure of optimal experience using ESM data (Hektner et al., 2007). Nonetheless, it still leaves open a series of questions that were already tackled in the EFM. First of all, both in Schmidt et al. (2007) and in the studies based on EFM, the challenges/skills variable is used as a condition for flow, not as a proxy. In the EFM, multiple elements of optimal experience are simultaneously taken into consideration, and all of them score significantly above average in channel 2 as theoretically expected (Fig. 4.2). Second, by creating a continuous challenges/skills variable (Schmidt et al., 2007), the problem of possibly confounding flow with other experiences (apathy, boredom, anxiety) remains open. Third, pooling some flow characteristics together does not allow researchers to analyze how the scores of single variables may vary according to activities and contexts. For example, data analyzed with EFM have shown that work is characterized by low levels of intrinsic motivation, even though it is commonly reported as a privileged opportunity for optimal experience (Csikszentmihalyi & LeFevre, 1989; Delle Fave & Massimini, 2005; Haworth & Hill, 1992). Finally, Schmidt et al. (2007) raised the important issue of the contributions of personality factors and contextual variables to optimal experience (Csikszentmihalyi & Larson, 1984; Wong & Csikszentmihalyi, 1991) which will be addressed in Chapter 5.

4.8 Latest Directions in Flow Methodology

Today's technological advancements offer flow researchers new instruments and methodologies to explore the intrinsic complexity of conscious states and subjective experience.

One line of research investigates the physiological markers of flow that would permit tracking the dynamics of optimal experience without disrupting it. Findings suggest that flow is associated with low salivary cortisol, which is related to lower levels of stress and lower blood pressure (Adam, 2005; Matias & Freire, 2009). In a laboratory study, the physiological parameters of professional musicians were assessed while they played the piano (Blom & Ullén, 2008; de Manzano et al., 2010). A significant relation was found between flow and heart period, blood pressure, heart rate variability, activity of the zygomaticus major muscle, and respiratory depth, pointing to the unique physiological pattern of flow.

Researchers have also begun to explore the neurophysiology of flow through Transcranial Magnetic Stimulation (TMS), a noninvasive mapping technique that allows researchers to see what regions of the brain are activated when a person performs a certain task, by suppressing the neural activity of those regions.

Research in this field is, however, in its infancy, with most neurophysiological data on flow still dating back to Hamilton's studies in the late 1970s—early 1980s. Hamilton assessed the attention patterns of individuals reporting and not reporting frequent flow experiences through evoked potentials, during a laboratory task. Results highlighted that participants who rarely experienced flow showed an increase in cortical activation, whereas those reporting flow frequently showed an activation decrease while concentrating on the task. These findings suggested that investment of attention seems to decrease mental effort (Csikszentmihalyi, 1990; Hamilton, 1976).

Another current line of research investigates flow as an ordered state of consciousness (Section 4.3.4). From the perspective of chaos theory, flow can be considered as an *attractor* in consciousness that fluctuates over time in a nonlinear dynamic fashion. This conceptualization was recently tested and confirmed by Ceja and Navarro (2009) in a sample of employees. Participants were monitored with ESM for 21 consecutive days, and data were submitted to complexity theory analyses for the identification of the nonlinear dynamics of flow: the program VRA 4.7 was used to run visual recurrence analysis and TISEAN 3.0.1 to perform surrogate data analysis.

These new research instruments and approaches, along with the more traditional single-administration questionnaires and experience sampling technique, promise to shed light on the multiple facets of optimal experience, furthering our scientific understanding of the ingredients of a good life (Seligman & Csikszentmihalyi, 2000).

4.9 Appendix

Date__________ Time beeped ___________Time you answered ___________

AS YOU WERE BEEPED:

What were you thinking about?[1]

Where were you?

What was the main thing you were doing?

Why were you doing it?[2] Because you wanted to ( )
Because you had to ( )
Because there was nothing else to do ( )

What else were you doing?

How well were you concentrating?[3] 0–12 scale

[1] Participants are asked to be as specific as possible when answering open-ended questions.

[2] Participants can tick more than one option.

[3] Likert-type scales range from 0 "not at all" to 12 "to the maximum".

Was it hard to concentrate?	0–12 scale
How self-conscious were you?	0–12 scale
Were you in control of the situation?	0–12 scale

DESCRIBE HOW YOU FELT AS YOU WERE BEEPED:

Alert	0–12 scale
Happy	0–12 scale
Apathetic	0–12 scale
Strong	0–12 scale
Lonely	0–12 scale
Cheerful	0–12 scale
Anxious	0–12 scale
Sociable	0–12 scale
Active	0–12 scale
Bored	0–12 scale
Involved	0–12 scale
Excited	0–12 scale
Sad	0–12 scale
Free	0–12 scale
Tired	0–12 scale
Friendly	0–12 scale
Creative	0–12 scale
Obliged	0–12 scale
Relaxed	0–12 scale
Clear ideas	0–12 scale

Was the activity you were doing an occasion for self-expression and action?[4]	0–12 scale
Considering your personal skills and abilities were you able to tackle the situation?	0–12 scale
Did you wish you had been doing something else? What?	0–12 scale
Was there anything at stake for you in the activity? What?	0–12 scale

[4]This question and the following one respectively measure the perceived challenges and skills in the activity (in Italian: "*L'attività che stavi svolgendo era per te stimolante e rappresentava un'occasione e un impegno per esprimerti ed agire?*", "*Considerando le tue abilità e capacità personali, eri in grado di far fronte alla situazione?*")

AS YOU WERE BEEPED

Who were you with?	
Did you wish you had been with somebody else? Whom with?	0–12 scale
Time was passing[5]	0–12 scale
Did you feel satisfied with yourself?	0–12 scale
Did you wish you had been somewhere else? Where?	0–12 scale
Did you feel any particular physical sensation? Which one/s?	0–12 scale
The sensation was: pleasant ( ) unpleasant ( )	
Was the activity you were doing important for some overall life goal? Which one/s?	0–12 scale

SINCE YOU WERE LAST BEEPED:

Has anything happened or have you done anything which could have affected the way you feel?
What?

It was: positive ( ) negative ( )

References

Adam, E. (2005). Memory emotion and cortisol levels in the everyday lives of working parents. In B. Schneider & L. Waite (Eds.), *Being together, working apart* (pp. 105–133). Cambridge: Cambridge University Press.

Asakawa, K., & Csikszentmihalyi, M. (1998). The quality of experience of Asian American adolescents in academic activities: An exploration of educational achievement. *Journal of Research on Adolescence*, *8*, 241–262.

Bakker, A. B. (2005). Flow among music teachers and their students: The crossover of peak experiences. *Journal of Vocational Behavior*, *66*, 26–44.

Bakker, A. B. (2008). The work-related flow inventory: Construction and initial validation of the WOLF. *Journal of Vocational Behavior*, *72*, 400–414.

Bassi, M., & Delle Fave, A. (2009). Daily experience and psychological selection in dyadic relationships: Monozygotic twins and best friends. In T. Freire (Ed.), *Understanding positive life: Research and practice on positive psychology* (pp. 65–84). Lisboa, Portugal: Climepsi Editores.

Bassi, M., & Delle Fave, A. (2010). Impact of extreme weather conditions on high-altitude climbers' goals and quality of experience. *Journal of Leisure Research*, *42*, 469–488.

[5]Likert-type scale ranging from 0 "slow" to 12 "fast".

Bassi, M., Sartori, R., & Delle Fave, A. (2010). The monitoring of experience and agency in daily life: A study with Italian adolescents. In M. Balconi (Ed.), *Neuropsychology of the sense of agency: From consciousness to action* (pp. 81–105). Dordrecht, NL: Springer.
Beylefeld, A. A., & Struwig, M. C. (2007). A gaming approach to learning medial microbiology: Students' experiences of flow. *Medical Teacher*, *29*, 933–940.
Blom, Ö., & Ullén, F. (2008). The psychophysiology of flow during music performance. *IV European Conference on Positive Psychology*. Book of Abstract, p. 55.
Bryk, A., & Raudenbush, S. (1992). *Hierarchical linear models*. Newbury Park, CA: Sage.
Cacioppo, J. T., & Berntson, G. G. (1994). Relationship between attitudes and evaluative space: A critical review, with emphasis on the separability of positive and negative substrates. *Journal of Personality and Social Psychology*, *76*, 839–855.
Calvo, C. T., Catuera, R. J., Ruano, F. J., Vaillo, R. R., & Gimeno, E. C. (2008). Psychometric properties of the Spanish versions of the flow state scale. *The Spanish Journal of Psychology*, *11*, 660–669.
Carli, M. (1986). Selezione psicologica e qualità dell'esperienza [psychological selection and quality of experience]. In F. Massimini & P. Inghilleri (Eds.), *L'esperienza quotidiana—teoria e metodo d'analisi* (pp. 285–303). Milano: Franco Angeli.
Ceja, L., & Navarro, J. (2009). Dynamics of flow: A nonlinear perspective. *Journal of Happiness Studies*, *10*, 665–684.
Chen, H. (2006). Flow on the net-detecting web users' positive affects and their flow states. *Computers in Human Behavior*, *22*, 221–233.
Chen, H., Wigand, R. T., & Nilan, M. S. (1999). Optimal experience of web activities. *Computers in Human Behavior*, *15*, 585–608.
Clarke, S. G., & Haworth, J. (1994). 'Flow' experience in the daily lives of sixth-form college students. *British Journal of Psychology*, *85*, 511–523.
Conner Christensen, T., Feldman Barrett, L., Bliss-Moreau, E., Lebo, K., & Kaschub, C. (2003). A practical guide to experience-sampling procedures. *Journal of Happiness Studies*, *4*, 53–78.
Conner, T. S., Tennen, H., Fleeson, W., & Feldman Barrett, L. (2009). Experience sampling methods: A modern idiographic approach to personality research. *Social and Personality Psychology Compass*, *3*, 1–22.
Csikszentmihalyi, M. (1975/2000). *Beyond boredom and anxiety*. San Francisco: Jossey Bass.
Csikszentmihalyi, M. (1990). *Flow: The psychology of optimal experience*. New York: Harper & Row.
Csikszentmihalyi, M. (1997a). Activity, experience and personal growth. In J. Curtis & S. Russell (Eds.), *Physical activity in human experience: Interdisciplinary perspectives* (pp. 59–88). Champaign, IL: Human Kinetics.
Csikszentmihalyi, M. (1997b). *Finding flow: The psychology of engagement wit everyday life*. New York: Basic Books.
Csikszentmihalyi, M., & Beattie, O. (1979). Life themes: A theoretical and empirical exploration of their origins and effects. *Journal of Humanistic Psychology*, *19*, 45–63.
Csikszentmihalyi, M., & Csikszentmihalyi, I. (Eds.). (1988). *Optimal experience: Psychological studies of flow in consciousness*. New York: Cambridge University Press.
Csikszentmihalyi, M., & Larson, R. W. (1984). *Being adolescent: Conflict and growth in the teenage years*. New York: Basic Books.
Csikszentmihalyi, M., & Larson, R. W. (1987). Validity and reliability of the experience sampling method. *Journal of Nervous and Mental Disease*, *175*, 526–536.
Csikszentmihalyi, M., Larson, R. W., & Prescott, S. (1977). The ecology of adolescent activity and experience. *Journal of Youth and Adolescence*, *6*, 281–294.
Csikszentmihalyi, M., & LeFevre, J. (1989). Optimal experience in work and leisure. *Journal of Personality and Social Psychology*, *56*, 815–822.
Delle Fave, A. (1996). Esperienza ottimale e fluttuazioni dello stato di coscienza: Risultati sperimentali [Optimal experience and fluctuation in the state of consciousness: Experimental results]. In F. Massimini, P. Inghilleri, & A. Delle Fave (Eds.), *La selezione psicologica umana—teoria e metodo d'analisi* (pp. 541–568). Milano: Coop. libraria I.U.L.M.

Delle Fave, A. (2004). A feeling of wellbeing in learning and teaching. In M. Tokoro & L. Steels (Eds.), *A learning zone of one's own* (pp. 97–110). Amsterdam: IOS Press.

Delle Fave, A. (2009). Development through disability. In G. W. Burns (Ed.), *Happiness, healing, enhancement* (pp. 88–99). Hoboken, NJ: Wiley.

Delle Fave, A., & Bassi, M. (2000). The quality of experience in adolescents' daily life: Developmental perspectives. *Genetic, Social, and General Psychology Monographs, 126*, 347–367.

Delle Fave, A., & Bassi, M. (2003). Italian adolescents and leisure: The role of engagement and optimal experience. In S. Verma & R. Larson (Eds.), *Examining adolescent leisure time across cultures: Developmental opportunities and risks. New directions in child and adolescent development* (pp. 79–93). San Francisco: Jossey-Bass.

Delle Fave, A., Bassi, M., & Massimini, F. (2003). Quality of experience and risk perception in high-altitude rock climbing. *Journal of applied sport psychology, 15*, 82–99.

Delle Fave, A., & Massimini, F. (1988). Modernization and the changing contexts of flow in work and leisure. In M. Csikszentmihalyi., I. Csikszentmihalyi (Eds.), *Optimal experience: Psychological studies of flow in consciousness* (pp. 193–213). New York: Cambridge University Press.

Delle Fave, A., & Massinimi, F. (1992). Experience sampling method and the measuring of clinical change: A case of anxiety syndrome. In M. W. deVries (Ed.), *The experience of psychopathology—investigating mental disorders in their natural settings* (pp. 280–298). Cambridge: Cambridge University Press.

Delle Fave, A., & Massimini, F. (2004a). The cross-cultural investigation of optimal experience. *Ricerche di Psicologia, 27*, 79–102.

Delle Fave, A., & Massimini, F. (2004b). Parenthood and the quality of experience in daily life: A longitudinal study. *Social Indicators Research, 67*, 75–106.

Delle Fave, A., & Massimini, F. (2005). The investigation of optimal experience and apathy: Developmental and psychosocial implications. *European Psychologist, 10*, 264–274.

de Manzano, Ö., Theorell, T., Harmat, L., & Ullén, F. (2010). The psychophysiology of flow during piano playing. *Emotion*, 10(3), 301–311

deVries, M. W. (Ed.). (1992). *The experience of psychopathology—investigating mental disorders in their natural settings*. Cambridge: Cambridge University Press.

Eckblad, G. (1981). *Scheme theory: A conceptual framework for cognitive-motivational processes*. London: Academic Press.

Ellis, G. D., Voelk, J. E., & Morris, C. (1994). Measurement and analysis issues with explanation of variance in daily experience using the flow model. *Journal of Leisure Research, 26*, 337–356.

Engeser, S., & Rheinberg, F. (2008). Flow, performance and moderators of challenge-skill balance. *Motivation and Emotion, 32*, 158–172.

Feldman Barrett, L. (1997). The relationships among momentary emotion experiences, personality descriptions, and retrospective ratings of emotion. *Personality and Social Psychology Bulletin, 23*, 1100–1110.

Fournier, J., Gaudreau, P., Demontrond-Behr, P., Visioli, J., Forest, J., & Jackson, S. A. (2007). French translation of the flow state scale-2: Factor structure, cross-cultural invariance, and associations with goal attainment. *Psychology of Sport and Exercise, 8*, 897–916.

Freire, T. (2006). Experiências óptimas e lazer: Sobre a qualidade da experiência subjectiva na vida diária [Optimal experiences and leisure: About the quality of subjective experience in daily life]. *Psicologia: Teoria, Investigação e Prática, 11*, 243–258.

Goldstein, H. (1987). *Multilevel models in educational and social research*. London: Griffin.

Guo, Y. M., & Poole, M. S. (2009). Antecedents of flow in online shopping: A test of alternative models. *Information Systems Journal, 19*, 369–390.

Hamilton, J. A. (1976). Attention and intrinsic rewards in the control of psychophysiological states. *Psychotherapy and Psychosomatics, 27*, 54–61.

Harré, R., & Secord, P. (1972). *The explanation of social behavior*. London: Basic Blackwell.

Haworth, J., & Hill, S. (1992). Work, leisure and psychological well-being in a sample of young adults. *Journal of Community and Applied Social Psychology*, *2*, 147–160.
Hektner, J. M. (1996). *Exploring optimal personality development: A longitudinal study of adolescents*. Doctoral dissertation, University of Chicago, Chicago.
Hektner, J. M., Schmidt, J., & Csikszentmihalyi, M. (2007). *Experience sampling method: Measuring the quality of everyday life*. Thousand Oaks, CA: Sage.
Hoover, M. C. (1983). *Individual differences in the relation of heart rate to self-reports*. Unpublished doctoral dissertation, University of Chicago, Chicago.
Hormuth, S. E. (1986). The sampling of experiences in situ. *Journal of Personality*, *54*, 262–293.
Hurlburt, R. T., & Akhter, S. A. (2006). The descriptive experience sampling method. *Phenomenology and the Cognitive Sciences*, *5*, 271–301.
Inal, Y., & Cagiltay, K. (2007). Flow experiences of children in an interactive social game environment. *British Journal of Educational Technology*, *38*, 455–464.
Jackson, S. A., & Eklund, R. C. (2002). Assessing flow in physical activity: The flow state scale-2 and dispositional flow scale-2. *Journal of Sport & Exercise Psychology*, *24*, 133–150.
Jackson, S. A., Kimiecik, J. C., Ford, S., & Marsh, H. W. (1998). Psychological correlates of flow in sport. *Journal of Sport & Exercise Psychology*, *20*, 358–378.
Jackson, S. A., & Marsh, H. W. (1996). Development and validation of a scale to measure optimal experience: The flow state scale. *Journal of Sport & Exercise Psychology*, *18*, 17–35.
Jackson, S. A., Martin, A. J., & Eklund, R. C. (2008). Long and short measures of flow: The construct validity of the FSS-2, DFS-2, and new brief counterparts. *Journal of Sport & Exercise Psychology*, *30*, 561–587.
Kawabata, M., Mallett, C. J., & Jackson, S. A. (2008). The flow state scale-2 and dispositional flow state scale-2: Examination of factorial validity and reliability for Japanese adults. *Psychology of Sport and Exercise*, *9*, 465–485.
Keller, J., & Bless, H. (2008). Flow and regulatory compatibility: An experimental approach to the flow model of intrinsic motivation. *Personality and Social Psychology Bulletin*, *34*, 196–209.
Keller, J., & Blomann, F. (2008). Locus of control and the flow experience: An experimental analysis. *European Journal of Personality*, *22*, 1–19.
Larson, R. W., & Delespaul, P. A. E. G. (1992). Analyzing experience sampling data: A guidebook for the perplexed. In M. deVries (Ed.), *The experience of psychopathology— investigating mental disorders in their natural settings* (pp. 58–78). Cambridge: Cambridge University Press.
Love Collins, A., Sarkisian, N., & Winner, E. (2009). Flow and happiness in later life: An investigation into the role of daily and weekly flow experiences. *Journal of Happiness Studies*, *10*, 703–719.
Marsh, H. W., Martin, A. J., & Hau, K. T. (2006). A multiple method perspective on self-concept research in educational psychology: A construct validity approach. In M. Eid & E. Diener (Eds.), *Handbook of multimethod measurement in psychology* (pp. 441–456). Washington, DC: APA Press.
Martin, A. J., & Jackson, S. A. (2008). Brief approaches to assessing task absorption and enhanced subjective experience: Examining 'short' and 'core' flow in diverse performance domains. *Motivation and Emotion*, *32*, 141–157.
Massimini, F., & Carli, M. (1988). The systematic assessment of flow in daily experience. In M. Csikszentmihalyi, & I. Csikszentmihalyi (Eds.), *Optimal experience: Psychological studies of flow in consciousness* (pp. 266–287). New York: Cambridge University Press.
Massimini, F., Csikszentmihalyi, M., & Carli, M. (1987). Optimal experience: A tool for psychiatric rehabilitation. *Journal of Nervous and Mental Disease*, *175*, 545–549.
Massimini, F., Inghilleri, P., Delle Fave, A. (Eds.). (1996). *La selezione psicologica umana—teoria e metodo d'analisi* [Human psychological selection—Theory and method of analysis]. Milano: Coop. Libraria IULM.
Matias, G. P., & Freire, T. (2009). Experiência óptima e cortisol: A psicofisiologia no quotidiano [Optimal experience and cortisol: A psychophysiology in everyday life]. *Psychologica*, *50*, 233–248.

Mesurado, B. (2008). Factorial validity and reliability of optimal experience (flow) survey in children and teenagers. *Revista Iberoamericana de Diagnóstico y Evaluación Psicológica, 25*, 159–178.
Mesurado, B. (2009). Comparación de tres modelos teóricos explicativos del constructo experiencia óptimal o flow [Comparing three theoretical explanatory models of the flow construct]. *Interdisciplinaria, 26*, 121–137.
Moneta, G. B. (1990). *A modeling approach to the study of subjective experience: Everyday life variations as a function of perceived challenges and skills in the activity*. Unpublished doctoral dissertation, University of Chicago, Chicago.
Moneta, G. B. (2004). The flow model of intrinsic motivation in Chinese: Cultural and personal moderators. *Journal of Happiness Studies, 5*, 181–217.
Moneta, G. B., & Csikszentmihalyi, M. (1996). The effect of perceived challenges and skills on the quality of subjective experience. *Journal of Personality, 64*, 275–310.
Moneta, G. B., & Csikszentmihalyi, M. (1999). Models of concentration in natural environments: A comparative approach based on streams of experiential data. *Social Behavior and Personality, 27*, 603–638.
Nakamura, J., & Csikszentmihalyi, M. (2009). Flow theory and research. In S. J. Lopez & C. R. Snyder (Eds.), *Handbook of positive psychology* (pp. 195–206). New York: Oxford University Press.
Napa Scollon, C., Kim-Prieto, C., & Diener, E. (2003). Experience sampling: Promises and pitfalls, strengths and weaknesses. *Journal of Happiness Studies, 4*, 5–34.
Pace, S. (2004). A grounded theory of the flow experiences of web users. *International Journal of Human-Computer Studies, 60*, 327–363.
Pearce, J. M., Ainley, M., & Howard, S. (2005). The ebb and flow of online learning. *Computers in Human Behavior, 21*, 745–771.
Rheinberg, F., Manig, Y., Kliegl, R., Engeser, S., & Vollmeyer, R. (2007). Flow bei der arbeit, doch glück in der freizeit. Zielausrichtung, flow und glücksgefühle [Flow during work but happiness during spare time. Goals, flow experience and happiness]. *Zeitschrift für Arbeits- und Organisationspsychologie, 51*, 105–115.
Rheinberg, F., & Vollmeyer, R. (2003). Flow-erleben in einem computerspiel unter experimentell variierten bedingungen [Flow experience in a computer game under experimentally varying conditions]. *Zeitschrift für Psychologie, 211*, 161–170.
Rheinberg, F., Vollmeyer, R., & Engeser, S. (2003). Die erfassung des flow-erlebens [The assessment of flow experience]. In J. Stiensmeier-Pelster & F. Rheinberg (Eds.), *Diagnostik von selbstkonzept, lernmotivation und selbstregulation* (pp. 261–279). Goettingen: Hogrefe.
Russell, J. A., & Carroll, J. M. (1999). On the bipolarity of positive and negative affect. *Psychological Bulletin, 125*, 3–30.
Salanova, M., Bakker, A. B., & Llorens, S. (2006). Flow at work: Evidence for an upward spiral of personal and organizational resources. *Journal of Happiness Studies, 7*, 1–22.
Schimmack, U. (2003). Affect measurement in experience sampling research. *Journal of Happiness Studies, 4*, 79–106.
Schmidt, J., Shernoff, D., & Csikszentmihalyi, M. (2007). Individual and situational factors related to the experience of flow in adolescence: A multilevel approach. In A. D. Ong & M. van Dulmen (Eds.), *The handbook of methods in positive psychology* (pp. 542–558). Oxford: Oxford University Press.
Schüler, J. (2007). Arousal of flow—experience in a learning setting and its effects on exam-performance and affect. *Zeitschrift für Pädagogische Psychologie, 21*, 217–227.
Seifert, T., & Hedderson, C. (2010). Intrinsic motivation and flow in skateboarding: An ethnographic study. *Journal of Happiness Studies, 11*, 277–292.
Seligman, M. E. P., & Csikszentmihalyi, M. (2000). Positive psychology: An introduction. *American Psychologist, 1*, 5–14.
Shernoff, D. J., Csikszentmihalyi, M., Schneider, B., & Shernoff, E. S. (2003). Student engagement in high school classrooms from the perspective of flow theory. *School Psychology Quarterly, 18*, 158–176.

Sherry, J. L. (2004). Flow and media enjoyment. *Communication Theory*, *14*, 328–347.

Stone, A. A., Kessler, R. C., & Haythornwaite, J. A. (1991). Measuring daily events and experiences: Decisions for the researcher. *Journal of Personality*, *59*, 575–607.

Swarup, S., & Delle Fave, A. (1999). From India to Europe: Cultural change and the quality of experience. In A. Delle Fave, F. Meli (eds.), *Modernization and cultural identity* (pp. 103–120). Milano: Edizioni Dell'Arco.

Tennen, H., Suls, J., Affleck, G. (Eds.). (1991). Special issue: Personality and daily experience. *Journal of Personality*, *59*, 313–662.

Trull, T. J., & Ebner-Priemer, U. W. (2009). Using experience sampling methods/ecological momentary assessment (ESM/EMA) in clinical assessment and clinical research: Introduction to the special section. *Psychological assessment*, *21*, 457–462.

Walker, C. J. (2010). Experiencing flow: Is doing it together better than doing it alone? *Journal of Positive Psychology*, *5*, 3–11.

Wong, M. M., & Csikszentmihalyi, M. (1991). Motivation and academic achievement: The effects of personality traits and the quality of experience. *Journal of Personality*, *59*, 539–574.

Chapter 5
The Phenomenology of Optimal Experience in Daily Life

5.1 The Family of Optimal Experiences

Thirty-five years of research on optimal experience in daily life provided useful information on its phenomenology. Analyses of the nine flow dimensions originally identified by Csikszentmihalyi (1975/2000) were performed across samples varying in cultural background, age, profession, and educational level (Asakawa, 2004; Chen, 2006; Csikszentmihalyi & Nakamura, 2010; Delle Fave & Massimini, 2003, 2004a, 2005a; Delle Fave, 2007; Hektner, Schmidt, & Csikszentmihalyi, 2007; Love Collins, Sarkisian, & Winner, 2009; Nakamura & Csikszentmihalyi, 2009; Rheinberg, Manig, Kliegl, Engeser, & Vollmeyer, 2007; Schmidt, Shernoff, & Csikszentmihalyi, 2007). In all these studies, optimal experience was recurrently described as a positive and gratifying state of consciousness. For exemplification purposes, we will again refer to the findings obtained from Italian adolescents, illustrated in Chapter 4. As show in Table 5.1, optimal experience (Channel 2 of the EFM) is characterized by effortless and focused attention, deep involvement, sense of control over the situation, positive affect, transformation of temporal experience—time is perceived as passing faster than usual—clear long-term goals and short-term stakes in the activity, and intrinsic motivation (measured through the variables "wish to do the activity" and "free").

Differently from expectations, participants reported being more self-conscious than they usually are. Additionally, the values of unselfconsciousness vary significantly across the eight channels of the EFM, thus showing little power of discrimination in relation to different experiential profiles. This finding can be attributed to the participants' reported difficulty in understanding the item "How self-conscious were you?" However, mixed results in the assessment of unselfconsciousness were also obtained through single-administration questionnaires using multiple items (Hektner et al., 2007; Jackson & Eklund, 2002). Further investigation is required to better define the role and meaning of this dimension of experience, since it is not unanimously perceived as negative (Coppa & Delle Fave, 2007; Delle Fave & Massimini, 2004a); on the opposite, in some situations participants describe self-consciousness as a process of self-control and self-monitoring that in no way disturbs the flow of the activity, being rather an integral component of it (see also Chapter 7).

A. Delle Fave et al., *Psychological Selection and Optimal Experience Across Cultures*, Cross-Cultural Advancements in Positive Psychology 2,
DOI 10.1007/978-90-481-9876-4_5, © Springer Science+Business Media B.V. 2011

Table 5.1 Quality of experience in channel 2 (optimal experience)

	Mean scores
Concentration	0.52**
Ease of concentration	0.17**
Unselfconsciousness	−0.12*
Control	0.57**
Involved	0.55**
Wish to do activity	0.26**
Free	0.34**
Happy	0.46**
Time	0.29**
Stakes	0.30**
Goals	0.31**
Challenges	1.17**
Skills	1.02**
N participants	178

Note. *T*-tests were performed to identify scores that were different from the mean (corresponding to zero). Significance levels are reported: *$p<0.01$; **$p<0.001$.

A closer look at ESM data highlighted that flow is a much more complex construct than first hypothesized, presenting some stable characteristics as well as variable features depending on the kind of associated activity. In a cross-cultural study conducted with Italian and Nepalese participants differing in age, occupation, and physical conditions, Delle Fave and Massimini (2005a) detected a stable cognitive core in optimal experience, represented by components such as high concentration and control of the situation. Affective, volitional, and motivational variables fluctuated around this cognitive core according to the associated activities. More specifically, wide cross-domain variations were detected in the values of volitional and motivational variables, in particular perceived goals and short-term desirability of the activity (wish to do the activity). Structured leisure activities, such as sports and hobbies, were associated with both short-term desirability, and positive, though not significant values of long-term goals. In productive activities—such as study and work—the perception of goals was prominent, but the activity desirability scored negative, though not significantly. Finally, passive entertainments—such as watching TV—were characterized by significantly high short-term desirability and significantly low values of perceived goals. As for affect, data juxtaposed productive activities to structured leisure and watching TV: The former were characterized by around-average values of happiness, and the latter presented significantly above-average scores.

Table 5.2 illustrates the quality of experience Italian adolescents associated with some common daily activities, on average and in channel 2 (optimal experience).

Across activities, findings faithfully replicate the results obtained by Delle Fave and Massimini (2005a). In addition, interactions were associated with high values of short-term desirability and affect, and low scores of perceived goals. While studying, participants reported below-average values of ease of concentration and

Table 5.2 Experiential profile of daily activities in a sample of Italian adolescents: average values and ratings in channel 2 (optimal experience)

	Studying		Sport and hobbies		Watching TV		Interactions	
	Average	Ch. 2	Average	Ch. 2	Average	Ch. 2	Average	Ch. 2
Concentration	0.12*	0.53**	0.33**	0.62**	0.01	0.53**	0.09*	0.42**
Ease of concentration	−0.43**	−0.20*	0.07	0.16	0.21**	0.37*	0.23**	0.39**
Control	−0.13**	0.45**	0.18*	0.54**	0.02	0.60**	0.14**	0.53**
Involved	−0.01	0.40**	0.38**	0.74**	−0.13*	0.38*	0.35**	0.62**
Wish to do activity	−0.41**	−0.05	0.34**	0.50**	0.18**	0.22	0.22**	0.44**
Free	−0.34**	−0.04	0.31**	0.55**	0.00	0.69**	0.25**	0.47**
Happy	−0.29**	0.03	0.34**	0.54**	0.02	0.55**	0.34**	0.80**
Time	−0.45**	−0.11	0.28**	0.68**	0.04	0.14	0.18**	0.40**
Stakes	0.47**	0.72**	0.10	0.53**	−0.40**	−0.04	−0.17**	0.07
Goals	0.52**	0.68**	0.08	0.56**	−0.36**	−0.21	−0.17**	0.06
N participants	182	105	144	63	193	47	192	113

Note. *T*-tests were performed to identify scores that were different from the mean (corresponding to zero). Significance levels are reported: $^{*}p < 0.01$; $^{**}p < 0.001$.

perceived time as passing as slower than usual, even if not significantly; during structured leisure (sports and hobbies), they reported average ease of concentration and the perception of higher time speed. On the contrary, it was easier for participants to concentrate while watching TV and interacting; time was perceived as passing as fast as usual while watching TV, but faster during interactions.

Similar differences across activities were obtained through the administration of FQ to respondents belonging to 11 different cultures in Asia, Africa, Europe, and North America (Delle Fave, 2007; Chapter 7). All these findings support Delle Fave and Massimini's suggestion that flow may not be a monolithic experience (2005a); rather, there could be a *family* of optimal experiences related to the characteristics of associated activity domains.

The impact of activity typology on optimal experience was also explored using hierarchical linear models (HLM). Schmidt et al. (2007) entered schoolwork, maintenance activities, paid work, and active leisure as situational factors (level 1 variables) along with the challenges/skills variable (geometric mean), and flow as dependent variable (a composite score of concentration, enjoyment, interest, involvement, and control). They detected a positive effect of the challenges/skills variable and of active leisure, as well as a negative effect of productive activities and maintenance on flow levels. Similarly, Table 5.3 reports data of an HLM analysis run on the sample of Italian adolescents previously considered. In the model, affective, motivational, and cognitive components of experience are the dependent

Table 5.3 Coefficients (and standard errors) of multilevel regression analysis

Dependent variable	Concentration	Ease of concentration	Control	Involved	Wish to do activity
Beep-level fixed effects					
Intercept	6.35***	10.02***	6.98***	5.84***	8.85***
	(0.14)	(0.11)	(0.13)	(0.12)	(0.13)
Channel 2	1.50***	0.60***	1.40***	1.59***	1.28***
	(0.09)	(0.07)	(0.07)	(0.09)	(0.13)
Study	0.64***	−1.06***	−0.36***	0.21*	−1.59***
	(0.08)	(0.07)	(0.07)	(0.09)	(0.12)
Sport and hobbies	0.95***	0.04	0.17	1.11***	1.35***
	(0.14)	(0.12)	(0.12)	(0.14)	(0.21)
Interactions	0.24**	0.35***	0.20*	0.96***	0.82***
	(0.09)	(0.08)	(0.08)	(0.09)	(0.13)
Watching TV	0.21*	0.35***	0.16	−0.07	0.94***
	(0.10)	(0.09)	(0.09)	(0.10)	(0.15)
Variance components					
σ^2_e	6.31	4.74	4.85	6.86	14.17
σ^2_{u0}	3.35***	2.18***	3.06***	2.34***	2.35***
N participants	199	199	199	199	199
N observations	71,498	7,483	7,478	7,515	7,538

Note. *$p < 0.05$; **$p < 0.01$; ***$p < 0.001$.

Table 5.3 (continued)

Dependent variable:	Free	Happy	Time	Stakes	Goals
Beep-level fixed effects					
Intercept	6.08***	6.19***	6.15***	1.75***	1.28***
	(0.15)	(0.13)	(0.08)	(0.12)	(0.11)
Channel 2	1.04***	1.20***	1.02***	1.40***	1.00***
	(0.08)	(0.08)	(0.09)	(0.11)	(0.10)
Study	−1.04***	−0.76***	−1.42***	1.87***	1.77***
	(0.08)	(0.08)	(0.08)	(0.10)	(0.09)
Sport & hobbies	0.55***	0.80***	0.77***	0.37*	0.33*
	(0.14)	(0.13)	(0.14)	(0.17)	(0.17)
Interactions	0.47***	0.68***	0.24**	−0.41***	−0.48***
	(0.09)	(0.08)	(0.09)	(0.10)	(0.10)
Watching TV	−0.07	0.17	−0.03	−1.13***	−0.83***
	(0.10)	(0.95)	(0.10)	(0.12)	(0.11)
Variance components					
σ^2_e	6.16	5.76	6.55	9.84	8.07
σ^2_{u0}	4.24***	2.95***	1.01***	2.26***	1.91***
N participants	199	199	199	199	199
N observations	7,500	7,543	7,542	7,504	7,478

Note. $^*p < 0.05$; $^{**}p < 0.01$; $^{***}p < 0.001$.

variables, while predictors are type of activity (study, sport and hobbies, interactions, and watching TV), and channel 2 of the EFM (based on the match between high challenges and high skills).

As expected, the variable channel 2 exerts a significant positive effect on all the dependent variables. In addition, findings substantially replicate Delle Fave and Massimini's results (2005a): Study has a positive effect on concentration, involvement, stakes and goals, and a negative effect on ease of concentration, control, wish to do the activity, free, happy, and time transformation. Sports and hobbies exert positive effects on all the variables except for ease of concentration and control, whose scores are not significant. Interactions have positive effects on all the variables, but goals and stakes; watching TV has a positive effect on concentration, ease of concentration, and wish to do the activity, and a negative effect on stakes and goals.

Findings consistent with the suggestion of a family of optimal experiences (Delle Fave & Massimini, 2005a) also stem from research on new technologies such as Web use and virtual reality (VR). Research in this domain identified telepresence as an important component of optimal experience in mediated activities, that is activities requiring a medium, such as the Web and VR (Chen, 2006; Gaggioli, Bassi, & Delle Fave, 2003; Hoffman and Novak, 1996; Skadberg & Kimmel, 2004). Telepresence refers to "the experience of presence in an environment by means of a communication medium" (Steuer, 1992, p. 76). The environment may be a real one such as a distant space viewed through a video camera, or a nonexistent environment such as an animated world in a video game. Telepresence is captured through items such as "I was more in the 'computer world' than the 'real world' around me", "I forgot about my immediate surroundings", and "I felt that using the Web made me forget where I was" (Novak, Hoffman, & Yung, 2000; see also the ITC-Sense of Presence Inventory, Lessiter, Freeman, Keogh, & Davidoff, 2001). Telepresence shows some characteristics of flow, such as complete involvement, focused attention, and loss of self-awareness. It is, however, specific to mediated activities, thus representing an activity-specific feature of optimal experience. Participants report: "I felt as though I was here but I wasn't in the real world. My mind was in cyberspace"; "I felt oblivious to my surroundings. Completely lost in thought at deciphering what I was looking at, reading, and visualizing what the results of such code would be"; "I feel as if I can shut out all around me and totally concentrate on my reading and surfing of the net. I feel the world is now open to me as never before" (Chen, Wigand, & Nilan, 2000, p. 274).

Studies have also shown that the quality of experience is sensitive to the intensity of the challenges/skills ratio across the rings of the EFM (Figure 4.1), in respect of the unique profile of each activity. Delle Fave and Bassi (2000) analyzed the quality of experience in channel 2 (optimal experience) and channel 6 (apathy) reported by a group of Italian teenagers in activities such as studying at home, classwork, watching TV, and structured leisure. The quality of experience tended to improve from ring 1 to ring 3 in channel 2, and to get worse in channel 6. In other studies, the effect of social contexts on optimal experience was investigated (Delespaul, Resi, & deVries, 2004; Delle Fave, Bassi, & Massimini, 2002; Inal & Cagiltay, 2007; Schmidt et al., 2007; Walker, 2010). Among children, adolescents, and university students results showed that, whatever activity is associated with optimal experience (productive or leisure activities), the quality of experience improves in the presence of other people—above all friends and peers—compared to when participants are alone (see also Chapters 7 and 10).

5.2 The Motivational Dimension of Optimal Experience

A crucial aspect of optimal experience that has been extensively investigated is intrinsic motivation. Csikszentmihalyi (1975/2000) first described flow as an autotelic experience, being an end in itself, and entailing doing something out of interest and enjoyment, with no expectation of external gain or reward. Empirical findings globally substantiated this aspect of flow, especially in association with games, sports or artistic and literary forms. These activities were developed over the centuries for the express purpose of enriching life with enjoyable complex experiences (Csikszentmihalyi, 1990; p. 51). However, accurate analyses again unveiled a far more complex picture. In particular, data showed that optimal experience can also be retrieved in the compulsory activities of productive life. Studies highlighted that even during work and schoolwork optimal experience is the most positive and complex state of consciousness (Csikszentmihalyi & LeFevre, 1989; Delle Fave & Massimini, 2005a; Haworth & Hill, 1992). However, in these tasks low levels of intrinsic motivation are reported. Similar results were actually obtained in the leisure domain. Mannell, Zuzanek, and Larson (1988) showed that freely chosen but extrinsically motivated activities produced the highest levels of flow, demanding more effort, and commitment than freely chosen and intrinsically motivated activities.

These findings can be profitably understood by taking into account Deci and Ryan's Self-Determination Theory (SDT; 1985, 2000). SDT distinguishes different types of motivation on the basis of the perceived locus of causality and degree of autonomy in behavior regulation (Deci & Ryan, 2000). Autonomous motivation represents the highest level of self-determination and involves the experience of volition and choice; controlled motivation represents the lowest level of self-determination and involves the experience of being pressured and coerced (Rigby, Deci, Patrick, & Ryan, 1992; Vansteenkiste, Lens, & Deci, 2006); amotivation is a state in which individuals lack the intention to behave, or the ability to regulate themselves with respect to a given behavior. Intrinsic motivation is autonomous by definition, and intrinsically motivated activities are undertaken for their inherent interest and enjoyment. On the contrary, extrinsic motivation characterizes activities performed to attain an outcome that is separable from the activity itself. However, extrinsic motivation is not invariantly controlled, as the initially external regulation of behaviors can be internalized to various degrees. In particular, through the processes of identification and integration, individuals achieve increasing levels of internalized regulation, autonomy, and self-determination. Motivation based on these two kinds of regulation, even though still extrinsic in nature, approximates intrinsic motivation and can have similar beneficial effects on performance and well-being (Deci & Ryan, 2000).

Adopting the SDT framework in a study conducted on swimmers, Kowal and Fortier (1999) showed that intrinsic motivation and self-determined extrinsic motivation were positively related to flow, whereas amotivation was negatively related to it. Among architecture students, Mills and Fullagar (2008) found a positive relation between flow in academic activities and intrinsic motivations of knowledge and accomplishment, a negative relation with amotivation, and no relation with extrinsic motivation. College students analyzed by Wong (2000) positively associated autonomy—relative to control—with academic experience and flow. In addition, recent ESM studies highlighted that optimal experience during work—among teachers—and during classwork—among students—was mostly associated with controlled motivation (Bassi & Delle Fave, 2009; Bassi, 2008). However, its experiential dimensions were less positive in association with controlled motivation than with autonomous motivation, with no significant difference between situations characterized by intrinsic motivation and extrinsic autonomous motivation.

These studies showed not only that flow may arise during compulsory activities, but also that flow-related productive activities can be associated with both autonomous motivation and controlled motivation. These apparently contrasting results are partly related to specific activity characteristics, as shown in the previous section (Delle Fave & Massimini, 2005a). According to Mills and Fullagar (2008), for example, external-motivating contingences typical of certain activities can account for the differences between results obtained by Kowal and Fortier (1999) with swimmers and their own results with architecture students. Additionally, Hektner and Asakawa (2000) maintained that students who are often in flow cannot sustain their efforts in most activities through intrinsic motivation alone, but also need extrinsic rewards and social recognition for their accomplishment.

Another possible explanation for the contrasting findings can be the level of analysis (state vs trait) (Bassi, 2008; Mills & Fullagar, 2008). When motivation and flow are measured as dispositional constructs, intrinsic motivation is primarily associated with flow; when they are assessed as situational constructs (such as through ESM), state extrinsic contingent factors can have a more relevant influence on experience.

Finally, findings can also be interpreted taking into account the dynamic characteristic of optimal experience (Section 3.4), and the process of internalization of the perceived locus of causality and degree of autonomy in behavior regulation (Deci & Ryan, 2000). Individuals may engage in an activity because they are initially forced to do so by the surrounding environment (family members, teachers). People often need external incentives to take the first steps in an activity that requires effort and attention (Csikszentmihalyi, 1990). Nevertheless, in the course of time, the activity can be perceived to be intrinsically rewarding, as an opportunity for optimal experience; thus a virtuous circle can be triggered in which challenges and skills are increased, on the one hand, and locus of causality is gradually internalized.

5.3 Factors Favoring Optimal Experience

One thing has been clear to flow researchers since the beginning, namely that optimal experience is a fleeting state that cannot be switched on at will. When asked to describe how it arises and if they do something to make it start, the majority of participants (80–90%) commonly refer that flow is a spontaneous experience (Bassi & Massimini, 2003; Massimini, Inghilleri, & Delle Fave, 1996). However, researchers have identified several factors that can favor the onset of optimal experience and direct people's psychological selection (Massimini & Delle Fave, 2000). These can be individual characteristics, social and cultural features, and the dynamic interplay between individuals and their environment.

5.3.1 Individual Characteristics

Studies have shown that biological predispositions and specific talents influence the orientations of psychological selection and the perceived opportunities for optimal experience. Research with talented teenagers (Csikszentmihalyi, Rathunde, & Whalen, 1993) highlighted the relationship between talents in specific domains, such as music or mathematics, and the selective engagement in these domains as opportunities for optimal experiences and skill cultivation. Among US adolescents, additional personal characteristics were identified: (a) gender—girls experienced greater flow than boys and (b) age—older students (12th graders) reported higher engagement than younger students (10th graders) (Schmidt et al., 2007; Shernoff & Csikszentmihalyi, 2009). Among the elderly (between 70 and 86 years of age), age showed a negative correlation with both the number of days in which flow was reported and the average quality of flow (Love Collins et al., 2009). Additionally, women were more likely to experience higher average quality of flow than men.

Also health conditions influence the opportunities for and the contents of optimal experiences, both in daily life and in the long term (see Chapter 14). Cross-cultural studies conducted among people with disabilities and chronic diseases have detected the impact of physical constraints on the access to activities and socialization contexts (Bassi, Steca, Delle Fave, & Caprara, 2007b; Delle Fave & Maletto, 1992; Delle Fave & Massimini, 2004b). However, the pattern of daily experience fluctuation and the features and frequency of optimal experience reported by the participants are not influenced by physical conditions per se. Different results were obtained in the domain of clinical psychology (see Chapter 14): Mental disorders can negatively affect the quality of daily experience, thus undermining the evaluation and exploitation of opportunities for optimal experience in daily life (Barge-Schaapveld, Nicolson, Berkhof, & deVries, 1999; Delle Fave & Massimini, 1992).

Several personality traits have been related to the retrieval of optimal experience. Among US adolescents, studies revealed a positive association of flow with self-esteem and optimism (Schmidt et al., 2007). This finding was confirmed by Delle Fave, Steca, Bassi, and Caprara (2009b) comparing Italian teenagers reporting optimal experiences in their lives with those not reporting it. Besides having higher ratings of self-esteem and optimism, participants reporting optimal experiences scored higher in four of the Big Five factors, namely energy, agreeableness, emotional stability, and openness. Among German college students, Keller and Blomann (2008) observed that individuals characterized by a strong internal locus of control (LOC) were more sensitive to the challenges/skills balance and experienced flow more often than individuals with a weak internal LOC. Among US workers, Eisenberger, Jones, Stinglhamber, Shanock, and Randall (2005) found that the combination of high skills and high challenges resulted in an enhanced experience at work for achievement-oriented employees, while employees low in need for achievement failed to experience high skills and high challenges more favorably than the other skills/challenges combinations. Finally, a relationship was found between motivational orientations and flow. Moneta (2004) identified a positive association with intrinsic motivation orientations among US teenagers and Chinese college students. Abuhamdeh and Csikszentmihalyi (2009) investigated intrinsic motivation orientations (IMO) as a moderator of the relationship between level of difficulty and enjoyment among US and European internet chess players, showing that individuals high in IMO enjoyed more difficult games than individuals low in IMO.

According to Csikszentmihalyi (1990, 1997; Csikszentmihalyi & Csikszentmihalyi, 1988), there is more in the individual predisposition to experience flow than single personality traits. The capacity to experience flow appears to be nearly universal. However, some people—defined *autotelic* individuals (Csikszentmihalyi & Csikszentmihalyi, 1988)—perceive challenges and involvement in a variety of daily situations, while other people do not. Autotelic individuals develop an active and creative relationship with their environment in which they spontaneously identify opportunities for concentration and engagement. The autotelic personality is distinguished by "meta-skills" which enable the individual to enter flow and stay in it. These meta-skills include a general curiosity and interest in life, persistence, and low self-centeredness (Nakamura & Csikszentmihalyi, 2009). Autotelic persons are not necessarily happier, but they are involved in more complex activities, and feel better about themselves as a result. Their psychic energy seems inexhaustible (Csikszentmihalyi, 1997). They pay more attention to what happens around them, and they are willing to invest more attention in things for their own sake, without expecting an immediate return.

One way to identify autotelic individuals is by computing the frequency with which they report flow over time (e.g., over 1 week monitored with ESM). In so doing, Adlai-Gail (1994) showed that US autotelic adolescents had more positive experiences in daily life and had more well-defined goals than their non-autotelic counterparts. Defining autotelic and non-autotelic individuals by their level of intrinsic motivation in high challenges/high skills situations, Abuhamdeh (2000) reported that US autotelic adults globally reported a more positive quality of daily experience, and perceived less stress and strain while in flow than while not in flow. The reverse was true of their non-autotelic counterparts. The autotelic personality was extensively studied by Asakawa (2004, 2010) among Japanese college students. Autotelic students reported higher levels of involvement, concentration, and perceived importance in daily activities. They also reported higher *jujitsu-kan*, the Japanese concept referring to a sense of fulfillment and psychological well-being.

The perception of daily activities as challenges and opportunities for optimal experiences is also related to self-efficacy beliefs, at least as far as the academic domain is concerned (Bassi, Steca, Delle Fave & Caprara, 2007a). Self-efficacy can vary with time and across different domains, and it is even possible to distinguish different kinds of self-efficacy within the same domain (e.g., to learn specific school subjects; Bandura 2006). Nevertheless, in general self-efficacy beliefs strongly mediate the effects of individual skills and competencies on performance and achievement, by supporting effort and endurance in case of failures (Bandura, 1997; Bandura, Barbaranelli, Caprara, & Pastorelli, 2001). In this respect, self-efficacy promotes active engagement in perceived high-challenge situations, thus fostering the occurrence of optimal experiences through skill refinement.

Through its influence on psychological selection, optimal experience contributes to shape the trajectory of individual development (Massimini & Delle Fave, 2000; Chapter 3). In this process, important individual factors come into play, namely meaning-making and goal-setting. As stated by Kegan (1994), in time individuals can attribute different meanings to the same situation, according to progressively more complex principles in organizing experience. The changes in meaning-making depend on the outcomes of the day-by-day interaction between the individual and the environment. From this perspective, meaning-making is a dynamic process, representing the way in which people actively organize their own experience in time around their values and beliefs, through goal-setting, definition of priorities, and action strategies. Values and priorities are not necessarily fixed entities either: They are related to specific developmental tasks and stages, to the exposure and acquisition of new information, to the organization criteria individuals adopt to integrate the new information into their previous *Weltanschauung* (Delle Fave, Bassi, & Massimini, 2009a).

Goals have been shown to play a crucial role in favoring optimal experience in all the samples analyzed. Clear goals about future career, for example, are reported by adolescents who perceive optimal experience in school-related activities (Asakawa & Csikszentmihalyi, 1998; Delle Fave & Massimini, 2005a; Hektner & Asakawa, 2000). Participants' intentions and goals also play an important role in Web activities (Chan & Ahern, 1999; Chen, 2006; Chen, Wigand, & Nilan, 1999): They guide people in surfing the net for information, playing a game, or engaging in a debate, thus narrowing down attention to important cues and away from distractions. The preferential association of optimal experience with goal-directed activities was also observed in an ESM study among Italian climbers in the Himalayan region (Bassi and Delle Fave, 2010). Long-term goals related to mountaineering allowed participants to keep focused in the face of adverse weather conditions and environmental perils, and to organize behavior and intentions in a structured way, thus favoring the retrieval of optimal experience.

5.3.2 Cultural and Contextual Features

The occurrence and cultivation of optimal experience are also influenced by prominently contextual factors, affecting individual behavior and psychological selection in a more or less direct and immediate way (Massimini & Delle Fave, 2000). As shown in Chapters 2 and 3, day by day people acquire cultural information from their social environment, and they replicate and transmit it during the course of their lives. The process of psychological selection is therefore partially regulated by the set of norms and rules that characterizes the cultural system and the social contexts individuals live in (Csikszentmihalyi & Massimini, 1985; Massimini et al., 1996). Specifically, cultures favoring autonomy—considered as a human need toward self-regulated action and coherence in the organism's behavioral aims—can facilitate the retrieval of optimal experience in daily contexts, compared to cultures in which external control predominates (Deci & Ryan, 2000; Massimini & Delle Fave, 2000; Schmidt et al., 2007). Similarly, contexts supporting individuals' ability to focus attention and to overcome distractions can foster individuals' long-term commitment to meaningful flow-related activities through the selective investment of psychic energy and personal resources (Csikszentmihalyi & Nakamura, 2010).

Cultures exert a crucial influence on individuals' psychological selection and on the discovery and cultivation of optimal activities through the proximal environment in the stage of development, especially the family. Family interaction patterns can facilitate or hamper the natural tendency of children to selectively reproduce rewarding activities (Hektner et al., 2007; Schmidt, 2003). In US, Japanese, and Italian samples, parents have been shown to represent models of engagement and commitment to self-determined goals (Asakawa & Csikszentmihalyi, 1998; Bassi & Delle Fave, 2006; Larson & Richards, 1994; Rathunde, 1997, 2001; Deci and Ryan 2000; Chapter 10). In particular, parents who provide the right balance of supportive and challenging environments can promote their children's optimal experience (Rathunde, 1997, 2001). Also parents with high levels of perceived parental self-efficacy can foster their children's psychosocial adaptation (Steca, Bassi, Caprara, & Delle Fave, 2010; Chapter 10). In addition, the combined effect of culture and family was highlighted in a cross-cultural study on Caucasian American and Asian American adolescents. Parents of Asian-American adolescents structured their children's lives to facilitate academic success, provided them with more autonomy in school activities, promoted optimal experiences, and favored internalization of cultural values (Asakawa, 2001; Asakawa & Csikszentmihalyi, 1998).

Cultural rules further contribute to define the range and variety of activities available to the individuals as potential opportunities for optimal experiences (Delle Fave & Massimini, 2004a). Some activities are more frequently associated with optimal activities than others. For example, the Italian adolescents previously considered prominently associated interactions and sports and hobbies with flow that with any other experience identified through the EFM (23.4 and 22.4% of the answers respectively). Also learning activities can promote flow, but they are often associated with apathy and boredom (see Chapter 11). On the opposite, maintenance activities—such as eating or taking care of personal hygiene—and watching TV are primarily associated with boredom (22.6 and 21.8% respectively) and apathy (18 and 22.5%).

The opportunity of being exposed to more or less challenging and complex environments during daily life influences the quality of experience individuals associate with daily activities. For example, in the work domain, activities such as planning, problem solving, and work evaluation provide opportunities for optimal experience (Nielsen & Cleal, 2010). By contrast, the enrolment in repetitive and automatized tasks strongly limits the availability of occasions for optimal experiences. In these conditions, optimal experiences can be found outside the work context, in leisure, family or social relations; however, the great amount of daily life revolves around low-challenge and alienating tasks (Delle Fave & Massimini, 1991). Similarly, data gathered among people with physical disabilities highlighted that the environmental opportunities available to them are often not matched with their own potentials, skills, and resources (Delle Fave & Massimini, 2005b).

Besides challenges, another activity characteristic that favors the onset of optimal experience is structure: Activities presenting clear rules and providing feedback to individuals' actions are more likely to be associated with optimal experience. This was observed in the contrast between free time activities such as sports, hobbies, on the one hand, and activities such as watching TV or doing nothing, on the other (Delle Fave & Bassi, 2003). It was also observed in the investigation of Web activities, with interface usability allowing individuals to understand the structure and thus the use of a Web site (Pace, 2004).

5.4 Optimal Experience and Related Constructs: Similarities and Differences

The in-depth analysis of the phenomenology of optimal experience has allowed researchers to distinguish between flow and similar constructs, such as peak experience or involvement. It has also spurred the investigation of the relationship between flow and other positive-psychology constructs, such as psychological well-being and satisfaction with life (see Chapter 1).

5.4.1 Peak Experience

Optimal experience has been assimilated to *peak experience* (Privette & Bundrick, 1991; Privette, 1983). This construct was first developed by Maslow (1971) who described it as a state of extreme joy, deep feeling of fulfillment, and loss of self in a mystical and transpersonal dimension. Peak experiences are related to the need for self-actualization, and are described as highly relevant and meaningful for the individual. They are quite rare events, which arise unexpectedly and "capture" the person regardless of her will or intention. Moreover, few people report peak experiences in their lives: In Maslow's pioneer studies, only one out of 3,000 participants described it.

In recent years, optimal experience is still often misrepresented as an extreme condition (Bakker, 2005), even though empirical findings on peak experience and on flow identified several differences between these two states (Delle Fave & Bassi, 1998; Delle Fave et al., 2009b):

(1) Unlike peak experiences, optimal experience is not an extreme condition. It is characterized by a complex and positive balance between the emotional, cognitive, and motivational components of the psychic system (Figure 4.2). It involves a harmonious feeling of global well-being, arising from the synchronic interplay of high cognitive investment, substantially positive mood and motivation in the short and/or in the long term.
(2) Optimal experience is mainly characterized by concentration and involvement, rather than by happiness and joy, typical features of peak experiences. The emotional components are only partially relevant, and they widely vary according to the associated activities, as shown above.
(3) Differently from peak experiences, in optimal experience participants do not report loss of self-awareness in an ecstatic dimension. Rather, they perceive engagement and control of the situation. The loss of self-consciousness associated with optimal experience has to be understood as a complete absorption in the activity that leaves the person free of concerns about her own behavior,

self-image, or social judgment. The action naturally flows and the person is not worried about outcomes or external evaluations of her performance.

(4) Optimal experience is not prominently associated with leisure activities or recreational tasks, as assumed by Privette and Bundrick (1991). Compulsory activities such as work and studying can promote the onset of optimal experience by virtue of the engagement and concentration they require (see also Chapters 8 and 11). Concerning leisure, not all the recreational activities provide opportunities for optimal experience per se (Chapter 9). Sports, games, arts, and hobbies are often associated with optimal experience in that they merge enjoyment and intrinsic motivation with concentration, goal-setting, and intentional effort toward specific skill acquisition. They have been defined "serious leisure", in contrast with "casual" or "unserious leisure" (Stebbins, 1997). Their crucial aspect is structure, that is a clear set of rules and procedures which foster agency, engagement, and autonomous action toward meeting challenges and pursuing goals.

(5) Far from being an unusual or rare condition, optimal experience is part of the daily experience of individuals: In a cross-cultural study with 1,106 participants, the vast majority of participants (953, 86.2%) reported optimal experiences in their lives, and associated it with one or more activities (Delle Fave, 2007). Similar findings from a cross-cultural sample will be illustrated in Chapter 7. Our sample of Italian teenagers reported optimal experiences in 16% of all the ESM forms, in line with findings from other studies (Delle Fave and Massimini, 2005a).

(6) Differently from peak experience, flow is not characterized by passive immersion in an uncontrollable condition of transcendence. Absorption in the ongoing task and merging of action and awareness are reported, but they are supported by active engagement and intentionality.

(7) Finally, both peak experience and optimal experience are spontaneously occurring events, e.g., they cannot be induced at will. However, peak experiences arise in unpredictable situations and circumstances, whereas in order for optimal experiences to occur, the individual has to engage in an activity. It can be a purely intellectual task or it can involve the whole body (Hunter & Csikszentmihalyi, 2000). In any case, concentrating on a specific stimulus represents a necessary trigger to induce optimal experiences.

5.4.2 *Enduring and Situational Involvement*

Involvement is a popular concept in psychology, especially in the marketing and leisure domains (Havitz & Mannell, 2005; Huang, 2006). It is often used as an umbrella term encompassing similar but distinct dimensions that account for perseverance and long-term commitment in certain activities (Muncy & Hunt, 1984). In particular, it comprises *enduring involvement* and *situational involvement*. Enduring involvement represents an ongoing concern with an activity or product that transcends situational influences, and is thus relatively stable (Houston & Rothschild,

1978; Richins & Bloch, 1986). It comprises aspects such as interest in the product or activity, enjoyment, personal relevance, and self-reference or the extent to which the product or activity is related to the consumer's self-concept and self-expression. By contrast, situational involvement reflects temporary feelings of heightened involvement that accompany a particular situation (Celsi & Olson, 1988; Houston & Rothschild, 1978). Being sensitive to events, situational involvement is characterized by focused attention, goal-directedness, personal relevance, and by perceived risk since, in situations that involve uncertainty, consumers are more concerned about their behavior in order to avoid negative consequences.

Based on the descriptions above, Huang (2006) claimed that involvement and flow present overlapping characteristics. Not only is involvement advocated as an experiential component of flow, features such as focused attention, enjoyment, goal-directedness, and interest are shared by both the constructs of involvement and optimal experience. Analyzing unique as well as overlapping characteristics among Web consumers, Huang (2006) empirically showed that flow, enduring involvement and situational involvement are highly correlated constructs in the Web environment. The variables attention focus, control, curiosity, perceived risk, enjoyment, interest, self-reference, and personal relevance were entered into a second-order confirmatory factor model. Results identified attention focus and control as unique features of optimal experience, self-reference for enduring involvement, and perceived risk for situational involvement. The remaining variables were shared between the constructs; in particular, flow shared enjoyment with enduring involvement, curiosity with situational involvement, and interest with both.

From a different perspective, Havitz and Mannell (2005) proposed that flow, enduring and situational involvement be independent constructs. In a study using ESM, situational involvement and flow were assessed among individuals engaged in leisure and non-leisure activities. Flow evaluation was based on mood (happy and irritable) and focus of attention, while the measures of challenges and skills were omitted. Situation involvement was evaluated in terms of interest, enjoyment, self-relevance, and self-reference. Enduring involvement was measured with the same situational items 3–4 months after the ESM session. Structural equation modeling suggested that in both leisure and non-leisure activities, situational involvement mediated the relationship between enduring involvement and flow, so that the greater the enduring involvement a person had for a particular activity, the higher her situational involvement in any specific episode of that activity, and in turn, the higher the level of flow that was experienced.

The merit of the studies reported above (Havitz & Mannell, 2005; Huang, 2006) was to provide initial clarifications on the differences and relationships between the flow and involvement. However, additional research is needed in which all flow characteristics—and not just a few—are contrasted with enduring and situational involvement features, and various activity domains are taken into consideration.

Finally, meditation states have also been assimilated with flow. Given the complexity of this topic, and its culture-related implications, Chapter 6 will be entirely devoted to it.

5.4.3 Hedonic and Eudaimonic Constructs

To date, few studies have been carried out on the relationship of optimal experience with hedonic and eudaimonic constructs of well-being.

Chen, Ye, Chen, and Tung (2010) examined the role of satisfaction with an event as a mediator in the relation between flow and life satisfaction among spectators of an acrobatic show performed in Taiwan by the Cirque du Soleil team. Flow items ("I lose track of time", "I have a high level of concentration", "I forget personal problems", and "I feel fully involved") showed significantly positive correlations with satisfaction with the show (in terms of performance quality and service quality), and with the five items of the Satisfaction with Life Scale (SWLS; Diener, Emmons, Larn, & Griffin, 1985). In particular, moderate correlation scores (ranging between 0.10 and 0.25) between flow and SWLS items were obtained. In addition, structural equation modeling supported the prediction of the mediation of satisfaction with the event between flow and life satisfaction.

A positive correlation between flow and satisfaction with life was also identified by Asakawa (2010) among Japanese college students (partial $r = 0.21$). In another study measuring flow with FQ (Section 5.3.1), Delle Fave et al., 2009a compared life satisfaction scores of Italian teenagers reporting optimal experiences in their lives with scores of teenagers not reporting flow. No significant difference was detected between the two groups of participants. However, adolescents reporting flow scored higher in positive affect and lower in negative affect (measured by PANAS, Watson, Clark, & Tellegen, 1988) than their counterparts. Among US undergraduate students, Rogatko (2009) showed that participants with high levels of optimal experience measured through the Flow State Scale 2 (Section 4.3.3) reported higher increases in positive affect after performing a flow-inducing activity than individuals reporting low levels of flow.

Concerning other eudaimonic constructs of well-being, in the study by Delle Fave et al. (2009b) described above, participants with flow reported higher ratings of all the components of psychological well-being (Section 1.3.2; Ryff, 1989), namely personal growth, self-acceptance, purpose in life, autonomy, positive social relations, and environmental mastery than their counterparts. In a study with US college students, Steele and Fullagar (2009) showed that flow correlated positively with psychological well-being ($r = 0.30$). They further showed that flow completely mediated the relation between academic work characteristics (role clarity, professor support for autonomy, and feedback) and psychological well-being. A study conducted among Japanese college students (Asakawa, 2004, 2010) also highlighted significant positive correlations between optimal experience and the constructs of will for meaningful life and *jujitsu-kan* ($r = 0.34$ and $r = 0.20$, respectively).

Altogether, findings show modest correlations between flow and satisfaction with life, as theoretically expected of distinct hedonic and eudaimonic constructs (Chapter 4; Gallagher, Lopez, & Preacher, 2009; Linley, Maltby, Wood, Osborne, & Hurling, 2009). In particular, affect is not a predominant feature of optimal experience, as shown above. Increase in positive affect and decrease in negative affect can be consequences of performing optimal activities. Reflecting on the involvement in the task that has just been carried out and on the perception of successfully investing high personal abilities in opportunities for growth and self-expression can enhance positive affect and reduce negative feeling states.

On the contrary, optimal experience as a state of full concentration and engagement in meaningful and challenging activities can play an important role in the construction of eudaimonic well-being by sustaining skill development in daily tasks, by feeding back on personal goals and intention, by enhancing positive affect and reducing negative affect in relation to personal achievements. Future research is needed to outline the role of optimal experience in a more articulate picture of human happiness in which eudaimonic and hedonic constructs are integrated for the development of a full life (Seligman, 2002).

References

Abuhamdeh, S. (2000). *The autotelic personality: An exploratory investigation.* Unpublished manuscript, University of Chicago.

Abuhamdeh, S., & Csikszentmihalyi, M. (2009). Intrinsic and extrinsic motivational orientations in the competitive context: An examination of person–situation interactions. *Journal of Personality, 77*, 1615–1635.

Adlai-Gail, W. (1994). *Exploring the autotelic personality.* Doctoral dissertation, University of Chicago, Chicago.

Asakawa, K. (2001). Family socialization practices and their effects on the internalization of educational values for Asian and White American adolescents. *Applied Developmental Science*, 5, 184–194.

Asakawa, K. (2004). Flow experience and autotelic personality in Japanese college students: How do they experience challenges in daily life? *Journal of Happiness Studies, 5*, 123–154.

Asakawa, K. (2010). Flow experience, culture, and well-being: How do autotelic Japanese college student feel, behave, and think in their daily lives? *Journal of Happiness Studies, 11*, 205–223.

Asakawa, K., & Csikszentmihalyi, M. (1998). The quality of experience of Asian American adolescents in activities related to future goals. *Journal of Youth and Adolescence, 27*, 141–163.

Bakker, A. B. (2005). Flow among music teachers and their students: The crossover of peak experiences. *Journal of Vocational Behavior, 66*, 26–44.

Bandura, A. (1997). *Self-efficacy: The exercise of control.* New York: Freeman.

Bandura, A. (2006). Guide for constructing self-efficacy scales. In F. Pajares & T. Urdan (Eds.), *Self-efficacy beliefs of adolescents* (Vol. 5, pp. 307–337). Greenwich, CT: Information Age Publishing.

Bandura, A., Barbaranelli, C., Caprara, G. V., & Pastorelli, C. (2001). Self-efficacy beliefs as shapers of children's aspirations and career trajectories. *Child Development, 72*, 187–206.

Barge-Schaapveld, D. Q. C. M., Nicolson, N. A., Berkhof, J., & deVries, M. W. (1999). Quality of life in depression: Daily life determinants and variability. *Psychiatry Research, 88*, 173–189.

Bassi, M. (2008). Optimal experience, motivational orientations and the work paradox among teachers. Paper presented at *4th European Conference on Positive Psychology*, Book of Abstracts, 59. Opatija, Croatia, 2–4 July.

Bassi, M., & Delle Fave, A. (2006). The daily experience of Italian adolescents' in family interactions. Gender and developmental issues. In A. Delle Fave (Ed.), *Dimensions of well-being: Research and intervention* (pp. 172–190). Milano: Franco Angeli.

Bassi, M., & Delle Fave, A. (2009). Self-determination and optimal experience at school: Joining perspectives. Paper presented at *1st International Positive Psychology Conference*, Book of Abstracts, 43. Philadelphia, US, 18–21 June.

Bassi, M., & Delle Fave, A. (2010). Impact of extreme weather conditions on high-altitude climbers' goals and quality of experience. *Journal of Leisure Research, 42*, 469–488.

Bassi, M., & Massimini, F. (2003). Immigrati africani a milano: Qualità dell'esperienza tra passato e presente [African immigrants in Milano: Quality of experience between past and present]. In A. Delle Fave (Ed.), *L'inizio del viaggio. Esperienze di immigrazione e progetti di accoglienza a milano* (pp. 155–186). Milano: Arcipelago Edizioni.

Bassi, M., Preziosa, A., & Pozzoli, S. (2007b). Experience sampling method e lo studio dell'esperienza quotidiana: Implicazioni per l'intervento. In A. Delle Fave (Ed.), *La condivisione del benessere. Il contributo della psicologia positiva* (pp. 169–189). Milano: Franco Angeli.

Bassi, M., Steca, P., Delle Fave, A., & Caprara, G. V. (2007a). Academic self-efficacy beliefs and quality of experience in learning. *Journal of Youth and Adolescence, 36*, 301–312.

Celsi, R. L., & Olson, J. C. (1988). The role of involvement in attention and comprehension processes. *Journal of Consumer Research, 15*, 210–224.

Chan, T. S., & Ahern, T. C. (1999). Targeting motivation—adapting flow theory to instructional design. *Journal of Educational Computing Research, 21*, 151–163.

Chen, H. (2006). Flow on the net-detecting web users' positive affects and their flow states. *Computers in Human Behavior, 22*, 221–233.

Chen, H., Wigand, R. T., & Nilan, M. S. (1999). Optimal experience of web activities. *Computers in Human Behavior, 15*, 585–608.

Chen, H., Wigand, R. T., & Nilan, M. S. (2000). Exploring web users' optimal flow experiences. *Information Technology & People, 13*, 263–281.

Chen, L. H., Ye, Y. C., Chen, M. Y., & Tung, I. W. (2010). Alegría! Flow in leisure and life satisfaction: The mediating role of event satisfaction using data from an acrobatics show. *Social Indicators Research, 99*, 301–313. Published online 9 February 2010.

Coppa, R., & Delle Fave, A. (2007). Pratica religiosa ed esperienza ottimale: Una prospettiva eudaimonica [religious practice and optimal experience: A eudaimonic perspective]. In A. Delle Fave (Ed.), *La condivisione del benessere. Il contributo della psicologia positiva* (pp. 73–93). Milano: Franco Angeli.

Csikszentmihalyi, M. (1975/2000). *Beyond boredom and anxiety*. San Francisco: Jossey Bass.

Csikszentmihalyi, M. (1990). *Flow: The psychology of optimal experience*. New York: Harper & Row.

Csikszentmihalyi, M. (1997). *Finding flow: The psychology of engagement wit everyday life*. New York: Basic Books.

Csikszentmihalyi, M., & Csikszentmihalyi, I. (Eds.) (1988). *Optimal experience: Psychological studies of flow in consciousness*. New York: Cambridge University Press.

Csikszentmihalyi, M., & LeFevre, J. (1989). Optimal experience in work and leisure. *Journal of Personality and Social Psychology, 56*, 815–822.

Csikszentmihalyi, M., & Massimini, F. (1985). On the psychological selection of bio-cultural information. *New Ideas in Psychology, 3*, 115–138.

Csikszentmihalyi, M., & Nakamura, J. (2010). Effortless attention in everyday life: A systematic phenomenology. In B. J. Bruya (Ed.), *Effortless attention* (pp. 179–189). Boston: The MIT Press.

Csikszentmihalyi, M., Rathunde, K., & Whalen, S. (1993). *Talented teenagers: The roots of success and failure*. New York: Cambridge University Press.

Deci, E. L., & Ryan, R. M. (1985). *Intrinsic motivation and self-determination in human behavior*. New York: Plenum Press.

Deci, E. L., & Ryan, R. M. (2000). The "what" and "why" of goal pursuits: Human needs and the self-determination of behavior. *Psychological Inquiry, 11*, 227–268.

Delespaul, P. A. E. G., Resi, H. T., & deVries, M. W. (2004). Ecological and motivational determinants of activation: Studying compared to sports and watching TV. *Social Indicators Research, 67*, 129–143.

Delle Fave, A. (2007). Individual development and community empowerment: Suggestions from studies on optimal experience. In J. Haworth & G. Hart (Eds.), *Well-being: Individual, community, and societal perspectives* (pp. 41–56). London: Palgrave McMillan.
Delle Fave, A., & Bassi, M. (1998). Esperienza di flow e sviluppo della complessità nel comportamento umano [Flow experience and development of complexity in human behavior]. *Informazione in Psicologia, Psicoterapia, Psichiatria, 32/33*, 32–47.
Delle Fave, A., & Bassi, M. (2000). The quality of experience in adolescents' daily life: Developmental perspectives. *Genetic, Social, and General Psychology Monographs, 126*, 347–367.
Delle Fave, A., & Bassi, M. (2003). Italian adolescents and leisure: The role of engagement and optimal experience. In S. Verma & R. Larson (Eds.), *Examining adolescent leisure time across cultures: Developmental opportunities and risks: New directions in child and adolescent development* (pp. 79–93). San Francisco: Jossey-Bass.
Delle Fave, A., Bassi, M., & Massimini, F. (2002). Quality of experience and daily social context of Italian adolescents. In A. L. Comunian & U. P. Gielen (Eds.), *It's all about relationships* (pp. 159–172). Lengerich: Pabst Science Publishers.
Delle Fave, A., Bassi, M., & Massimini, F. (2009a). Experiencia óptima y evolución humana [Optimal experience and psychological selection]. In C. Vasquez & G. Hervas (Eds.), *La ciencia del bienestar: Fundamentos de una psicología positiva* (pp. 209–230). Madrid: Alianza Editorial.
Delle Fave, A., & Maletto, C. (1992). Processi di attenzione e qualità dell'esperienza soggettiva [Attention processes and quality of subjective experience in blind individuals]. In D. Galati (Ed.), *La psicologia dei non vedenti. Processi cognitivi, affettivi e strategie adattativi* (pp. 321–353). Milano: Franco Angeli.
Delle Fave, A., & Massimini, F. (1991). Modernization and the quality of daily experience in a southern Italy village. In N. Bleichrodt & P. J. D. Drenth (Eds.), *Contemporary issues in cross–cultural psychology* (pp. 110–119). Amsterdam: Swets & Zeitlinger B.V.
Delle Fave, A., & Massimini, F. (1992). Experience sampling method and the measuring of clinical change: A case of anxiety syndrome. In M. W. deVries (Ed.), *The experience of psychopathology—investigating mental disorders in their natural settings* (pp. 280–298). Cambridge: Cambridge University Press.
Delle Fave, A., & Massimini, F. (2003). Optimal experience in work and leisure among teachers and physicians: Individual and bio-cultural implications. *Leisure Studies, 22*, 323–342.
Delle Fave, A., & Massimini, F. (2004a). The cross-cultural investigation of optimal experience. *Ricerche di Psicologia, 27*, 79–102.
Delle Fave, A., & Massimini, F. (2004b). Bringing subjectivity into focus: Optimal experiences, life themes and person-centered rehabilitation. In P. A. Linley & S. Joseph (Eds.), *Positive psychology in practice* (pp. 581–597). London: Wiley & Sons.
Delle Fave, A., & Massimini, F. (2005a). The investigation of optimal experience and apathy: Developmental and psychosocial implications. *European Psychologist, 10*, 264–274.
Delle Fave, A., & Massimini, F. (2005b). The relevance of subjective wellbeing to social policies: Optimal experience and tailored intervention. In F. Huppert, B. Keverne, & N. Baylis (Eds.), *The science of wellbeing* (pp. 379–404). Oxford: Oxford University Press.
Delle Fave, A., Steca, P., Bassi, M., & Caprara, G. V. (2009b). Optimal experience in adolescence: Bridging personality and well-being. Paper presented at 2nd *Applied Positive Psychology Conference*, Book of Abstracts, 24. Warwick, UK, 1–3 April.
Diener, E., Emmons, R. A., Larn, R. J., & Griffin, S. (1985). The satisfaction with life scale. *Journal of Personality Assessment, 49*, 71–75.
Eisenberger, R., Jones, J. R., Stinglhamber, F., Shanock, L., & Randall, A. T. (2005). Flow experiences at work: For high need achievers alone? *Journal of Organizational Behavior, 26*, 755–775.
Gaggioli, A., Bassi, M., & Delle Fave, A. (2003). Quality of experience in virtual environments. In G. Riva, F. Davide, & W. A. Ijsselsteijn (Eds.), *Being there: Concepts, effects and measurements of user presence in synthetic environments* (pp. 121–135). Amsterdam: IOS Press.

Gallagher, M. W., Lopez, S. J., & Preacher, K. J. (2009). The hierarchical structure of well-being. *Journal of Personality*, *77*, 1025–1049.
Havitz, M. E., & Mannell, R. C. (2005). Enduring involvement, situational involvement, and flow in leisure an non-leisure activities. *Journal of Leisure Research*, *37*, 152–177.
Haworth, J., & Hill, S. (1992). Work, leisure and psychological well-being in a sample of young adults. *Journal of Community and Applied Social Psychology*, *2*, 147–160.
Hektner, J. M., & Asakawa, K. (2000). Learning to like challenges. In M. Csikszentmihayi & B. Schneider (Eds.), *Becoming adult: How teenagers prepare for the world of work*. New York: Basic Books.
Hektner, J. M., Schmidt, J., & Csikszentmihalyi, M. (2007). *Experience sampling method: Measuring the quality of everyday life*. Thousand Oaks, CA: Sage.
Hoffman, D., & Novak, T. P. (1996). Marketing in hypermedia computer-mediated environments: Conceptual foundations. *Journal of Marketing*, *60*, 50–68.
Houston, M. J., & Rothschild, M. J. (1978). Conceptual and methodological perspectives on involvement. In S. C. Jain (Ed.), *Research frontiers in marketing: Dialogues and directions* (pp. 184–187). Chicago: American Marketing Association.
Huang, M. H. (2006). Flow, enduring, and situational involvement in the web environment: A tripartite second-order examination. *Psychology & Marketing*, *23*, 383–411.
Hunter, J., & Csikszentmihalyi, M. (2000). The phenomenology of body-mind: The contrasting cases of flow in sports and contemplation. *Anthropology of Consciousness*, *11*, 5–24.
Inal, Y., & Cagiltay, K. (2007). Flow experiences of children in an interactive social game environment. *British Journal of Educational Technology*, *38*, 455–464.
Jackson, S. A., & Eklund, R. C. (2002). Assessing flow in physical activity: The flow state scale-2 and dispositional flow scale-2. *Journal of Sport & Exercise Psychology*, *24*, 133–150.
Kegan, R. (1994). *In over our heads*. Cambridge: Cambridge University Press.
Keller, J., & Blomann, F. (2008). Locus of control and the flow experience: An experimental analysis. *European Journal of Personality*, *22*, 1–19.
Kowal, J., & Fortier, M. S. (1999). Motivational determinants of flow: Contributions from self-determination theory. *Journal of Social Psychology*, *139*, 355–368.
Larson, R. W., & Richards, M. H. (1994). *Divergent realities: The emotional lives of mothers, fathers, and adolescents*. New York: Basic Books.
Lessiter, J., Freeman, J., Keogh, E., & Davidoff, J. (2001). A cross-media presence questionnaire: The ITC-sense of presence inventory. *Presence*, *10*, 282–297.
Linley, P. A., Maltby, J., Wood, A. M., Osborne, G., & Hurling, R. (2009). Measuring happiness: The higher order factor structure of subjective and psychological well-being measures. *Personality and Individual Differences*, *47*, 878–884.
Love Collins, A., Sarkisian, N., & Winner, E. (2009). Flow and happiness in later life: An investigation into the role of daily and weekly flow experiences. *Journal of Happiness Studies*, *10*, 703–719.
Mannell, R. C., Zuzanek, J., & Larson, R. (1988). Leisure states and "flow" experiences: Testing perceived freedom and intrinsic motivation hypothesis. *Journal of Leisure Research*, *20*, 289–304.
Maslow, A. (1971). *The farther reaches of human nature*. New York: Viking Press.
Massimini, F., & Delle Fave, A. (2000). Individual development in a bio-cultural perspective. *American Psychologist*, *55*, 24–33.
Massimini, F., Inghilleri, P., & Delle Fave, A. (Eds.). (1996). *La selezione psicologica umana—teoria e metodo d'analisi* [Human psychological selection—Theory and method of analysis]. Milano: Coop. Libraria IULM.
Mills, M., & Fullagar, C. J. (2008). Motivation and flow: Toward an understanding of the dynamics of the relation in architecture students. *Journal of Psychology*, *142*, 533–553.
Moneta, G. B. (2004). The flow model of intrinsic motivation in Chinese: Cultural and personal moderators. *Journal of Happiness Studies*, *5*, 181–217.

Muncy, J. A., & Hunt, S. D. (1984). Consumer involvement: Definitional issues and research directions. *Advances in Consumer Research*, *11*, 15–19.

Nakamura, J., & Csikszentmihalyi, M. (2009). Flow theory and research. In S. J. Lopez & C. R. Snyder (Eds.), *Handbook of positive psychology* (pp. 195–206). New York: Oxford University Press.

Nielsen, K., & Cleal, B. (2010). Predicting flow at work: Investigating the activities and job characteristics that predict flow states at work. *Journal of Occupational Health Psychology*, *15*, 180–190.

Novak, T. P., Hoffman, D., & Yung, Y. (2000). Measuring the flow construct in online environments: A structural modeling approach. *Marketing Science*, *19*, 22–42.

Pace, S. (2004). A grounded theory of the flow experiences of web users. *International Journal of Human-Computer Studies*, *60*, 327–363.

Privette, G. (1983). *Peak experience*, peak performance, and flow: A comparative analysis of positive human experiences. *Journal of Personality and Social Psychology*, *45*, 1361–1368.

Privette, G., & Bundrick, C. M. (1991). *Peak experience*, peak performance, and flow: Correspondence of personal descriptions and theoretical constructs. In A. Jones, & R. Crandall (Eds.), Handbook of Self-Actualization (Special Issue). *Journal of Social Behavior and Personality*, *6*, 169–188.

Rathunde, K. (1997). Parent-adolescent interaction and optimal experience. *Journal of Youth and Adolescence*, *26*, 669–689.

Rathunde, K. (2001). Family context and the development of undivided interest: A longitudinal study of family support and challenge and adolescents' quality of experience. *Applied Developmental Science*, *5*, 158–171.

Rheinberg, F., Manig, Y., Kliegl, R., Engeser, S., & Vollmeyer, R. (2007). Flow bei der arbeit, doch glück in der freizeit. Zielausrichtung, flow und glücksgefühle [flow during work but happiness during spare time. Goals, flow experience and happiness]. *Zeitschrift für Arbeits- und Organisationspsychologie*, *51*, 105–115.

Richins, M., & Bloch, P. H. (1986). After the new wears off: The temporal context of product involvement. *Journal of Consumer Research*, *13*, 280–285.

Rigby, C., Deci, E., Patrick, B., & Ryan, R. (1992). Beyond the intrinsic-extrinsic dichotomy: Self-determination in motivation and learning. *Motivation and Emotion*, *16*, 165–185.

Rogatko, T. P. (2009). The influence of flow on positive affect in college students. *Journal of Happiness Studies*, *10*, 133–148.

Ryff, C. D. (1989). Happiness is everything, or is it? Explorations on the meaning of psychological well-being. *Journal of Personality and Social Psychology*, *57*, 1069–1081.

Schmidt, J. (2003). Correlates of reduced misconduct among adolescents facing adversity. *Journal of Youth and Adolescence*, *32*, 439–452.

Schmidt, J., Shernoff, D., & Csikszentmihalyi, M. (2007). Individual and situational factors related to the experience of flow in adolescence: A multilevel approach. In A. D. Ong & M. van Dulmen (Eds.), *The handbook of methods in positive psychology* (pp. 542–558). Oxford: Oxford University Press.

Seligman, M. E. P. (2002). *Authentic happiness: Using the new positive psychology to realize your potential for lasting fulfillment*. New York: Free Press.

Shernoff, D., & Csikszentmihalyi, M. (2009). Flow in schools. Cultivating engaged learners and optimal learning environments. In R. Gilman, E. Huebner, & M. Furlong (Eds.), *Handbook of positive psychology in schools* (pp. 131–145). New York: Taylor & Francis.

Skadberg, Y. X., & Kimmel, J. R. (2004). Visitors' flow experience while browsing a web site: Its measurement, contributing factors and consequences. *Computers in Human Behavior*, *20*, 403–422.

Stebbins, R. A. (1997). Serious leisure and well-being. In J. T. Haworth (Ed.), *Work, leisure, and well-being* (pp. 117–130). London: Routledge.

Steca, P., Bassi, M., Caprara, G. V., & Delle Fave, A. (2010). Parents' self-efficacy beliefs and their children's psychosocial adaptation during adolescence. *Journal of Youth and Adolescence*, published online 4 March 2010.

Steele, J. P., & Fullagar, C. J. (2009). Facilitators and outcome of student engagement in a college setting. *Journal of Psychology*, *143*, 5–27.

Steuer, J. (1992). Defining virtual reality: Dimensions determining telepresence. *Journal of Communication*, *42*, 73–93.

Vansteenkiste, M., Lens, W., & Deci, E. (2006). Intrinsic versus extrinsic goal contents in self-determination theory: Another look at the quality of academic motivation. *Educational Psychologist*, *41*, 9–31.

Walker, C. J. (2010). Experiencing flow: Is doing it together better than doing it alone?. Journal of Positive Psychology, 5, 3–11.

Watson, D., Clark, L. A., & Tellegen, A. (1988). Development and validation of brief measures of positive and negative affect: The PANAS scale. *Journal of Personality and Social Psychology*, *54*, 1063–1070.

Wong, M. (2000). The relations among causality orientations, academic experience, academic performance, and academic commitment. *Personality and Social Psychology Bulletin*, *26*, 315–326.

Chapter 6
Optimal Experience and Meditation: Western and Asian Approaches to Well-Being

6.1 Flow and Meditation: A Controversial Issue

Various Western scholars have argued that optimal experience is a state of meditation, or—on the opposite—that the experience of meditation is a form of optimal experience (Kristeller & Rikhye, 2008; Bermant et al. in press). Meditation is a practice originally developed in India, as a substantial component of the ideal human developmental pathway, and it is grounded in a well-defined philosophical and spiritual perspective. Flow experience, even though recognized as a universal aspect of human psychological functioning, has been investigated, operationalized, and interpreted in the perspective of Western scientific psychology.

In order to appropriately discuss similarities and differences between flow and meditation, the cultural contexts in which the study of the two experiences emerged have to be taken into account. In particular, in order to provide an adequate definition of meditation, it is necessary to briefly outline its cultural and conceptual background.

This chapter does not aim at offering even a superficial overview of all the knowledge and wisdom traditions developed in the Indian subcontinent throughout the centuries. The topic is extremely complex, and a vast amount of excellent literature is available on it. We also cannot adequately provide details on the different types of meditation techniques that have been developed throughout the centuries, mainly within the Hindu and Buddhist traditions. We rather pursue a much more limited goal, namely the comparison of flow experience with the experience of meditation in its major aspects, as they were described in some of the classical works of ancient India. To this purpose, it is-however-important to first outline some basic conceptualizations developed in the Indian traditions as concerns consciousness and cognitive processes.

6.2 Consciousness Studies in the Indian Tradition

In the history of Indian culture various philosophical systems addressed the issue of human origin, destiny, and relationship with the universe. In particular, Indian

A. Delle Fave et al., *Psychological Selection and Optimal Experience Across Cultures*, Cross-Cultural Advancements in Positive Psychology 2,
DOI 10.1007/978-90-481-9876-4_6, © Springer Science+Business Media B.V. 2011

culture developed a systematic and astonishingly deep knowledge about human consciousness and psychological functioning. Most of the assumptions and conceptualizations formalized throughout the centuries by the various schools and traditions that flourished in the subcontinent have been confirmed by the findings of the scientific Western psychology.

However, in India the investigation of psychological functions and structures did not represent an independent knowledge domain. On the contrary, it was substantially related to ethics and spirituality (Kuppuswami, 1977; Rao, 2008). The main Indian philosophical traditions—Hinduism, Buddhism, and Jainism—paid prominent attention to the psychological functioning, with the aim of helping individuals to attain liberation from suffering through their emancipation from the constraints and entrapments of passions and attachment to worldly objects.

Indian psychological investigation stemmed from all the nine major ancient thought systems. Six of these systems are grouped together as Astika, or orthodox, in that they assume the truthfulness and authority of the Vedas—the oldest scriptures of India, considered *apaurusheya*, divine in origin. The other three systems are labeled as Nastika, or heterodox, in that they do not recognize Vedic knowledge as the ultimate truth. The Astika group includes Mimamsa (the teachings directly derived from the Vedas), Upanishads and Advaita Vedanta, Samkhya, Yoga, Nyaya, and Vaisesika. The Nastika group comprises Jainism, Buddhism, and Lokayata. The core difference among these two groups of theories is the recognition or denial of a universal and eternal consciousness principle, respectively (Swami Prabhavananda, 1977).

Despite this and other differences in metaphysical and theoretical assumptions, the ultimate goal of all these traditions was to show pathways to achieve an inner state of bliss and peace, as well as balance and equanimity of attitudes and behavior in daily activities and relationships.

For the specific purposes of this chapter, we will adopt a somehow rough approach, since we are well aware of the impossibility to address all the issues related to the comparison of concepts derived from two complex cultural traditions. Therefore, we will specifically focus on few major concepts developed within some of the Indian knowledge traditions belonging to the Astika group. These concepts can help us understand optimal experience from a different epistemological perspective and compare it with the experience of meditation, providing a theoretical background to such a comparison.

6.2.1 Levels of Consciousness and Mind Functioning

According to the Samkhya conceptualization, the universe stemmed from the interaction between the *Purusha*—the consciousness principle, passive and unchangeable—and the *Prakriti*—the material principle, active and dynamic. This interaction led to the differentiation of all living entities. Both principles—eternal consciousness and material nature—are therefore embodied in each living being. This implies the ontological identity between the individual soul (*Ātman*) and the universal consciousness principle (*Brahman*), both eternal and unchangeable. Ātman is present in every living being, and after the death of the body it migrates in another being, carrying the impressions (*samskaras*) of the previous lives.

As described in the Upanishads, within the mind–body system the Ātman plays the role of witness, taking no active part in the interaction of the individual with the environment. The Ātman is therefore pure consciousness, and in essence it is happiness and bliss, *ananda*. However, humans can hardly experience this original condition of bliss due to a set of sheaths (*kosha*) which cover, like layers of an onion, this core essence. *Annamaykosha* is the most external sheath, and it refers to the physical body. *Prānamayakosha* is related to breathing and vital energy. *Manomayakosha* includes the basic psychological functions, such as sensation, perception, emotions, experience fluctuation, and routine information processing. *Vijnānamayakosha* refers to higher cognitive and metacognitive functions, such as intellect, intuition, and discrimination. It directly covers the core, *Ānandamayakosha*, the pure consciousness.

Individuals differ according to the prominence they give to different koshas, by relating their essential identity to a particular set of functions and dimensions (Swami Chinmayananda, 1992). The majority of people tend to identify themselves with the first three koshas, thus being conditioned by positive and negative emotions, attachment to external objects and mind fluctuations (Kiran Kumar, 2006).

The ceaseless contact with external and internal stimuli makes the mind wander like a "restless monkey" from one activity to the other, from one thought to the other. *Citta vrtti* represents the mind fluctuations across different feelings, thoughts, and experiences. This dependency of the individual on the attraction or repulsion which originates from the interaction of the mind with environmental objects or inner triggers—such as images, expectations, and memories—ultimately causes suffering. This suffering has two main sources: pleasure and pain. On the one hand, it derives from the transient nature of the enjoyment of pleasurable objects and situations, which generates further desire, craving and longing for these objects. On the other hand, unpleasant and painful states cannot be always avoided, and they directly produce suffering (Swami Prabhavananda, 1977). This view of mind is substantially shared by all Indian philosophical systems.

According to the Upanishads, the individual is therefore entrapped into a web of unstable and ultimately distressing fluctuations of experience within the manomayakosha. Human evolution is considered as the progressive actualization of the levels of consciousness associated to the different koshas. People should strive to transcend the limitations of the first three sheaths and the associated self-definitions, moving toward the experience of ānanda (Kiran Kumar, 2003). The main goal of human beings is to get rid of the constraints of sensory attractions and mind fluctuations, and to identify with the state of perfect happiness and bliss which characterize Ātman.

Patanjali's Yoga Sūtras specifically describe the process leading to liberation through the experience of identification with the Ātman, as well as the eight steps required to attain it (Feuerstein, 1998). The first five steps are just preparatory practices. The process starts with prescriptions on daily behavior, *Yama* and *Niyama*.

They respectively refer to the realm of morality and ethics, with and emphasis on actions to be avoided (such as injuring, lust, and lying) and to the realm of religious behaviors (such as cleanliness, self-control, contentment, study, and devotion to God). After having developed these habits, a person can train the body through *āsanas* and *prānāyama*, postures and breathing exercises. The fifth preparatory step is *prathyāhāra*, the practice of focusing the attention inward, thus dissociating the mind from the sensory channels and withdrawing it from the external world (Rao & Paranjpe, 2008).

The three subsequent steps are concentration (*dhāranā*), meditation (*dhyāna*), and the complete absorption and loss of self-awareness (*samādhi*), which implies the total eradication of mental states (*niruddha*). Concentration allows individuals to overcome the unceasing flux of citta vrtti, by intentionally restraining the attention on one single object (*ekāgratā*). When this intentional pin-pointed attention gets prolonged in time, the individual enters the state of meditation, described in the Yoga Sūtras as the unbroken flow of attention on a single stimulus, which leads the person to become oblivious to all other sensations and impressions. All thoughts and psychological contents, sensory systems and mind are withdrawn from both external objects and internal images and products. This is the precondition for finally attaining samādhi, the state of identification with the permanent, unchangeable, and eternal self, the pure consciousness without object, which represents the essence of the individual.

In samādhi the distinction between subject and object is removed, there is stability and freedom from thoughts and mind fluctuations. Samādhi is impossible to describe through words, since it is a state of absolute subjectivity, in which the knower, the object of knowledge, and the act of knowing merge into a single entity (Sinha, 1958).

The Bhagavad Gitā—Lord Krishna's teachings to the warrior Arjuna within Mahabharata, one of the great Indian epics—made all these concepts accessible to a broader audience and applicable to ordinary people's life. By virtue of the universality of its philosophical content, Bhagavad Gitā has become very popular also in the West through innumerable translations and commentaries. Its core concept is the pursuit of non-attachment (*anāsakti*), a condition of mental balance and equanimity in dealing with life events without being emotionally affected by their positive or negative features and consequences (Swami Chinmayananda, 1992). The ideal of anāsakti embodies spiritual growth as well as action orientation. To be detached does not mean to withdraw from life demands and duties. Rather it implies to perform any action with dispassion, without concerns for failure or success, loss or gains (Pande & Naidu, 1992).

Moving from this core concept, Bhagavad Gitā provides different pathways to pursue mental equanimity and liberation from attachment and senses constraints: besides *Jñāna Yoga* (the way of intuitive knowledge and meditation practice) individuals can follow *Karma-Yoga* (the way of selfless action), or *Bhakti Yoga* (the way of devotion and surrender to God's will).

In particular, Karma-Yoga can be practiced by any person living an active life within a social context. As reported above, it involves performing actions without any concern for their outcomes, be they positive or negative (*niskāma karma*). When action is performed without attachment to its fruits, the individual realizes that actions belong to the world of mind and senses, which are only the superficial layer of reality. "Through right actions, undertaken without any self-dissipating anxiety for the fruits of those actions, a *Karma-Yogin* can reach an indescribable peace, arising out of the sense of steadfastness within him [. . .]. Peace is an unbroken sense of joy and it is the fragrance of an integrated personality" (Swami Chinmayananda, 1975, p. 304).

Depending on one's stage of psychological development, people may pursue desires (*kāma*), wealth (*artha*), personal and collective values (*dharma*), and liberation (*moksha*). The pursuit of desires and wealth to the exclusion of pursuit of values and of liberation is a sign of lower level of evolution. Therefore, well-being and good life can be achieved through minimization, restraint, and detachment from need fulfillment rather than through maximization, indulgence, and striving for need fulfillment. Such conceptions involve surrendering rather than controlling and holding on. Self-realization is accorded greater prominence than self-actualization (Kiran Kumar, 2003).

6.3 Flow and Meditation: Differences and Analogies

In order to appropriately draw a comparison between flow and meditation, a substantial ambiguity in terminology has first to be removed. Flow is an experience, which can be associated to a vast range of activities, while the term "meditation" is used to identify both an action and an experience. A variety of meditation practices were developed through history. They can be broadly grouped in the two categories of concentrative meditation, which requires the narrowing of attention on one single object, and mindfulness meditation, which aims at enhancing non-judgmental awareness of sensory and mental events (Goleman, 1988).

When discussing similarities or overlapping aspects of flow and meditation, researchers should therefore carefully consider what they are referring to: activities or associated experiences? It could be easily argued that the comparison should involve the experiences, with their psychological dimensions. However, such comparison is somehow problematic if we take into account one critical aspect, common to both experiences: their multidimensionality. In optimal experience variations in its emotional and motivational features were systematically observed across activities (Delle Fave & Massimini, 2005; Delle Fave, 2007; Chapters 5 and 7), and different kinds of mental functions come into play during different meditation strategies (Ivanovski & Malhi, 2007).

Nevertheless, due to the complete lack of investigations on this topic, we will engage in a first comparative endeavor. In our opinion, a comparison between Flow and the experience reported during the practice of meditation is possible, and it can be useful to disentangle the two conditions. Speaking about meditation, we will mainly refer to the concentrative meditation practice, first systematized in Patanjali's Yoga-Sūtras. This choice is based on the consideration that both experiences share a crucial component, which deeply contributes to shape them: concentration and pin-pointed attention. However, the analysis has to be conducted at different levels: the epistemological level, the neurophysiological level, and the phenomenological one.

In addition, when addressing the motivations and meanings underlying the two conditions, a distinction should be made between experience and activity, since both can be motivational drives. People can aim at performing specific activities, regardless of the associated experience, and/or they can aim at achieving peculiar states of consciousness, regardless of the associated activity. People can attribute relevance and meanings to activities, to the associated experiences, or to both. Other chapters of this book address some of these issues in relation to flow, at the theoretical level (see Chapters 3 and 5) and at the level of application in various life domains (see Chapters 8, 9, and 15).

6.3.1 The Epistemological Perspective

From the epistemological point of view, meditative experience and flow are grounded in substantially different perspectives. In the Indian tradition, the practice of concentration is one of the steps to attain liberation from the web of human conditionings and passions, which prevents individuals from attaining the supreme state of bliss, the experience of identification with the Ātman. Thus, the aim of systematic concentration practice is the attainment of a transcendent state, in which the individual is free from any kind of contingent constraints and worldly pursuits.

The practice of concentration and meditation is based on well-defined rules and techniques, which were developed within the different systems and schools, but which share the common goal of calming the mind and freeing consciousness from sorrows and desires. Moreover, concentration and meditation are not goals per se, rather they represent the gateway to access a higher state—samādhi—in which any consciousness content disappears, only subjectivity remains, and the individual self, with its time and space limitations, is replaced by the eternal Ātman.

While only few people actually reach samādhi, nevertheless the constant practice of meditation promotes mental health and well-being through the progressive liberation of the individual from the citta vrtti, the emotional ties and fluctuations which bind humans to the ups and downs of life, making them conditioned by external events and past experiences. The ideal developmental pathway traced by all Indian psychological systems—regardless of their specificities and metaphysical backgrounds—leads to freedom from change and becoming, from the relativity and precariousness of daily experiences, from the attachment to goals and memories which are grounded in this relativity, and which therefore prevent individuals from developing higher psychological faculties and from attaining ānanda, blissful happiness.

From the perspective of Flow Theory, which is grounded in Western culture and scientific psychology, concentration can be triggered by any kind of daily activity, provided that it is sufficiently challenging to capture individual's attention and to foster mobilization of personal skills. This assumption, which was supported by empirical findings, locates optimal experience within the mind fluctuation process—citta vrtti—taking place in the Manomayakosha, as one of the various mental states potentially arising from the interaction between the individual psychological system and external or inner objects.

The universality and relevance of flow to individual functioning was also supported through cross-cultural findings, primarily focusing on the structure of the activities that promote optimal experience, and on the development they foster through goal-setting and skill enhancement, thus providing individuals with practical orientation and purposes in life. Moreover, optimal experience does not automatically bring about well-being and development. Its outcomes vary according to the features of the associated activities and their role within the value system of the individuals and of their social environment (Delle Fave, 2009; Chapters 7 and 15).

Therefore, a key difference lies between the two conditions. The experience of meditation preludes to the attainment of more complex and universal states of consciousness, helping the person transcend the space, time, individual and cultural boundaries. Flow experience, on the opposite, is considered the most complex and rewarding state individuals can achieve during daily life, and it allows the person to build competencies within culturally meaningful domains. From the psychological point of view, mediation is a way, flow is an aim. From the cultural point of view, meditation helps individuals attain a detached, stable, and equanimous attitude toward the mutable world of events and interactions. This, however, does not mean to become passive and disengaged from daily duties and commitments, rather to approach them all with balance and wisdom. Flow—when associated with socially sanctioned activities—helps people taking active and enthusiastic part in their cultural context. The dimension of detachment and balance cultivation is not part of the picture, as it is expected due to the different historical and cultural background of the two concepts.

Incidentally, the detached attitude toward action expressed in Karma Yoga could apparently seem analogous to intrinsic motivation in flow. However, there is a core difference between the two conditions: niskāma karma is the result of an intentional detachment effort; intrinsic motivation is an emerging feature of optimal experience related to the rewarding interplay between challenges and skills.

6.3.2 The Neurophysiological Perspective

Throughout the last three decades, researchers have attempted to detect the neurophysiological underpinnings of meditation, especially after empirical findings showed that its practice can reduce anxiety, pain, and stress-related symptoms (Ivanovski & Malhi, 2007; Murphy, Donovan, & Taylor, 1999). The attempt is quite demanding, since the wide variety of meditation techniques that have been increasingly integrated into medical and psychotherapeutic treatments (Andresen, 2000; Baer, 2003) can generate different outcomes in the brain functions. As previously outlined, authors usually distinguish between the two broad categories of concentrative meditation (which requires the narrowing of attention on one single object) and mindfulness meditation (which aims at enhancing non-judgmental awareness of sensory and mental events). Since treatment programs often use a mixture of techniques derived from both approaches, it is very difficult to disentangle the effect of one or the other aspects of the practice. Telles and Naveen (2004) detected changes in auditory evoked potentials. Lutz et al. (2004) described a generalized increase of synchronization of gamma waves among experienced meditators. Davidson et al. (2003) detected significant activation increases in the left-side anterior regions, associated with reduced anxiety and enhanced positive affect among participants practicing mindfulness meditation. However, as clearly highlighted by Kristeller and Rikhye (2008), most studies are based on evidence from small samples, and investigate specific meditative practices, that can deeply differ from each other, providing opposite findings. For example, Yoga Nidra (which is based on imagery and withdrawal from action) promotes deep relaxation and a decreased activation, while mindfulness meditation leads to an activation increase.

As thoroughly reported in Chapter 3, the neurophysiological investigation of flow is still in its infancy. Dietrich (2004) hypothesized a state of transient hypofrontality, which suppresses the explicit conscious analytical functions, except for executive attention which enables the one-pointedness of mind. More recently, Weber et al. (2009) suggested that flow can be related to the synchronization of brain waves oscillations and an increase of prefrontal activation, which allows for effortless and effective information processing, also involving pleasure and reward circuits. Nevertheless, like in studies on meditation, neurophysiological findings on flow have been obtained on small samples of participants, mainly performing mental tasks. Due to the wide variety of activities associated with optimal experience, we can easily hypothesize that brain patterns of activation vary according to the specific task performed. Therefore, apparent contradictions in findings should not be surprising.

Such a scattered evidence does not allow us to draw any conclusion about similarities and differences in the biological correlates of flow and meditation states. However, it rises a caveat: any future study on the neurophysiological processes involved in the two conditions has to take into account the typology of associated practice or activity, making generalizations not only problematic, but also potentially misleading.

6.3.3 The Phenomenological Perspective

From the phenomenological point of view, meditative experience and flow involve different onset mechanisms, and are characterized by different cognitive, emotional, and motivational features.

As concerns the *factors promoting the onset* of the experience, most meditation techniques require specific postures (āsanas) and a silent and quiet environment. The body should be kept in a comfortable position, and concentration is pursued with conscious effort and active removal of distracting thoughts. Attention is focused on a single and often very simple stimulus—be it the flame of a candle, the forehead center between the eyebrows, the breathing movements, the steps during a walk, an inner visual representation. All these conditions and actions are not integral part of the usual daily activities, unless one intentionally decides to daily practice them.

In the case of flow, no presumptive specificity of the environmental setting can be defined, since any activity—and the same activity in different settings—can foster the onset of this experience. However, the task should be characterized by some peculiar features: it should be complex, highly structured, and challenging enough to promote active engagement and the mobilization of individual skills toward a well-defined objective. When all these prerequisites are present, Flow arises spontaneously though unpredictably, without effort and intentionality. Usually, people "find themselves" in flow, they do not consciously pursue it, although they recognize its positive features and implications.

As concerns *cognitive aspects*, the practice of meditation implies in the first stage the active focus of attention on one single object or thought, and the removal of any other content and thought from the mind. This process generally requires intentional effort, since attention spontaneously and impulsively moves toward other external objects or thoughts (Kuppuswami, 1985). In the second stage the information processing stops. The mind is still and silent, it ignores the stimuli that ceaselessly arise outside and inside, and it observes without any judgment or emotional attachment the target object or thought. External behavior is absent; the body is usually motionless and completely relaxed. Finally, in the last stage self-consciousness is lost and the person's identification with the individual ego (*ahamkhāra*) disappears. The role of control is prominent during the first two stages, but its function is to maintain the attention focused. On the contrary, no control can be exerted on the situation: the practice of meditation implies a merging of the consciousness into a higher dimension in which the only possible attitude of the individual is surrendering, and not controlling. "Until the mind is perfectly naked, it has no entry into the Bliss of Truth" (Swami Chinmayananda, 1975, p. 424).

On the contrary, flow experience is characterized by an efficient and constant processing of information (as described in Chapter 3) in response to a perceived challenge arising from the environment or from the internal contents of consciousness. Concentration flows steadily and effortlessly, and attention is focused of the task at hand; behavior coherently follows this processing, continuously adjusting to the changing requirements of the task through the active control of the situation and the mobilization of the person's mental and physical skills and abilities. This is true of any activity: playing tennis, solving a mathematical equation, writing a work report, playing a musical instrument, or interacting with one's own children. The mind and the body jointly and appropriately respond to the task demands, and the merging of action and awareness arises from this harmonious flux of thought and behavior. Of course, according to the nature of the activity the interplay between body and mind can change. As highlighted by Hunter and Csikszentmihalyi (2000) during sports and physical activities the mind works in the background to support the body action, while the opposite is true of primarily mental tasks. Like in the Gestalt phenomenon of reversible figures, the background and the figure become alternatively mind or body, according to the required task.

Bhagavad Gitā and Yoga Sūtras describe constant training and non-attachment as the two key methods to develop concentration of attention. In other terms, this kind of concentration depends on habit formation, and it can be cultivated only through detachment from passions and desires (Kuppuswami, 1985). It therefore develops differently from the focused attention characterizing flow experience, which is basically triggered by the attraction of the mind toward a challenging, interesting, and appealing activity. Vyasa, who compiled one of the most famous commentaries of the Yoga Sūtras, specified that in daily life we can concentrate for some time on one object, making the mind steady and temporarily absorbed in the task at hand (Rao & Paranjpe, 2008). Similarly, very strong emotions and passions promote pin-pointed attention. However, the aim of meditation is to achieve a continuous one-pointedness of attention, regardless of activity features or external conditions.

As concerns *emotions*, a deep feeling of bliss is associated with meditative states. However, the prominent feelings are calmness, stillness, and evenness of mind. Excitement or elation is not compatible with this condition, in which steadiness and stability predominate on any kind of peak perception.

Emotions do not necessarily play a prominent role in flow as well. In Chapter 5 we highlighted that feelings of excitement, enjoyment and pleasure may arise during optimal experience, but they do not basically characterize it. Positive emotions are rather related to the features of the ongoing task: relational and recreational activities are associated with intense positive feelings, while in intellectual and highly complex psychophysical task participants report average levels of emotional variables (see also Chapter 7).

As concerns *motivation*, analogies and divergences can be detected between the experience of meditation and flow experience at three different levels. The first level refers to the immediate desirability of the associated activity (the wish to do it here and now). The second level refers to the goals a person pursues in doing the associated activity, and at this level we can further distinguish between short-term goals—results and outcomes of the activity—and long term goals—general life accomplishments related to the activity. The third level refers to the potential of the experience itself as a motivational engine to promote the cultivation of the associated activities.

Indian writings on meditation, in particular Patanjali's Yoga-Sūtras, clearly stress the need of persevering in meditation practice through discipline. The Bhagavad Gita provides details on the related difficulties, such as laziness, failure to control the wandering mind, attraction toward more appealing tasks (Chapter 12; Radhakrishnan, 1960). The activity of meditation is not considered immediately desirable per se, but it represents a powerful instrument to pursue a chief long-term goal, namely to build up "a free individual who takes into account the limitations engendered by the bodily needs, the sense stimuli and the limited social norms and becomes more universalistic in his outlook [....]. The individual becomes creative in the real sense of the term and not a mere creature of needs, habits, and social norms" (Kuppuswami, 1985, p. 219).

The short-term goals embedded in the practice of meditation, as reported above, are very clearly specified for each of the three stages: dhāranā, dhyāna, and niruddha. Finally, as concerns the motivational power of the experience of meditation per se, "the sum total of pleasures of the whole world is nothing when compared to the bliss derived through concentration and meditation" (Swami Sivananda, 1986, p. 43).

Both immediate activity desirability and the perception of goals are simultaneously at work in shaping Flow experience. However, during a specific optimal activity these dimensions do not necessarily show a joint fluctuation in perceived values: this is related to the meaning people attribute to the activity.

As concerns desirability, for example, it is important to distinguish between mandatory and freely chosen tasks. School and work activities, with their valence of duty and imposition, are perceived as generally undesirable, even when they are associated with flow experience. This finding has been detected through retrospective questionnaires, as well as through experience sampling procedures: while experiencing flow in studying or work, participants report average values of the wish to do the activity (Delle Fave & Massimini, 2005; Shernoff & Csikszentmihalyi, 2009; Chapters 8 and 11). Conversely, freely chosen activities such as hobbies, amateur sports, and interactions with friends are usually perceived as highly desirable per se, and their desirability hits significantly above average values during optimal experience.

The perception of long-term goals in flow experience is prominently related to the perceived meaning and relevance of the ongoing activity for the individual's life projects (Steger, Frazier, Oishi, & Kaler, 2006). Study and work, though less desirable than leisure, are associated with a significantly higher perception of life goals, compared with recreational activities (Delle Fave & Bassi, 2003; Delle Fave, 2009; Chapter 9). The perception of short-term goals is instead related to the immediate outcome of the optimal activity: performing a surgery operation, expressing one's creativity in arts, solving a mathematical problem, reaching the peak of a mountain, discovering the end of the story while watching a movie or reading a book. It therefore does not substantially vary across activities. Rather, pursuing specific goals while performing an activity is actually an essential component of optimal experience, as first described by Csikszentmihalyi (1975/2000) and subsequently confirmed by most studies. It guides the flow of action and awareness toward an outcome.

Finally, flow experience is usually characterized by intrinsic motivation. People report to perform the ongoing activity by virtue of the enjoyment derived from it, free from concerns about success and social recognition. The proximal goals of the activity, even though crucial components of flow, can play the double role of directing attention, and of supporting the unfolding of the experience (Nakamura & Csikszentmihalyi, 2009). The positive features of this peculiar and complex state of consciousness promote the active investment of time and effort in the practice and cultivation of the associated activities. This progressively leads to an increase in skills and competencies, and to the search for higher challenges in order to support the engagement, concentration, and involvement that characterize optimal experience in the long run.

Given this premises, both meditation and flow activities can be practiced regardless of their overall perceived desirability, which may increase during the activity by virtue of the associated positive experience. However, optimal experience can also arise during activities—such as autonomously chosen leisure or interactions with beloved ones—which are intrinsically desirable, do not require regular practice, and can be performed according to the person's wish.

As concerns goals, short-term ones are an intrinsic component of both meditation and flow activities, since they play the role of orienting behavior and supporting concentration on the task. Long-term goals instead radically differ in meditation practice and in optimal activities. The former aims at the person's attainment of a stable condition of evenness and serene detachment from worldly passions. The latter promote the refinement of skills in specific domains and the orientation of psychological selection along defined developmental pathways.

As concerns the motivational power of the experience per se, the intrinsic reward due to the positive psychological features of both flow and meditation states supports their replication through the cultivation of associated activities.

6.4 Meditation, Flow, and Human Development

At the end of this brief and tentative excursus, we can ask ourselves: Is there any relationship between meditation states, as described in the Indian writings, and the experience of flow? Or better, can we detect a connection between the two conditions, within the developmental pathway of human beings?

Flow and meditation are rooted into two different cultural traditions, which define and describe psychological functioning, mind activities, and the pursuit of well-being through different conceptualization and from different perspectives. Flow is grounded in the Western individualistic and pragmatic tradition. Meditation was developed in the collectivistic and spiritual tradition of Asian cultures. Consistently with their cultural specificity, these two states have been attributed different roles in the pathway of human development.

As repeatedly outlined throughout this book, the onset of optimal experience is related to the perception of engaging challenges to be faced with adequate personal skills. This implies a dynamic process of change with time: the active investment of time and effort in the practice and cultivation of optimal activities progressively leads to an increase in skills and competencies, and to the search for higher challenges in order to support the engagement, concentration, and involvement that characterize optimal experience. This process gives rise to a virtuous cycle fostering the ceaseless acquisition of increasingly complex information and the refinement of related competencies. Thus, optimal experience can be considered the "psychic compass" supporting the developmental trajectory each individual autonomously builds and follows throughout life (Massimini & Delle Fave, 2000). In time, the preferential cultivation of optimal activities promotes individual differentiation and growing complexity (i.e., internal order and integration). Given the interdependence of individuals and culture, the growth of complexity involves constructive information exchange with the environment. This process supports development, that is the harmonization of individual life theme with environmental opportunities for action. By pursuing optimal experiences, individuals can creatively devote themselves to the cultivation of specific activities, discovering innovative goals, and thus spreading new information. With the support of optimal experience, the human ability to create and to select opportunities for action that enhances psychic complexity can be considered the basis of cultural change (Smith, Christopher, Delle Fave, & Bhawuk, 2002; Chapter 3).

Within the Indian tradition, the constant practice of meditation is a key instrument to overcome the narrow mind-related self-definitions and the attachment to sensory objects, thus attaining identification with the pure consciousness. This is the chief aim of the spiritual wisdom tradition of India. The Baghavad Gitā conveys a clear message concerning this topic: the achievement of goals and the fulfillment of desires provide joy and elation; however, it also gives rise to the need for obtaining more, or to achieve higher goals in the same domains. Bhawuk (2008) proposed an interesting model to explain this uninterrupted chain of striving, enjoying, and striving again, showing that desire is the center of human emotions, cognitions, and behavior.

Regardless of the chosen pathway, from the Indian perspective the highest stage in human evolution is the dis-identification from the individual self, and from the false identity created by the attachment to worldly objects. This can be pursued through the constant practice of meditation, through devotion and religious practice, as well as through Karma Yoga, the selfless commitment to right action and behavior. From the Western perspective instead, productivity and tangible outcomes of one's own individual actions are prominently valued, even at the spiritual and religious levels of the Judaic–Christian tradition. Well-being is defined as optimal *functioning*, and it is contextualized within the web of daily interactions, activities, and social roles. In the original description provided by Rogers, optimal functioning entails qualities such awareness of one's strengths and weaknesses, perception of purpose and meaning in life, openness to change, and trust in relationships and cooperation (Rogers, 1963), which are based on the evaluation of psychological qualities and features belonging to the realm of mind, to the manomayakosha. More recently, the pursuit of goals and purposes has been identified as one of the key components of psychological well-being (Ryff & Singer, 1996).

A crucial divergence therefore can be outlined between the ultimate aim of flow and the ultimate aim of meditation. Flow experience fosters development through the activation of a chain of desires—though, in most cases, a virtuous one: search for higher challenges, skill refinement, setting of increasingly complex goals, and so on. This process surely promotes development, and when involving meaningful and socially accepted activities, it also allows the person to actively contribute to the well-being of the other members of society. However, it confines this developmental process within the realm of the world objects. Meditation, as well as the practice of niskāma karma, frees the person from the boundaries of such world realm, projecting the individual consciousness toward transcendence.

This clearly highlights that flow and meditation refer to different levels of psychological analysis, and that the cultural representation of these two states affects the meaning attributed to them and their applications in intervention. In Asian tradition, as per our knowledge, despite the extremely articulated explorations of psychological functions, flow is not described as a peculiar experience per se. Considering its features of deep concentration and absorption, it could be interpreted as one of the spontaneous experiences of integration and complexity that arises during daily life, providing the individual with an unintentional and transient glimpse into higher-order levels of consciousness and identity (Kiran Kumar, 2006). In the West, meditation practice is mainly used for its practical outcomes. It is a powerful tool to enhance concentration abilities and attain better performances in the training of sport and music professionals. It has found useful applications in medicine and psychotherapy to help people manage stress, anxiety, and physical pain. However, its connection with high-order levels of consciousness is basically overlooked.

These considerations highlight the difficulty to appropriately understand and use concepts derived from other cultural traditions. But they also suggest the added value of integrating the complementary contribution of different cultures to the common pursuit of human development. Through the identification and operationalization of flow, Western scholars have shed light on the virtuous mechanisms of daily life experience fluctuation. Through the analysis of consciousness dimensions that transcend daily experience, Asian scholars have traced pathways toward a more complete understanding of human potential.

References

Andresen, J. (2000). Meditation meets behavioural medicine. The story of experimental research on meditation. *Journal of Consciousness Studies*, *7*, 17–74.

Baer, R. A. (2003). Mindfulness training as a clinical intervention: A conceptual and empirical review. *Clinical Psychology Science and Practice*, *10*, 125–143.

Bermant, G., Talwar, C., & Rozin, P. (in press). To celebrate positive psychology and extend its horizons. In K. Sheldon, T. Kashdan, & M. Steger (Eds.), *Integrated psychology: Linking positive psychology and the negative*. New York: Oxford University Press.

Bhawuk, D. P. S. (2008). Anchoring cognition, emotion and behavior in desire: a model from the Bhagavad Gitā. In K. R. Rao, A. C. Paranjpe, & A. K. Dalal (Eds.), *Handbook of Indian psychology* (pp. 390–413). New Delhi: Cambridge University Press India.

Chinmayananda, S. (1975). *The holy Geeta. A commentary*. Bombay: Central Chinmaya Mission Trust.

Chinmayananda, S. (1992). *Discourses on the taittiriya Upanishad*. Bombay: Central Chinmaya Mission Trust.

Csikszentmihalyi, M. (1975/2000). *Beyond boredom and anxiety*. San Francisco: Jossey Bass.

Davidson, R. J., Kabat-Zinn, J., Schumacher, J., Rosenkranz, M., Muller, D., Santorelli, S. F., et al. (2003). Alterations in brain and immune function produced by mindfulness meditation. *Psychosomatic Medicine*, *65*, 564–570.

Delle Fave, A. (2007). Individual development and community empowerment: Suggestions from studies on optimal experience. In J. Haworth & G. Hart (Eds.), *Well-being: Individual, community, and societal perspectives* (pp. 41–56). London: Palgrave McMillan.
Delle Fave, A. (2009). Optimal experience and meaning: Which relationship? *Psychological Topics, Special issue on positive psychology, 18*, 285–302.
Delle Fave, A., & Bassi, M. (2003). Adolescents' use of free time in Italy: The role of engagement and optimal experience. In S. Verma, R. W. Larson (Eds.), *Examining adolescent leisure time across cultures: Developmental opportunities and risks. New directions for child and adolescent development series* (pp. 79–93). San Francisco: Jossey Bass.
Delle Fave, A., & Massimini, F. (2005). The investigation of optimal experience and apathy: Developmental and psychosocial implications. *European Psychologist, 10*, 264–274.
Dietrich, A. (2004). Neurocognitive mechanisms underlying the experience of flow. *Consciousness and Cognition, 13*, 746–761.
Feuerstein, G. (1998). *The yoga-sutra of Patanjali. A new translation and commentary*. Rochester, VT: Inner Traditions International.
Goleman, D. (1988). *The meditative mind: The varieties of meditative experience*. New York: Tarcher/Perigee Books.
Hunter, J., & Csikszentmihalyi, M. (2000). The phenomenology of body-mind: The contrasting cases of flow in sports and contemplation. *Anthropology of Consciousness, 11*, 5–24.
Ivanovski, B., & Malhi, G. S. (2007). The psychological and neurophysiological concomitants of mindfulness forms of meditation. *Acta Neurppsychiatrica, 19*, 76–91.
Kiran Kumar, S. K. (2003). An Indian conception of well-being. In J. Henry (Ed.), *Proceedings of European positive psychology conference* (pp. 72–79). Leicester: British Psychological Society.
Kiran Kumar, S. K. (2006). The role of spirituality in attaining well-being: Approach of Sanātana dharma. In A. Delle Fave (Ed.), *Dimensions of well-being* (pp. 538–551). Milano: Franco Angeli.
Kristeller, J. L., & Rikhye, K. (2008). Meditative traditions and contemporary psychology. In K. R. Rao, A. C. Paranjpe, & A. K. Dalal (Eds.), *Handbook of Indian psychology* (pp. 506–538). New Delhi: Cambridge University Press India.
Kuppuswami, B. (1977). *Dharma and society*. New Delhi: McMillan.
Kuppuswami, B. (1985). *Elements of ancient Indian psychology*. Delhi: Konark Publishers.
Lutz, A., Greischar, L. L., Rawlings, B., Ricard, M., & Davidson, R. J. (2004). Long-tem meditators self-induce high amplitude gamma synchrony during mental practice. *Proceedings of the National Academy of Sciences, 10*, 16369–16373.
Massimini, F., & Delle Fave, A. (2000). Individual development in a bio-cultural perspective. *American Psychologist, 55*, 24–33.
Murphy, M., Donovan, S., & Taylor, E. (1999). *The physical and psychological effects of meditation: A review of contemporary research with a comprehensive bibliography, 1981–1996*. Sausalito, CA: Institute of Noetic Science.
Nakamura, J., & Csikszentmihalyi, M. (2009). Flow theory and research. In S. J. Lopez & C. R. Snyder (Eds.), *Handbook of positive psychology* (pp. 195–206). New York: Oxford University Press.
Pande, N., & Naidu, R. K. (1992). Anāsakti and health: A study on non-attachment. *Psychology and Developing Societies, 4*, 89–104.
Prabhavananda, S. (1977). *Spiritual heritage of India*. Madras: Sri Ramakrishna Math.
Radhakrishnan, S. (1960). *Bhagavad Gitā*. London: Allen & Unwin.
Rao, K. R. (2008). Prologue: Introducing Indian psychology. In K. R. Rao, A. C. Paranjpe, & A. K. Dalal (Eds.), *Handbook of Indian psychology* (pp. 1–18). New Delhi: Cambridge University Press India.
Rao, K. R., & Paranjpe, A. C. (2008). Yoga psychology: Theory and application. In K. R. Rao, A. C. Paranjpe, & A. K. Dalal (Eds.), *Handbook of Indian psychology* (pp. 186–216). New Delhi: Cambridge University Press India.

Rogers, C. (1963). The actualizing tendency in relation to "motives" and to consciousness. In M. R. Jones (Ed.), *Nebraska symposium on motivation, 11* (pp. 1–24). Lincoln: University of Nebraska Press.
Ryff, C. D., & Singer, B. (1996). Psychological well-being: Meaning, measurement, and implications for psychotherapy research. *Psychotherapy and Psychosomatics*, *65*, 14–23.
Shernoff, D., & Csikszentmihalyi, M. (2009). Flow in schools. Cultivating engaged learners and optimal learning environments. In R. Gilman, E. Huebner, & M. Furlong (Eds.), *Handbook of positive psychology in schools* (pp. 131–145). New York: Taylor & Francis.
Sinha, J. (1958). *India psychology—cognition* (Vol. 1). Calcutta: Sinha Publishing House.
Sivananda, S. (1986). *Concentration and meditation*. Rishikesh: Yoga-Vedanta Forest Academy Press.
Smith, K. D., Christopher, J. C., Delle Fave, A., & Bhawuk, D. P. S. (2002). Post-Newtonian metatheories in the natural sciences and in cross-cultural psychology. In P. Boski, F. J. R. van de Vijver, & A. M. Chodynicka (Eds.), *New directions in cross-cultural psychology* (pp. 107–125). Warsaw: Wydawnictwo Intytutu Psychologii PAN.
Steger, M. F., Frazier, P., Oishi, S., & Kaler, M. (2006). The meaning of life questionnaire: Assessing the presence of and search for meaning in life. *Journal of Counseling Psychology*, *53*, 80–93.
Telles, S., & Naveen, K. V. (2004). Changes in middle latency auditory evoked potentials during meditation. *Psychological Reports*, *94*, 398–400.
Weber, R., Tamborini, R., Westcott-Baker, A., & Kantor, B. (2009). Theorizing flow and media enjoyment as cognitive synchronization of attentional and reward networks. *Communication Theory*, *19*, 397–422.

Part II
Applications

Chapter 7
Optimal Experience Across Cultures

7.1 Psychology and Cultures

The foundations of psychology as a quantitative and experimental discipline were set in Europe and in the United States during the second half of the nineteenth century. Theories and inquiry instruments were built according to western behavior, standards, and world outlooks. Scholars aimed at analyzing and understanding human psychological traits—which were considered universal features—by examining small and selected samples of European and North American subjects, be they children, young people or elderly, males or females. The results gathered on cognitive functions, learning patterns, developmental rates - and phases were taken as standard findings for cross-cultural investigations. In other words, tests and theories originating in the western countries were applied tout court to other cultural contexts. A large percentage of non-western individuals showed poor performances in psychological tasks or in providing the answers to the questionnaires. Thus, the leading role of a civilized west, made of intellectually developed individuals, could be scientifically supported. The white men had to accomplish the mission of spreading knowledge, inspiring the rest of the world populations with their models of individual behavior, social relations, and institutions.

During the second half of the previous century several efforts were made to unveil the biases embedded in the theoretical and evaluation instruments of psychological research. This awareness, which however is far from being common to all psychologists even today, stems from cultural studies. The work of social scientists, and in particular of anthropologists (Romney & D'Andrade, 1964), highlighted the prominent role of culture in influencing the psychological development of individuals. The features of the biocultural environment—in terms of survival strategies, ecological requirements, social structure, opportunities for learning—can support or hamper the growth of specific abilities and cognitive functions in the individual. Thus, each psychological study cannot overlook the cultural background subjects have been raised in during childhood and are exposed to during adulthood.

The use of western standards and theories for the investigation of human behavior has been labeled as the etic approach (Berry, 1969). It is assumed that any circumscribed observation concerning human behavior can be automatically generalized to

A. Delle Fave et al., *Psychological Selection and Optimal Experience Across Cultures*, Cross-Cultural Advancements in Positive Psychology 2,
DOI 10.1007/978-90-481-9876-4_7, © Springer Science+Business Media B.V. 2011

all members of the species, regardless their cultural roots. This lack of concern for cultural differences led to serious distortion of psychological data, with even more serious consequences in terms of ethnic discrimination. Just to give few, very famous examples, the use of western-based intelligence scales with African-American participants still recently supported all kinds of racist interpretations (Herrnstein & Murray, 1994). This contributed to heavily impairing the chances of integration of minority citizens in the western social, educational, and cultural systems. The attribution of low performance in intelligence tests to genetic inheritance has consequences that only "mislead about race" (Block, 1995), if we do not take into account the effects of the environment on the development of individual abilities.

The same bias was found in the comparative evaluation of cognitive development in children. The Binet–Simon scale, developed at the beginning of last century to assess children's intelligence, deeply oriented the study of human psychological development, regardless of the cultural and family background the children were raised in. Problems soon arose, when the rate of cognitive abilities was to be evaluated in cultures where children were not exposed to western formal education. Some scholars claimed, "intelligence tests are about academic learning because this is the primary criterion that establishes the validity of the tests for children and adolescents" (Ackerman, 1996, p. 228). The same kind of bias can be ascribed to the Piagetian theory and its related research tools, which had a tremendous impact on the progress of developmental studies, on one side, being however ethno-centered, on the other side (Gardner, 1982).

Similarly, for decades psychoanalytic approaches were used worldwide to interpret human behavior in the most diverse realms, such as literary critique, individual development, and creativity. Again, an ethnocentric perspective applied a western-based notion of primary relationships, values, and pathology to the rest of the world. The problem was even more remarkable in the case of psychoanalytical psychotherapy, which was often employed in non-western countries. Cultural differences have been often overlooked in this approach to counseling. In most Asian and African societies family relations, sexuality, and personality development are rooted in a set of cultural customs and beliefs often opposite to the western ones. This has created great difficulties and misunderstandings at the therapeutic level, either producing patients' psychosocial maladjustment, or their refusal of the therapeutic approach. As a matter of fact, any psychotherapeutic intervention has to be aimed at supporting the integration of the patient in his/her cultural system, thus respecting the features of social relations and individual identity accepted in the social context (Laungani, 1992; Marsella & Pedersen, 1981).

During the last 40 years, the development of cross-cultural psychology has been a great advancement in dealing with these issues. A growing number of scholars have started to pay attention to the role of culture in affecting individual behavior and psychological functions. Systematic research studies have been conducted at the cross-cultural level on the most various topics, from human development to cognition, and social as well as clinical psychology. In the same period biocultural theories were developed, in the attempt to detect the mechanisms underlying the evolution and changes of cultures in time (see Chapter 2). Super and Harkness

(1986) formalized the concept of developmental niche, as the set of biocultural factors (genetic traits, rearing practices, parental roles, educational patterns) which contribute to child development.

Psychologists have shown growing awareness about the role of culture in shaping human beings. The process of enculturation (Herskovitz, 1948), defined as the acquisition of behavioral rules that allow individuals to become integrated members of their social community, has been highlighted as one of the basic features of human development. As reported in Chapter 2, cultural differences in value systems involve the weight and the meaning attributed to collective norms, daily activities, and social roles (Triandis, 1994). Specific activities or behaviors do not necessarily have the same meaning or function in different cultures.

The mainstream approach in cross-cultural research is centered on a basic concept: The detection of psychological differences related to cultural traits can help discovering the universal common features of human beings. This is the so-called universalistic, or derived etic perspective: It assumes that all members of our species, however deeply influenced by their cultural heritage, share common psychological mechanisms and features, which the study of differences could highlight. Standardized research tools and quantitative assessments, originally developed in one culture, can be adequately modified to be employed in other cultures. The evaluation of the differences in the results takes into account the cultural background of the participants.

However, this approach is not accepted by all scholars. A large number of researchers maintain that the cultural influence is so pervasive on humans that the most correct perspective in interpreting individual behavior should give primacy to the specific values and rules of the original culture. This perspective is endorsed by cultural psychology, whose approach has been labeled as emic: Any evaluation in psychology should refer to standards and expectations typical of the particular culture. Cross-cultural comparisons based on quantitative investigations and on experimental tools have a limited relevance. The relations between individual behavior and cultural instructions can be better understood within the specific cultural system, and qualitative analyses are thus more suited to get significant results (Cohen & Kitayama, 2007; Stigler, Shweder, & Herdt, 1990).

An even more radical emic perspective characterizes the more recently emerging field of indigenous psychologies (Kim & Berry, 1993). Researchers in this field are concerned with the study of traditional interpretations of human behavior, which most cultures all over the world have developed throughout the centuries and sometimes the millennia. The history of each society is characterized by a set of values, beliefs, and practices related to mental health, psychological functioning, individual behavior. The complex structure of Indian philosophical and religious system is based on precise assumptions about the components and mechanisms of human mind (see also Chapter 6). The healing ceremonies of Native Americans stem from a unique interpretation of the interplay between individual psychic functioning and environment. Each culture has a codified and exhaustive set of instructions concerning psychological and behavioral issues. Starting from this observation, a global psychological characterization of individuals can be drawn, which can even contradict the assumptions of western studies, giving rise to alternative visions of mankind and human behavior. In order to solve the twofold problem of scientific ethnocentrism and cross-cultural equivalence, Yang (2000) has proposed a "cross-cultural indigenous approach" (CCI), moving from qualitative mono-cultural studies as a basis to envisage cross-culturally appropriate and focused research.

7.1.1 Cultural Dimensions of Psychological Processes

During the last few decades, cross-cultural studies and theories have repeatedly addressed the issue of defining two complex and multifaceted concepts such as individualism and collectivism, that turned to be very useful for understanding differences between cultures (Bond & Smith, 1996; Smith & Bond, 1999; Triandis, Chan, Bhawuk, Iwao, & Sinha, 1995). Broadly speaking, collectivistic cultures emphasize the prominence of social norms and rules in directing individual behavior. On the contrary, for individualistic cultures the person is the primary unit of the society; thus they foster their members' independence and autonomy (Eaton & Louw, 2000; Hofstede, 1980; Kagitçibasi, 1997; Kim, Triandis, Kagitçibasi, Choi, & Yoon, 1994). Individualistic societies emphasize personal initiative and resources in dealing with the environment, and the imperative of asserting individual control, freedom, and autonomy within all kinds of interpersonal relationships: family, work, society as a whole. In many respects, post-modernism is the result of this process. Collectivistic societies, on the contrary, give priority to social harmony: Individuals tend to modify their behavior to adjust to group and context features, rather than trying to change them (Diaz-Guerrero, 1979; Han, 2008; Leung, Fernandez-Dols, & Iwawaki, 1992; Morling, Kitayama, & Miyamoto, 2002; Weisz, Rothbaum, & Blackburn, 1984). Idiocentrism is more common in urban societies, as well as in multicultural and cosmopolitan contexts, characterized by a variety of behavioral norm systems available to individual choice (Hofstede, 1980).

Individualism and collectivism can be further distinguished according to the dimension of horizontality/verticality (Singelis, Triandis, Bhawuk, & Gelfand, 1995; Triandis et al., 1995). Vertical individualistic cultures (such as the United States) are characterized by greater inequalities than horizontal ones (for example, Australia). Analogously, vertical collectivistic societies are characterized by a deeply rooted class hierarchy (for example, India with its caste system) than horizontal ones (such as the kibbutz communities in Israel).

Related to the distinction between individualistic and collectivistic societies is the identification of two specific patterns of self-construal proposed by Markus and Kitayama (1991): the independent self-construal and the interdependent one. In collectivistic cultures individuals build their self-definition according to interpersonal and group dimensions: Goals are settled within the community; social behavior is grounded in shared norms; the quality of relationships and other people's needs are crucially important. In individualistic cultures people use subjective cues and dimensions to define themselves; goals are prominently personalized; individual attitudes and tendencies substantially influence social behavior and relationships.

Brewer and Gardner (1996) further distinguished between the relational and the collective dimension of interdependence, the former referring to interpersonal relations, while the latter to the relation between the self and significant in-groups (Gabriel & Gardner, 1999; Somech, 2000). More recently, the multidimensionality of this construct has been highlighted by Hardin and her colleagues (2004).

Parenting practices and socialization strategies promote the development of these culture-specific attitudes and behavioral patterns from early childhood (De Vos, 1985; Hsu, 1985; Shweder & Bourne, 1984). Investigating the impact of cultural values and socialization patterns on individual and group behavior is therefore an essential prerequisite to understand and contextualize cross-cultural differences in cognitive information processing, emotional repertoire, and motivational mechanisms. In particular, the development of an independent or interdependent self-identity deeply influences individual experience in its various components (Markus & Kitayama, 1991).

At the cognitive level, variation in cultural values may promote the development and adoption of different control strategies in the individual adaptation to the environment. Indirect and collective control strategies are predominant in societies focused on the preservation of interpersonal harmony through the avoidance of conflicts between individuals (Triandis, 1994; Yamaguchi, 2001). Collective control allows for the sharing of responsibility among individuals participating in the same task, thus maintaining harmony even in case of failure or negative outcomes (Latané & Darley, 1970). On the opposite, cultures valuing autonomy promote the adoption of a direct control strategy: Individuals act as main characters and are entitled to independently introduce changes in their environment. As concerns dissonance-related behaviors, concerns about personal competence and efficacy are primarily threatening in individualistic cultures, while in collectivistic societies individuals are primarily worried by possible rejection by others (Kitayama, Snibbe, Markus, & Suzuki, 2004). As a consequence, a person raised in a collectivistic context does not perceive cognitive dissonance in adjusting to others' behavior: Cognitive coherence in individual terms is a western construct that turns to be inadequate to understand human behavior in other cultural contexts (Fiske, Kitayama, Markus, & Nisbett, 1998).

Several studies comparing East Asian and European-American participants showed that the former (belonging to a collectivistic culture) prominently paid attention to contextual aspects in perceiving and describing objects and events (Hedden et al., 2002; Ji, Peng, & Nisbett, 2000; Masuda & Nisbett, 2001), and in memory recollection tasks (Han, Leichtman, & Wang, 1998), giving more emphasis to situational attributes than European-American participants, who focused their attention on object-specific features in perception and memory tasks, and to self-descriptions in remembering events. Similarly, people from collectivistic cultures tend to relate individual behavior to circumstances and contextual aspects more than to stable personal dispositions, thus endorsing change, contradiction, and nonlinear development of events as substantial aspects of reality and as explanatory aspects of behavior, through a holistic thinking pattern opposed to the prominently analytic one characterizing western cultures (Ji, Nisbett, & Su, 2001).

The importance attributed to personal feelings and motivations also varies across cultural systems; it is a product of the hierarchy of values that individuals develop during their life, according to ideal models and social values acquired through the learning process. This is the reason why self-serving and self-enhancement motivations are traditionally praised in western countries and less emphasized in collectivistic societies (Ho & Chan, 2009; Kitayama, Takagi, & Matsumoto, 1995). Such attitude led, for example, to the strong personalization of the artistic and scientific works in European history. On the contrary, in several Asian societies the names of painters, sculptors, architects, and scientists have never been recorded. Nevertheless, these individuals enriched human cultural heritage with their masterpieces and discoveries.

Finally, as discussed in Chapter 1, conceptualizations and psychological aspects of happiness and well-being have deep cultural roots (Diener, Oishi, & Lucas, 2004; Park, Peterson, & Seligman, 2006; Ryan & Deci, 2001; Uchida, Norasakkunkit, & Kitayama, 2004). Cultures shape individuals' well-being, not only providing a meaning-making system for daily events and interactions, but also fostering or limiting opportunities for growth and self-expression. As concerns optimal experience, our research group has collected a relevant amount of cross-cultural evidence on the features and developmental role of flow. In this chapter we will try to address some general issues, while the following chapters will be devoted to the analysis of the structural and contextual dimensions of optimal experience, and of its potential for intervention within specific domains.

7.2 Flow and Psychological Selection Across Cultures

The hypothesized universality and relevance of optimal experience to individual and cultural functioning needs to be supported by cross-cultural findings. Moreover, in order to understand the potential of optimal experience in fostering personal growth and culture empowerment, it is important to investigate the associated activities and their long-term role in the individuals' lives and at the cultural level. It cannot be assumed that all opportunities for optimal experience have the same consequences on the development of persons and communities.

In this chapter, we will generally address the above-mentioned issues by means of empirical evidence obtained from adult and adolescent participants belonging to different cultures, who completed flow questionnaire and life theme questionnaire (Delle Fave, 2007).

We will first merge results provided by 870 adult participants, 379 women and 491 men, aged 15–78 (average age 35). Among them, 354 (40.7% of the sample) belonged to non-western, prominently Asian cultures. They came from India (36 women and 16 men), Indonesia (32 women and 31 men), Iran (10 women and 17 men), West Africa (Ivory Coast and Ghana, 13 men), North Africa (Morocco and Tunisia, 3 women and 10 men), Philippines (11 women), Somalia (6 women and 6 men), and Thailand (20 women and 4 men). This group also comprised European and North American citizens who nevertheless were members of cultural minorities, preserving their original language, lifestyle, and values: This was true of Navajos living in Arizona and New Mexico (51 women and 28 men) and Rom Gypsies settled in Italy (32 women and 28 men). The western sample comprised 516 Italian participants (59.3% of the sample), living in urban and rural areas, and engaged in a variety of traditional and modern jobs. The job distribution was substantially similar in both groups: Each of them included farmers, craftsmen, shopkeepers, tailors, factory blue collar workers, housemaids, clerks, housewives, college students, production and sale managers, financial consultants, academicians, nurses, and teachers.

7.2.1 Optimal Activities Across Cultures

The majority of participants in the adult sample (736, 84.6% of the global sample) reported optimal experiences in their lives, and associated it with one or more activities. In previous studies, optimal activities were grouped into various functional categories (Csikszentmihalyi, 1997; Delle Fave & Massimini, 2004). For sake of clarity and synthesis, we will adopt a broader grouping criterion based on the identification of general life domains: productive activities, free time, interactions, and introspection. More in depth analyses will be performed within specific domains in other chapters of this volume.

Table 7.1 summarizes the domain distribution of optimal activities reported by the western and non-western participants. In both groups, each participant provided two activities on average. The same table also illustrates the distribution of the selected optimal activities: As described in Chapter 4, in the flow questionnaire each participant was invited to select from her list the activity associated with the most pervasive optimal experience.

The global domain distribution of optimal activities shows substantial similarities between groups: free time (sport, hobbies, reading, relaxed leisure, and the use of media) and productive activities (work and study) largely predominated. Interactions referred to parenting and spending time with family, as well as to socializing with friends. Introspection included thinking (about present, past, and future events), daydreaming, enjoying solitude, prayer, and meditation. A significant difference between western and non-western participants was detected

Table 7.1 Percentage distribution of optimal activities across cultures

	Optimal activities		Selected optimal activities	
Categories	Western	Non-western	Western	Non-western
Productive activities	37.3	37.0	40.4	42.6
Leisure	46.7	39.2	46.6	35.9
Interactions	11.0	13.1	10.3	10.7
Introspection	5.0	10.7	2.7	10.7
N answers	992	617	438	298

instead in the distribution of selected optimal activities ($\chi^2 = 24.0$, $p<0.0001$). The difference was mainly due to the lower percentage of non-western participants quoting free-time activities ($\chi^2 = 6.8$, $p<0.01$), and the higher percentage of participants selecting introspection in this same group ($\chi^2 = 10.5$, $p<0.01$). As concerns the activity distribution by gender, no difference emerged within each group.

A closer analysis of the selected optimal activities highlighted some peculiarities. In the productive domain, 227 participants quoted work, and 71 quoted study and learning activities. Volunteering health care activities were quoted by six participants, and were also included in this domain. Work prominently comprised traditional activities such as farming, housework, and handicrafts, which were indicated by 167 participants (73.6% of those who selected work as pervasive optimal activity). This category also included 13 participants who quoted teaching and nursing. Modern office and factory work were instead selected by 60 participants. Considering that 368 of the participants (42.3%) worked in offices and factories, this finding is quite interesting, though not surprising. As repeatedly shown in several studies, in order to be associated with optimal experience an activity should provide opportunities for creativity, autonomy, and skill development, either embedded in the task structure itself, or related to peculiarly engaging situations (e.g., "when I have to deal with something new;" "when the work requires concentration;" "when there is a problem to solve;" "in the project phase"). In the following section and in Chapter 8 we will more systematically address the theoretical issues and findings concerning the relationship between flow and work. Here we only anticipate that—considering the distinctive features of optimal experience reported in Chapter 3—the lower task automation and the higher workers' autonomy characterizing traditional professions seems to enhance the chances for attaining optimal experience while performing them.

Analogously, among the 309 participants who selected free-time activities as opportunities for the most pervasive optimal experiences, over half (167, 54%) quoted structured leisure (Kleiber, Larson, & Csikszentmihalyi, 1986), namely tasks characterized by well-defined rules and contents, requiring specific competencies and skill cultivation. These activities included sports and physical exercise (selected by 88 participants) and arts, hobbies, and games (79 participants). Reading books and journals was selected by 89 participants. Unstructured leisure was indicated by 33 participants: It comprised relaxing activities such as resting, lying on the beach, enjoying holidays, going for a stroll, and listening to music. Finally, 20 participants selected watching TV.

A limited number of participants (77, 10.5% of the total sample) identified interactions as opportunities for the most pervasive optimal experiences. They mostly referred to family and couple relationships (69% of the answers within the domain) and to a lesser extent to socialization with friends and significant others.

Introspection was quoted as prominent opportunity for flow by an even smaller percentage of participants (44, 6% of the total sample). As previously reported, this percentage mostly comprised non-western participants (72.7%). It referred to reflections on self and life, to plans and projects, memories and daydreaming; it also comprised prayer and meditation, quoted by Indonesian and Thai participants. A closer analysis of the relationship between religion and flow will be proposed in Chapter 12.

It is worth reporting that only two western participants quoted shopping and buying objects as opportunities for optimal experience, consistently with other studies (see, for example, Kasser & Ryan, 1996; Myers, 2000) highlighting that material goods and extrinsic rewards do not foster per se well-being and optimal states.

7.2.2 Optimal Experience Across Activities and Cultures

Table 7.2 shows the psychological features of optimal experience across domains, and in the two cultural groups. Optimal experience showed a recurrent structure across activity categories. In almost all domains, variables scored above 6, confirming theoretical assumptions and previous empirical evidence. The only exception was detected in the values of unselfconsciousness. In the studies with ESM and flow questionnaire conducted among western non-US participants, this variable showed wider fluctuations than expected from theoretical assumptions and evidence gathered among North American samples (Csikszentmihalyi, 1997; Csikszentmihalyi, Rathunde, & Whalen, 1993). Mixed results were obtained also in other single-administration questionnaires using multiple items (Hektner, Schmidt, & Csikszentmihalyi, 2007). As reported in Chapter 4, further investigation is required to better define the role and meaning of self-consciousness, since many participants did not consider self-monitoring as a negative aspect of the experience, especially during the performance of intellectual tasks (Delle Fave & Massimini, 2004). In these situations, perceiving moment-by-moment control on one's own action and behavior seems to support flow, instead of disturbing it (see also Chapters 6 and 12).

In spite of the recurrent structure of flow experience, a nonparametric ANOVA comparison detected significant differences across domains for most of the variable values: involvement ($F = 3.6$, $p < 0.05$), clear feedback ($F = 3.3$, $p < 0.05$), wish doing the activity ($F = 11.1$, $p < 0.0001$), excitement ($F = 7.5$, $p < 0.0001$), ease of concentration ($F = 5.0$, $p < 0.01$), unselfconsciousness ($F = 4.1$, $p < 0.01$), enjoyment ($F = 3.3$, $p < 0.05$), relaxation ($F = 7.3$, $p < 0.0001$), clear goals ($F = 3.0$, $p < 0.05$), control of the situation ($F = 3.4$, $p < 0.05$), and challenges ($F = 10.9$, $p < 0.0001$). The values of concentration and skills did not vary significantly across domains.

A post hoc Scheffe's test with significance detected for alpha being equal to 0.05 allowed for disentangling specific pairwise differences between domains. More specifically, productive activities and interactions shared significantly higher values of challenges compared with the two other domains. Interactions and leisure were associated with significantly higher values of wish to do the activity than productive activities and introspection. Relaxation and unselfconsciousness scored significantly higher in leisure than in productive activities, while the values of enjoyment and

Table 7.2 Optimal experience during selected optimal activities among western and non-western participants

Variables	Productive activities (W = 177, NW=127)		Leisure (W = 204, NW=107)		Interactions (W = 45, NW=32)		Introspection (W = 12, NW=32)	
	W *M* (*sd*)	NW *M* (*sd*)	W *M* (*sd*)	NW *M* (*sd*)	W *M* (*sd*)	NW *M* (*sd*)	W *M* (*sd*)	NW *M* (*sd*)
Involvement	6.5 (1.3)	7.2 (1.4)	6.8 (1.5)	6.9 (1.8)	7.4 (1.2)	7.4 (1.0)	7.2 (0.8)	6.7 (2.1)
Clear feedback	6.9 (1.2)	7.0 (1.7)	6.7 (1.8)	6.7 (1.8)	7.2 (1.5)	7.2 (1.0)	6.8 (1.5)	6.3 (2.4)
Intrinsic motivation	6.7 (1.7)	6.8 (2.0)	7.5 (1.2)	7.1 (1.8)	7.7 (0.8)	7.4 (1.2)	7.3 (2.3)	6.3 (2.4)
Excitement	7.2 (1.3)	7.5 (1.1)	7.7 (0.8)	7.8 (0.6)	7.8 (0.5)	7.7 (0.6)	7.6 (0.8)	7.4 (1.4)
Ease of concentration	5.7 (2.5)	6.1 (2.8)	6.2 (2.3)	6.6 (2.3)	6.9 (2.0)	6.8 (2.2)	4.8 (3.3)	5.8 (3.1)
Unselfconsciousness	4.7 (2.9)	5.2 (2.7)	5.5 (2.9)	6.2 (2.6)	4.3 (3.0)	7.1 (1.6)	3.9 (3.0)	5.1 (3.1)
Enjoyment	6.8 (1.6)	7.2 (1.7)	6.9 (1.5)	7.4 (1.2)	7.4 (1.1)	7.7 (0.6)	6.4 (1.5)	6.9 (1.5)
Concentration	6.3 (1.7)	6.8 (1.6)	6.2 (2.0)	6.9 (1.9)	6.9 (1.6)	7.0 (1.4)	6.6 (1.9)	6.1 (2.6)
Relaxation	5.9 (2.3)	6.2 (2.6)	6.8 (1.8)	6.8 (2.2)	6.5 (2.3)	6.6 (2.5)	7.1 (1.4)	5.6 (2.6)
Clear goals	7.1 (1.4)	7.3 (1.4)	6.7 (2.0)	7.2 (1.5)	6.7 (1.9)	7.4 (1.0)	7.0 (1.2)	6.4 (2.4)
Control of situation	6.5 (1.5)	7.2 (1.2)	6.6 (1.8)	7.3 (1.4)	6.8 (1.3)	7.2 (0.8)	5.9 (2.3)	6.0 (2.5)
Challenges	6.7 (1.2)	6.5 (2.0)	6.3 (1.8)	5.7 (2.6)	7.3 (0.8)	7.2 (0.9)	6.5 (1.6)	5.6 (2.5)
Skills	6.6 (1.4)	6.4 (1.7)	6.5 (1.6)	6.2 (1.9)	6.7 (1.1)	6.5 (1.8)	6.4 (1.2)	6.1 (2.1)

Note: W = N. of western participants; NW = N. of non-western participants.

ease of concentration were significantly higher in interactions than in productive activities. No relevant pairwise differences were detected for concentration, clear feedbacks, clear goals, and skills.

A GLM procedure was then used to investigate the relative contribution of culture and activity domain in determining variable differences. Adopting the Type 3 SS criterion, culture accounted for overall significant differences of involvement ($F = 16.1$, $p < 0.0001$), excitement ($F = 8.0$, $p < 0.01$), enjoyment ($F = 4.5$, $p < 0.05$), concentration ($F = 4.2$, $p < 0.05$), relaxation ($F = 4.1$, $p < 0.05$), and control of the situation ($F = 14.1$, $p < 0.001$) with non-western participants scoring higher than western ones for all these variables.

Comparisons between the two cultural groups were subsequently conducted through the nonparametric Wilcoxon procedure to detect their similarities and differences in optimal experience within each specific activity domain. The ratings of perceived challenges and skills did not differ significantly between the two groups in any domain. In productive activities non-western participants scored significantly higher than western ones for most variables: involvement ($Z = 4.9$, $p < 0.0001$), excitement ($Z = 2.9$, $p < 0.01$), ease of concentration ($Z = 2.9$, $p < 0.01$), enjoyment ($Z = 3.7$, $p < 0.0001$), concentration ($Z = 2.3$, $p < 0.05$), relaxation ($Z = 2.0$, $p < 0.05$), clear goals ($Z = 2.5$, $p < 0.05$), and control of the situation ($Z = 4.3$, $p < 0.0001$). On the opposite, only few group differences were detected in the leisure domain, with non-western participants reporting significant higher values of enjoyment ($Z = 3.1$, $p < 0.01$), concentration ($Z = 3.4$, $p < 0.001$), and control of the situation ($Z = 3.5$, $p < 0.001$). During interactions, only unselfconsciousness scored significantly higher among non-western participants ($Z = 4.1$, $p < 0.0001$), while no group differences were detected as concerned introspection.

These comparisons highlighted the peculiar experiential features of flow across domains and cultures. A closer analysis of each domain will help clarify some of these findings.

7.2.2.1 Flow in Productive Activities

As concerns work, traditional activities were quoted as occasions for flow more frequently than office and factory tasks by both cultural groups. More specifically, among the 141 western participants who selected work as opportunity for the most pervasive optimal experiences, 68.1% quoted traditional activities such as handicrafts, cooking, farming, and gardening. Among the 86 non-western participants who performed the same selection, an even higher percentage (82.6%) referred to traditional activities. Interestingly enough, among western participants (but not among non-western ones) significant differences were detected in the features of flow according to the selected work activity (Table 7.3) with higher values reported in traditional occupations for several variables: wish to do the activity ($Z = 2.5$, $p < 0.05$), excitement ($Z = 2.9$, $p < 0.01$), ease of concentration ($Z = 2.5$, $p < 0.05$), unselfconsciousness ($Z = 3.4$, $p < 0.001$), and relaxation ($Z = 3.6$, $p < 0.001$).

The globally better quality of experience associated with work by non-western participants can be at least partially explained by the very high percentage of

Table 7.3 Optimal experience in different productive activities among western and non-western participants

	Traditional work (W = 96, NW = 71)		Modern work (W = 45, NW = 15)		Study (W = 31, NW = 40)	
Variables	W *M* (*sd*)	NW *M* (*sd*)	W *M* (*sd*)	NW *M* (*sd*)	W *M* (*sd*)	NW *M* (*sd*)
Involvement	6.7 (1.3)	7.3 (1.2)	6.5 (1.4)	7.1 (1.6)	5.7 (1.2)	7.0 (1.5)
Clear feedback	7.1 (1.1)	7.4 (1.1)	6.9 (1.5)	6.9 (1.6)	6.5 (1.1)	6.3 (2.2)
Intrinsic motivation	7.1 (1.3)	7.0 (1.9)	6.2 (2.0)	6.9 (1.6)	5.9 (1.9)	6.3 (2.3)
Excitement	7.6 (0.9)	7.8 (0.6)	7.1 (1.4)	7.6 (1.1)	6.1 (1.6)	7.0 (1.7)
Ease of concentration	6.3 (2.2)	7.0 (2.0)	5.1 (2.8)	6.9 (2.5)	4.9 (2.2)	4.0 (3.1)
Unselfconsciousness	5.4 (2.6)	6.1 (2.3)	3.5 (3.1)	5.1 (3.0)	4.5 (2.8)	3.6 (2.6)
Enjoyment	7.0 (1.2)	7.6 (1.2)	6.6 (1.6)	7.1 (1.5)	6.1 (2.2)	6.4 (2.4)
Concentration	6.7 (1.6)	7.2 (1.2)	6.5 (1.6)	7.2 (1.3)	4.8 (1.5)	5.7 (2.1)
Relaxation	6.7 (1.8)	6.6 (2.3)	5.1 (2.5)	6.7 (2.6)	4.8 (2.4)	4.9 (2.8)
Clear goals	7.3 (1.2)	7.6 (1.1)	7.3 (1.4)	7.2 (1.5)	6.5 (1.8)	6.7 (1.8)
Control of situation	6.9 (1.3)	7.4 (1.1)	6.6 (1.5)	7.1 (1.3)	5.5 (2.0)	6.8 (1.4)
Challenges	6.8 (1.1)	6.6 (1.9)	6.6 (1.5)	7.3 (2.0)	6.3 (1.1)	6.1 (2.3)
Skills	6.9 (1.1)	6.7 (1.6)	6.6 (1.5)	6.8 (1.7)	5.9 (1.6)	5.6 (1.7)

Note: W = N. of western participants; NW = N. of non-western participants.

participants who selected traditional activities in this group. Investigations have showed the negative effects of modernization on individual psychological selection (Delle Fave & Massimini, 1988, 1991). Technology and automation have led to the standardization of behavior and of its products, to restrictions in individual initiative, to a decrease in the variation of activity structure and outcomes. Energy and artifact consumption prevail on the creative transformation and effective use of environmental resources (Oskamp, 2000). Efforts to humanize work through changes at the organizational and structural levels often clash with individual needs and cultural values (Hui & Luk, 1997). Nevertheless, as discussed in detail in Chapter 8, work represents a substantial opportunity for optimal experience, and the awareness of its potential has brought scholars and practitioners to thorough investigation of individual and social strategies to improve the quality of work life across professions and cultures.

In the domain of productive activities, significant cross-cultural differences were detected in the features of flow during learning tasks (Table 7.3) with higher values reported by non-western participants for involvement ($Z = 3.9$, $p < 0.0001$), excitement ($Z = 2.8$, $p < 0.01$), concentration ($Z = 2.6$, $p < 0.05$), and control of the situation ($Z = 2.9$, $p < 0.01$). The extensive bulk of studies conducted on flow and learning across countries, and among youth living in a wide variety of conditions (see Chapters 11 and 15) will show in detail how these differences can be related to the interplay between the collective meaning attributed to education, the more or less selective access to school, and the individual process of psychological selection.

7.2.2.2 Flow in Leisure

As shown in Table 7.4, leisure activities were overall associated with peculiarly high values of wish to do the activity and excitement, as expected on the basis of their free choice nature. The distinction between structured and relaxed leisure was reflected in the features of the associated optimal experience. A nonparametric ANOVA comparison of leisure activities detected significant differences in the values of perceived challenges and enjoyment in favor of sports and hobbies among both western participants ($F = 3.4$, $p < 0.01$ and $F = 5.1$, $p < 0.01$, respectively) and non-western participants ($F = 10.0$, $p < 0.0001$ and $F = 3.4$, $p < 0.05$, respectively). Involvement scored highest during hobbies for both groups ($F = 3.6$, $p < 0.05$ among westerners and $F = 2.8$, $p < 0.05$ among non-westerners). On the contrary, by virtue of their less demanding nature, reading and unstructured activities were associated with higher levels of unselfconsciousness by western participants ($F = 3.7$, $p < 0.01$), while non-western participants unanimously associated unstructured tasks with the extreme value of the relaxation scale ($F = 4.6$, $p < .01$). It is worthy reminding that only 20 participants (16 of them belonging to the western group) quoted watching TV as an optimal activity, mainly referring to sport events and soap operas. This result confirms the widespread finding that, in spite of its daily fruition across cultures, TV does not provide relevant opportunities for optimal experience (Delle Fave & Massimini, 2004, 2005; Kubey & Csikszentmihalyi, 1990).

According to the associated activities, the twofold role of leisure across cultures—as an opportunity for enjoyable engagement or for pleasant relaxation—clearly emerges from these findings. This evidence is consistent with the wide variety of data gathered in several studies to investigate optimal experience in structured and relaxed leisure activities; a more detailed exploration of this topic will be provided in Chapter 9.

7.2.2.3 Flow in Interactions

Interactions were associated with the most globally positive experience, with substantially overlapping ratings among both western and non-western participants. This finding can be related to the global recruitment of all the various components of optimal experience that characterizes interactions: Relational ties imply an affective dimension which elicits positive emotions such as excitement, enjoyment, and relaxation; they are based on the need for relatedness, thus being intrinsically motivated; they are selected and cultivated in lifelong perspective, thus representing meaningful and long-term challenges recruiting individuals' attention and cognitive resources (as discussed in detail in Chapter 10).

However, a remarkably low percentage of participants reported this activity as an opportunity for flow. This finding can be interpreted from two different perspectives. The first one is methodological, and it concerns the research tool. The three sentences used in the flow questionnaire to evoke optimal experiences (see Chapter 3) with their emphasis on "doing something," on individuality ("I," "my" are recurrent words), and on psychological isolation ("the world seems to be cut

Table 7.4 Optimal experience in leisure among western and non-western participants

	Sport (W = 64, NW = 24)		Hobbies (W = 46, NW = 33)		Reading (W = 54, NW = 35)		Relaxed leisure (W = 22, NW = 11)	
Variables	W *M* (*sd*)	NW *M* (*sd*)	W *M* (*sd*)	NW *M* (*sd*)	W *M* (*sd*)	NW *M* (*sd*)	W *M* (*sd*)	NW *M* (*sd*)
Involvement	6.4 (1.5)	6.9 (1.7)	7.3 (1.2)	7.6 (1.0)	6.6 (1.7)	6.6 (2.1)	7.0 (1.1)	6.1 (2.1)
Clear feedback	6.4 (1.5)	6.7 (1.6)	6.7 (2.2)	7.1 (1.7)	6.8 (1.8)	6.4 (1.9)	6.5 (2.0)	6.3 (2.8)
Intrinsic motivation	7.5 (1.2)	7.0 (2.0)	7.5 (0.9)	7.3 (1.6)	7.5 (1.0)	7.2 (1.4)	7.5 (1.7)	6.5 (2.8)
Excitement	7.8 (0.7)	7.8 (0.4)	7.7 (0.7)	7.9 (0.3)	7.6 (0.9)	7.7 (0.7)	7.9 (0.5)	7.5 (1.3)
Ease of concentration	6.0 (2.6)	5.9 (3.1)	5.9 (2.6)	7.1 (1.7)	6.3 (2.1)	6.2 (2.5)	6.6 (2.1)	7.8 (0.4)
Unselfconsciousness	4.5 (2.9)	5.7 (3.0)	5.4 (3.0)	6.6 (2.1)	6.2 (2.6)	5.7 (2.9)	6.0 (3.1)	8.0 (0.0)
Enjoyment	7.3 (1.0)	7.6 (0.9)	7.4 (1.2)	7.8 (0.5)	6.4 (1.9)	6.9 (1.5)	6.8 (1.4)	7.3 (1.5)
Concentration	6.0 (1.9)	6.9 (2.0)	6.5 (2.1)	7.1 (1.9)	6.5 (1.6)	6.5 (2.1)	6.0 (2.5)	7.1 (1.1)
Relaxation	6.7 (1.7)	5.8 (3.2)	6.4 (2.2)	7.7 (0.7)	6.8 (1.9)	6.6 (2.1)	7.4 (1.4)	8.0 (0.0)
Clear goals	6.8 (1.7)	6.8 (1.4)	6.7 (2.2)	7.5 (0.8)	6.7 (2.1)	7.3 (1.2)	6.2 (2.5)	7.0 (2.8)
Control of situation	6.7 (1.4)	7.0 (2.0)	6.6 (2.1)	7.6 (0.7)	6.7 (1.8)	7.1 (1.5)	6.2 (2.4)	7.8 (0.7)
Challenges	6.5 (1.6)	7.4 (0.7)	6.9 (1.5)	6.7 (2.2)	5.9 (2.1)	4.4 (2.3)	5.9 (2.0)	5.2 (3.8)
Skills	6.2 (1.6)	6.8 (1.4)	7.0 (1.1)	7.0 (1.2)	6.5 (1.9)	6.6 (2.0)	6.0 (2.1)	5.9 (2.7)

off from me") primarily induce people to think about individual tasks. The second perspective refers to the structure of daily relationships, and to their social and psychological aspects. Interactions comprise a wide variety of activities, ranging from intense discussions to relaxed small talk, in some cases involving physical contact, and varying in contents and communication patterns according to the cultural context and to the social status of the interlocutors (Fiske & Fiske, 2007; Hinde, 1979; Omark, Strayer, & Freedman, 1980; Smith, 2001). Variations can be also detected according to sample features, especially participants' age: Adolescents invest their attention and resources on peer interactions more than adults; adults perceive parenting activities as highly challenging and rewarding, while children perceive family as a low-challenging and relaxed context. Finally, the individual and cultural meanings attributed to relationships can influence the associated quality of experience.

A more detailed discussion about relationships, flow, and psychological selection across cultures will be proposed in Chapter 10. Here we only point out that all participants—regardless of the individualistic or collectivistic features of their culture—reported interactions as opportunities for flow in similar percentage, and described the experience in the same way. The higher values of unselfconsciousness detected among non-western participants confirm previous ESM findings (Asakawa & Csikszentmihalyi, 2000) derived from the comparison between Asian-American adolescents and European-American ones. It can be related to the prevalence of interdependent self-construal in collectivistic cultures (Markus & Kitayama, 1991).

7.2.2.4 Flow and Psychological Selection

Table 7.5 shows some synthetic results derived from the administration of the life theme questionnaire to western and non-western participants. More specifically, it

Table 7.5 Percentage distribution of positive influences, challenges, and goals across cultures

	Positive influences		Present challenges		Future goals	
Categories	Western	Non-western	Western	Non-western	Western	Non-western
Productive activities	21.9	15.8	43.6	29.6	31.9	24.4
Family	45.3	50.1	20.5	32.8	31.7	37.4
Leisure	7.6	4.2	2.6	1.4	4.1	1.9
Social relations	17.3	11.8	6.5	6.3	4.4	6.4
Personal growth	7.2	17.7	18.3	14.1	19.2	15.9
Material goods	0.6	0.4	8.5	15.8	8.8	14.0
N answers	1,390	543	567	348	856	471

Note: N western participants = 516; N non-western participants = 251.

illustrates the percentage distribution of answers referring to positive life influences, present challenges, and future goals in the two groups.

In both groups family was prominent among positive influences, followed by productive activities and social relations. As for present challenges and future goals, productive activities prevailed in both groups, followed by personal growth and by material goods. However, referring to present life western participants put greater emphasis on productive activities, which accounted for almost 50% of their challenges, while the answers of non-western participants were distributed more homogeneously across these major categories.

A different perspective on these findings can be obtained by comparing the number of participants quoting each activity category in the two groups. This kind of analysis highlighted that a significantly higher percentage of non-western participants (36.7% vs. 21.3% of the western ones) quoted family among present challenges ($\chi^2 = 20.5$, $p < 0.0001$) and among future goals (52.2% vs. 44.2%, $\chi^2 = 4.3$, $p < 0.05$). A significant difference was also detected for the present and future relevance of material goods, quoted among present challenges by 21.2% of the non-western participants, compared with 8.3% of the western ones ($\chi^2 = 25.2$, $p < 0.0001$), and among future goals by 21.1% of the non-western participants, compared with 14% of the western ones ($\chi^2 = 6.3$, $p < 0.05$). This last result can easily be explained through the lower level of affluence and the lack of welfare policies characterizing the countries in which most non-western participants live.

After this global overview of the results, we would like to run a final analysis, in the attempt to link the findings derived from the two questionnaires. More specifically, we will investigate the joint recurrence of the major life domains as opportunities for flow and as components of the life theme (positive influences, present challenges, and future goals) among participants in the two cultural groups. Table 7.6 provides a synthesis of these findings, showing the percentage of participants who reported four different levels of congruence (progressively recruiting more dimensions among those explored through the answers to the questionnaires) in the two groups. Productive activities were quoted as both present challenges and

Table 7.6 Percentage of participants reporting domain congruence across dimensions of psychological selection

	Congruence level 1 challenges/goals		Congruence level 2 LT		Congruence level 3 flow/challenges/goals		Congruence level 4 flow and LT	
Categories	W	NW	W	NW	W	NW	W	NW
Productive activities	26.4	24.3	13.8	8.0	10.5	10.4	6.4	3.6
Family	13.4	25.5	12.6	20.7	2.5	4.8	2.1	4.0
Social relations	0.8	1.2	0.4	0.4	0.6	0.4	–	–
Personal growth	8.0	6.4	0.8	1.6	–	–	0.4	–

Note: LT = Positive influences + challenges + goals; W = Western participants (N = 516); NW = Non-western participants (N = 251).

future goals (congruence level 1) in similar percentages of participants across cultures; analogously, around 10% of the participants in both groups referred to them as optimal activities, as well as present and future targets of resource investment (congruence level 3). However, the percentage of western participants reporting work as a recurrent element of the life theme (congruence level 2) was significantly higher ($\chi^2 = 5.4, p < 0.05$).

As for family, its lifelong relevance was prominently highlighted by non-western participants, both across the answers to the life theme questionnaire (congruence levels 1 and 2), and as both a flow activity and a component of the life theme (congruence levels 3 and 4). At the congruence levels 1 and 2, participants' percentages significantly differed in the two groups ($\chi^2 = 17.3, p < 0.0001$; and $\chi^2 = 8.6, p < 0.01$. respectively).

The other domains were recurrent in a very limited percentage of participants in both groups. Leisure-related findings were not reported in the table due to exiguous number of participants (prominently western ones) reporting this domain as a component of their life theme.

In sum, these findings provide a complex picture in which each of the various life domains shows a specific pattern. Productive activities showed the more pervasive impact on the lifelong resource investment and skill cultivation across cultures. Leisure, while providing frequent opportunities for flow experience, did not emerge as a significant lifelong focus of attention. The opposite was true of family, a major long-term concern, but an infrequent context of optimal experiences.

What do these results suggest as concerns the role of optimal experience in daily life and in the long-term perspective of psychological selection? First of all, they confirmed the cross-cultural recurrence of flow, and its consistent psychological features. Second, they showed domain-related variations in the features of flow, which proved to be stable across cultures. Third, they highlighted the complex relationship pattern between flow and psychological selection. This relationship seems to be modulated by two different elements: (a) the structure of flow activities and their potential in recruiting individual attention and concentration during their performance; (b) the meaning and relevance of flow activities in the lifelong perspective. These two elements are not always consistent with each other: structured leisure activities provide flow but they are not relevant components of the life theme; on the contrary, family interactions are rarely associated with optimal experience, but they represent a major core of long-term resource investment. Work seems to be the only domain in which the two elements are combined. Findings derived from other studies conducted with ESM suggested this trend (Delle Fave & Massimini, 2005).

7.3 Adolescence Across Cultures: Finding Flow, Building the Future

The investigation of the opportunities for flow in daily life and within the process of psychological selection during adolescence is particularly interesting, in that during this life stage individuals start developing awareness of their identity and of the social roles they are expected and wish to play in the future.

The findings presented here derive from three different groups of adolescents. The first one included 58 Navajo teenagers (34 girls and 24 boys aged 14–19), attending Ganado High School—a prominently western-style institution—and coming from traditional joint families (additional details on these participants will be provided in Chapter 13). The second group of adolescents comprised 40 girls aged 14–20, coming from a rural area in the Karimojong region of Uganda, and enrolled in a boarding school run by Catholic nuns. Participants in the third group were 102 adolescents (61 girls and 41 boys aged 15–19), students at different public high schools and living in an urban neighborhood of Central Italy. Finally, the fourth groups comprised 48 teenagers from Nepal (29 girls and 19 boys aged 13–17), attending different high schools in Kathmandu, the capital city of the country.

As a preliminary finding, it is worth noticing that the four groups differed in the percentage of participants reporting flow in their daily life. Among the adolescents attending Ganado high school, 37 (63.8%) identified this experience, while all Ugandan girls except one did. Participants reporting optimal experience accounted for 62.7% of the Italian adolescents, and for 70.8% of the Nepalese ones. The lower incidence of flow recognition among children and adolescents, in comparison with adults, was verified in other samples as well (Bassi & Delle Fave, 2004; Chapter 11).

As concerns optimal activities, Table 7.7 shows the results obtained from each of the four groups. Overall, a significant difference was detected across selected optimal activity categories as concerns the percentage distribution of participants from the four groups ($\chi^2 = 42.5, p < 0.0001$). In particular, two different trends emerged from the answer distribution. Among Navajo and Italian adolescents, leisure prevailed as the most frequently cited opportunity for optimal experience, both within the general flow activity distribution and among the selected activities. On the contrary, Ugandan and Nepalese adolescents prominently quoted study in both cases. This general finding was supported by the cross-group differences detected in the participants' percentage distribution in the domains of study ($\chi^2 = 33.9, p < 0.001$ as cited flow activity; $\chi^2 = 27.2, p < 0.0001$ as selected one) and leisure ($\chi^2 = 8.3$, $p < 0.05$ as cited flow activity; $\chi^2 = 26.9, p < 0.0001$). The participants' percentage

Table 7.7 Adolescents across cultures: percentage distribution of optimal activities and selected optimal activities

	Navajo		Uganda		Italy		Nepal	
Categories	Total	Selected	Total	Selected	Total	Selected	Total	Selected
Study	14.1	8.7	41.9	53.9	35.2	26.5	45.6	58.8
Leisure	67.6	68.6	37.8	23.1	46.7	56.2	28.6	20.6
Interactions	11.3	17.1	5.4	10.3	18.0	17.3	12.9	8.8
Introspection	7.0	5.6	14.9	12.7	0.0	0	12.9	11.8
N answers	71	35	74	39	122	64	70	34

Table 7.8 Adolescents across cultures: percentage distribution of positive influences, challenges, and goals

	Positive influences			Present challenges			Future goals		
Categories	Uganda	Italy	Nepal	Uganda	Italy	Nepal	Uganda	Italy	Nepal
Productive activities	50.0	15.7	41.9	54.0	57.2	73.5	80.0	52.6	55.6
Family	6.0	36.3	23.4	–	8.0	17.0	7.8	33.3	10.4
Leisure	15.0	17.0	16.9	0.0	1.8	0.0	2.2	5.8	4.7
Social relations	12.0	24.3	7.3	12.0	4.5	3.0	0.0	3.3	9.4
Personal growth	17	6.7	10.5	22.0	13.4	8.9	7.8	3.8	18.9
Material goods				2.0	0.0	4.4	2.2	0.4	0.9
N answers	100	300	124	110	68	558	90	240	106

Note: LT = Positive influences + challenges + goals; N Ugandan participants = 40; N Italian participants = 102, N Nepalese participants = 48.

distribution also differed across groups as concerns introspection ($\chi^2 = 19.7$, $p < 0.001$ as cited flow activity; $\chi^2 = 12.7, p < 0.01$ as selected one), more frequently reported by Ugandan and Nepalese adolescents than by Italian and Navajo ones.

The results obtained through the administration of the life theme questionnaire provided specific information on the long-term resource investment of these adolescents. The comparison will be restricted to three groups, since these data had not been collected among Navajo students. As Table 7.8 shows, school and studying (included in the category "productive activities") were prominently quoted among positive influences by Ugandan and Nepalese teenagers ($\chi^2 = 42.0$, $p < 0.0001$), while an opposite trend was detected for family ($\chi^2 = 45.3$, $p < 0.0001$), and for social relations ($\chi^2 = 33.6$, $p < 0.0001$) that recruited the answers of a higher percentage of Italian participants.

Over half of the participants across cultures identified their most important present challenge with study; nevertheless, their percentage distribution differed across groups ($\chi^2 = 9.3$, $p < 0.01$). Compared with the other two groups, a higher percentage of Ugandan teenagers reported challenges related to personal growth, in particular achieving autonomy and independence: For these girls, education represented a key instrument to escape the constraints of the traditional female role within a joint family system and to pursue professional and personal projects. Nepalese adolescents distinguished themselves from the other groups by the relevance attached to family, mostly referring to the importance of fulfilling parents' academic expectations, due to the financial burden represented by their school attendance.

As for goals, academic and work achievements were predominant across cultures. Italian adolescents significantly differed from the other two groups in the emphasis given to family as a goal ($\chi^2 = 32.6$, $p < 0.0001$), mostly referring to having a satisfying couple relationship and building their own family. Finally, a significant difference was detected across groups in goals related to personal growth ($\chi^2 = 12.9, p < 0.01$), mostly due to the high percentage of Nepalese teenagers who reported them, referring to psychological development and to the cultivation of self awareness through meditation practice.

Finally, and through the same procedure adopted for the adult sample, we will investigate the joint recurrence of the major life domains as opportunities for flow and as components of the life theme. Table 7.9 illustrates the percentage distribution of participants across four different levels of congruence in the three groups. Productive activities recruited the majority of adolescents in all groups, as the core domain recurring across the different dimensions of the psychological selection process. It was quoted as both present challenges and future goals (congruence level 1) by similar percentages of participants across cultures. At the congruence level 2, a significant group difference was detected ($\chi^2 = 17.7, p < 0.0001$), related to the lower percentage of Italian teenagers referring to productive activities, compared with the other two groups. This trend was persistent at the other two congruence levels: level 3 ($\chi^2 = 11.8, p < 0.01$) and 4 ($\chi^2 = 18.0, p < 0.0001$). On the contrary, the percentage of Italian adolescents reporting family as a recurrent element of their psychological selection was significantly higher at the congruence level 1 ($\chi^2 = 7.6, p < 0.05$) and 2 ($\chi^2 = 6.2, p < 0.05$).

7.4 Culture and Optimal Experience: Some General Remarks

The findings presented in the previous pages highlighted both recurrent aspects and cultural specificities of optimal experience. We will discuss them taking into account the two different types of cultures in which the data were collected. In particular, Italian participants can be considered as members of an individualistic culture, promoting the development of independent self-construals. Participants coming from Asian and African countries, on the contrary, belong to collectivistic cultures, valuing social harmony over individuality, and supporting interdependence.

We would like to stress that our participants widely varied in age, educational level, and occupation. It is also worth underlining that the instruments used for data collection—flow questionnaire and life theme questionnaire—included both qualitative and quantitative evaluations. In fact, the most popular inventories used in flow research are built as scales (see Chapter 4): They do not allow for participants' comments and descriptions. This entails the risk of taking for granted that all over the world people build their conception of optimal experience on the opinion of western psychologists. On the contrary, the mixed-method nature of the current study potentially enables new findings and theoretical interpretations of optimal experience to be drawn on the basis of the qualitative data, and the formulation of further hypotheses based on the quantitative data (Creswell, 2008; Denzin & Lincoln, 2000).

In the adult groups, after reading the three quotations in the opening section of the flow questionnaire, the majority of participants spontaneously identified

Table 7.9 Percentage of adolescents reporting domain congruence across dimensions of psychological selection

	Congruence level 1 challenges/goals			Congruence level 2 LT			Congruence level 3 flow/challenges/goals			Congruence level 4 flow and LT		
Categories	Uganda	Italy	Nepal	Uganda	Italy	Nepal	Uganda	Italy	Nepal	Uganda	Italy	Nepal
Productive activities	65.0	57.8	75.0	65.0	30.4	56.3	42.5	17.7	37.5	42.5	10.8	25.0
Family	2.5	13.7	4.2	–	10.8	2.1	–	4.9	–	–	4.9	–
Personal growth	2.5	3.0	2.0	2.5	–	–						–

Note: LT = Positive influences + challenges + goals; Ugandan participants N = 40; Italian participants N = 102; Nepalese participants N = 48.

optimal experiences in their lives, associating to it the same number of activities on average. When asked to report the cognitive, motivational, and emotional aspects of flow, both groups converged in the description of a highly positive condition "beyond boredom and anxiety" (Csikszentmihalyi, 1975), characterized by positive engagement, autonomous involvement, and skill mobilization. These findings suggest that flow is a universally shared experience. However, non-western participants scored significantly higher than westerners in involvement, excitement, enjoyment, concentration, relaxation, and control of the situation.

The distribution of optimal activities across life domains and the associated experience showed both similarities and differences between groups. Work and leisure were prominently identified as optimal activities, while interactions and introspection were far less frequent. A similar distribution pattern was observed for selected optimal activities. However, the percentage of participants quoting work and introspection was significantly higher among non-westerners, while westerners reported a higher percentage of leisure-related activities. As concerns the experiential features of flow, significant differences across domains were consistent between groups: Interactions were unanimously associated with the most positive variable values; work scored high in perceived challenges, but low in unselfconsciousness, concentration effort, and wish to do the activity; leisure was especially connected to high levels of enjoyment and relaxation. However, except for interactions, the two groups differed in the domain-related features of flow in relation to the same variables identified in the overall comparison.

How can we interpret these cross-cultural differences in the features of flow? Why did non-western participants report a globally higher quality of experience? We can formulate some general hypotheses, all linked to cultural aspects, though in different terms. First, we hypothesize that the low emphasis on personal achievement and individual performance typical of collectivistic societies leaves individuals more free from preoccupations related to activity outcomes, thus allowing them to benefit more fully from the intrinsic motivation and enjoyable skill mobilization that characterize flow. Moreover, non-western participants also reported overall lower levels of self-consciousness than their western counterparts: This finding further supports our hypothesis. Second, most Asian traditions praise quietness of the mind and one-pointed attention. The higher levels of relaxation and concentration reported by non-westerners, again coupled with lower levels of self–consciousness, can be rooted in this traditional outlook, that is reflected in parenting practices and community rituals across most non-western countries. However, these hypotheses need to be confirmed by further studies, recruiting western and non-western participants from additional countries.

As concerns optimal experience and psychological selection across the four groups of adolescents, the most evident finding is the relationship between cultural meanings and individuals' long-term orientation. Evidence of this relationship emerged for the domains of study and family. In particular, the high cultural value attached to education in developing societies, and the benefits it provides to the limited amount of people who can access it, led the examined high-school students to preferentially and massively invest their resources in the pursuit of academic achievement. Conversely, Italian teenagers were more concerned with the construction of a family. This apparently surprising finding can be explained through the social norms and customs concerning the family domain in individualistic and collectivistic cultures. In the former, youths do not have to struggle for finding a partner, since arranged marriages are the rule, still today. On the opposite, in individualistic countries each person autonomously deals with this aspect of life. Both strategies have advantages and disadvantages. Apparently, free choice in partner selection is desirable and more gratifying than social imposition. However, the exponential percentage of divorces, the steady occurrence of family abuses, and the growing number of individuals living alone—and suffering from their condition—in western countries does not allow to take for granted the superiority of the individualistic approach to this crucial aspect of the human biocultural survival and reproduction.

Finally, we would like to stress that this cross-cultural investigation opens more questions rather than providing answers. But, to quote T.S. Eliot (1942/1995), "...as we grow older, the world becomes stranger, the pattern more complicated..." (p. 122). Flow research has reached his maturity, and this outcome is inevitable.

References

Ackerman, P. L. (1996). A theory of adult intellectual development: Process, personality, interests, and knowledge. *Intelligence*, *22*, 227–257.

Asakawa, K., & Csikszentmihalyi, M. (2000). Feelings of connectedness and internalization of values in Asian American adolescents. *Journal of Youth and Adolescence*, *29*, 121–145.

Bassi, M., & Delle Fave, A. (2004). Adolescence and the changing context of optimal experience in time: Italy 1986–2000. *Journal of Happiness Studies*, *5*, 155–179.

Berry, J. W. (1969). On cross-cultural comparability. *International Journal of Psychology*, *4*, 119–128.

Block, N. (1995). How heritability misleads about race. *Cognition*, *56*, 99–128.

Bond, R. A., & Smith, P. B. (1996). Culture and conformity: A meta-analysis of studies using ash's (1952) line judgement task. *Psychological Bulletin*, *119*, 111–137.

Brewer, M. B., & Gardner, L. W. (1996). Who is this "we"? Levels of collective identity and self-representation. *Journal of Personality and Social Psychology*, *71*, 83–93.

Cohen, D., & Kitayama, S. (2007). Cultural psychology. This stanza and the next. In S. Kitayama & D. Cohen (Eds.), *Handbook of cultural psychology* (pp. 847–851). New York: Guilford Press.

Creswell, J. W. (2008). *Research design: Qualitative, quantitative and mixed methods approaches* (3rd ed.). Thousand Oaks, CA: Sage Publications.

Csikszentmihalyi, M. (1975/2000). *Beyond boredom and anxiety*. San Francisco: Jossey Bass.

Csikszentmihalyi, M. (1997). *Finding flow: The psychology of engagement with everyday life*. New York: Basic Books.

Csikszentmihalyi, M., Rathunde, K., & Whalen, S. (1993). *Talented teenagers: The roots of success and failure*. New York: Cambridge University Press.

Delle Fave, A. (2007). Individual development and community empowerment: Suggestions from studies on optimal experience. In J. Haworth & G. Hart (Eds.), *Well-being: Individual, community, and societal perspectives* (pp. 41–56). London: Palgrave McMillan.

Delle Fave, A., & Massimini, F. (1988). Modernization and changing contexts of flow in work and leisure. In M. Csikszentmihalyi & I. Csikszentmihalyi (eds.), *Optimal experience. psychological studies of flow in consciousness* (pp. 193–213). New York: Cambridge University Press.

Delle Fave, A., & Massimini, F. (1991). Modernization and the quality of daily experience in a southern Italy village. In N. Bleichrodt & P. J. D. Drenth (eds.), *Contemporary issues in cross-cultural psychology* (pp. 110–119). Amsterdam: Swets & Zeitlinger B.V.
Delle Fave, A., & Massimini, F. (2004). The cross-cultural investigation of optimal experience. *Ricerche di Psicologia, 27*, 79–102.
Delle Fave, A., & Massimini, F. (2005). The investigation of optimal experience and apathy: Developmental and psychosocial implications. *European Psychologist, 10*, 264–274.
Denzin, N. K., & Lincoln, Y. (2000). *Handbook of qualitative research*. Thousand Oaks, CA: Sage.
De Vos, G. (1985). Dimensions of the self in Japanese culture. In A. Marsella, G. De Vos, & F. L. K. Hsu (Eds.), *Culture and self* (pp. 149–184). London: Tavistock.
Diaz-Guerrero, R. (1979). The development of coping style. *Human Development, 22*, 320–331.
Diener, E., Oishi, S., & Lucas, R. (2004). Personality, culture, and subjective well-being: Emotional and cognitive evaluations of life. *Annual Review of Psychology, 54*, 403–425.
Eaton, L., & Louw, J. (2000). Culture and self in South Africa: Individualism-collectivism predictions. *The Journal of Social Psychology, 140*, 210–217.
Eliot, T. S. (1942). *The four quartets*. In A. Tonelli (Ed.), *The waste land – four quartets. Parallel text edition*. Milano: Feltrinelli 1995.
Fiske, A. P., & Fiske, S. T. (2007). Social relationships in our species and cultures. In S. Kitayama & D. Cohen (Eds.), *Handbook of cultural psychology* (pp. 283–306). New York: Guilford Press.
Fiske, A. P., Kitayama, S., Markus, H., & Nisbett, R. E. (1998). The cultural matrix of social psychology. In D. T. Gilbert, S. T. Fiske, & G. Lindzey (Eds.), *The handbook of social psychology* (4th ed., Vol. 2, pp. 915-981). Boston: McGraw-Hill.
Gabriel, S., & Gardner, L. W. (1999). Are there „his“ and „hers“ types of interdependence? The implications of gender differences in collective versus relational interdependence for affect, behaviour, and cognition. *Journal of Personality and Social Psychology, 77*, 642–655.
Gardner, H. (1982). *Developmental psychology*. Boston: Little Brown.
Han, A. G. (2008). Building a harmonious society and achieving individual harmony. *Journal of Chinese Political Science, 13*, 143–164.
Han, J. J., Leichtman, M. D., & Wang, Q. (1998). Autobiographical memory in Korean, Chinese, and American children. *Developmental Psychology, 34*, 701–713.
Hardin, E. E., Leong, F. T. L., & Bhagwat, A. A. (2004). Factor structure of the self-construal scale revisited. *Journal of Cross-Cultural Psychology, 35*, 327–345.
Hedden, T., Park, D. C., Nisbett, R. E., Ji, L., Jing, Q., & Jiao, S. (2002). Cultural variation in verbal versus spatial neuropsychological function across the lifespan. *Neuropsychology, 16*, 65–73.
Hektner, J. M., Schmidt, J., & Csikszentmihalyi, M. (2007). *Experience sampling method: Measuring the quality of everyday life*. Thousand Oaks, CA: Sage.
Herrnstein, R. J., & Murray, C. (1994). *The bell curve*. New York: Free Press.
Herskovitz, M. J. (1948). *Man and his works: The science of cultural anthropology*. New York: Knopf.
Hinde, R. (1979). *Toward understanding relationships*. London: Academic Press.
Ho, S. S. M., & Chan, R. S. Y. (2009). Social harmony in Hong Kong: Level, determinants and policy implications. *Social Indicators Research, 91*, 37–58.
Hofstede, G. (1980). *Culture's consequences: International differences in work-related values*. London: Sage.
Hsu, F. L. K. (1985). The self in cross-cultural perspective. In A. Marsella, G. De Vos, & F. L. K. Hsu (Eds.), *Culture and self* (pp. 24–55). London: Tavistock.
Hui, H., & Luk, C. L. (1997). Industrial/organizational psychology. In J. W. Berry, M. H. Segall & C. Kagitçibasi (eds.), *Handbook of cross-cultural psychology* (Vol. 3, pp. 371–412). Boston: Allyn and Bacon.
Ji, L. -J., Nisbett, R. E., & Su, Y. (2001). Culture, change, and prediction. *Psychological Science, 12*, 450–456.
Ji, L. -J., Peng, K., & Nisbett, R. E. (2000). Culture, control, and perception of relationships in the environment. *Journal of Personality and Social Psychology, 78*, 943–955.

Kagitçibasi, C. (1997). Individualism and collectivism. In Berry, J. W., Segall, M. H., & Kagitçibasi, C., *Handbook of cross-cultural psychology, social behavior and applications* (Vol.3, pp. 1–49). Needam Heights, MA: Allyn & Bacon.

Kasser, T., & Ryan, R. M. (1996). Further examining the American dream: Differential correlates of intrinsic and extrinsic goals. *Personality and Social Psychology Bulletin, 22*, 280–287.

Kim, U., & Berry, J. W. (1993). *Indigenous psychologies*. Newbury Park, CA: Sage.

Kim, J. S., Triandis, H. C., Kagitçibasi, C., Choi, S., & Yoon, G. (1994). *Individualism and collectivism: Theory, method and applications*. Thousand Oaks, CA: Sage.

Kitayama, S., Snibbe, A. C., Markus, H. R., & Suzuki, T. (2004). Is there any "free"choice? Self and dissonance in two cultures. *Psychological Science, 15*, 527–533.

Kitayama, S., Takagi, H., & Matsumoto, D. (1995). Cultural psychology of Japanese self: Causal attributions of success and failure. *Japanese Psychological Review, 38*, 247–280.

Kleiber, D., Larson, R. W., & Csikszentmihalyi, M. (1986). The experience of leisure in adolescence. *Journal of Leisure Research, 18*, 169–176.

Kubey, R., & Csikszentmihalyi, M. (1990). *Television and the quality of life: How viewing shapes everyday experience*. Hillsdale, NJ: Erlbaum.

Latané, B., & Darley, J. M. (1970). *The unresponsive bystander: Why doesn't he help?* New York: Appleton-Century-crofts.

Laungani, P. (1992). Cultural variations in the understanding and treatment of neurotic disorders: India and England. *Counselling Psychology Quarterly, 5*, 231–244.

Leung, K. A. Y., Fernandez-Dols, J. M., & Iwawaki, S. (1992). Preference for methods of conflicts processing in two collectivist cultures. *International Journal of Psychology, 27*, 195–209.

Markus, R., & Kitayama, S. (1991). Culture and the self: Implications for cognition, emotion, and motivation. *Psychological Review, 98*, 224–253.

Marsella, A. J., & Pedersen, P. B. (1981). *Cross-cultural counseling and psychotherapy*. New York: Pergamon Press.

Masuda, T., & Nisbett, R. E. (2001). Attending holistically versus analytically: Comparing the context sensitivity of Japanese and Americans. *Journal of Personality and Social Psychology, 81*, 922–934.

Morling, B., Kitayama, S., & Miyamoto, Y. (2002). Cultural practices emphasize influence in the United States and adjustment in Japan. *Personality and Social Psychology Bulletin, 28*, 311–323.

Myers, D. (2000). The funds, friends, and faith of happy people. *American Psychologist, 55*, 56–67.

Omark, D. R., Strayer, F. F., & Freedman, D. G. (1980). *Dominance relations*. New York: Garland STPM Press.

Oskamp, S. (2000). A sustainable future for humanity? *American Psychologist, 55*, 496–508.

Park, N., Peterson, C., & Seligman, M. E. P. (2006). Character strengths in fifty-four nations and the fifty US states. *Journal of Positive Psychology, 1*, 118–129.

Romney, A. K., & D'Andrade, R. (Eds.) (1964). Transcultural studies in cognition. Special issue. *American Anthropologist, 66*, 3.

Ryan, R., & Deci, E. (2001). On happiness and human potentials: A review of research on hedonic and eudaimonic well-being. *Annual Review of Psychology, 52*, 141–166.

Shweder, R. A., & Bourne, E. J. (1984). Does the concept of the person vary cross-culturally? In R. A. Shweder, & R. A. LeVine (Eds.), *Culture theory: Essays on mind, self, and emotion* (pp. 158–199). Cambridge, England: Cambridge University Press.

Singelis, T. M., Triandis, H. C., Bhawuk, D. S., & Gelfand, M. (1995). Horizontal and vertical dimensions of individualism and collectivism: A theoretical and measurement refinement. *Cross-Cultural Research, 29*, 240–275.

Smith, P. B. (2001). Cross-cultural studies on social influences. In D. Matsumoto (Ed.), *The handbook of culture and psychology* (pp. 361–374). New York: Oxford University Press.

Smith, P. B., & Bond, M. H. (1999). *Social psychology across cultures*. Boston: Allyn & Bacon.

Somech, A. (2000). The independent and the interdependent selves: Different meanings in different cultures. *International Journal of Intercultural Relations, 24*, 161–172.

Stigler, J. W., Shweder, R. A., & Herdt, G. (1990). *Cultural psychology*. Cambridge: Cambridge University Press.
Super, C. M., & Harkness, S. (1986). The developmental niche: A conceptualization at the interface of child and culture. *International Journal of Behavioral Development*, *9*, 545–569.
Triandis, H. C. (1994). *Culture and social behaviour*. New York: McGraw-Hill.
Triandis, H. C., Chan, D. K. S., Bhawuk, D., Iwao, S., & Sinha, J. B. P. (1995). Multimethod probes of allocentrism and idiocentrism. *International Journal of Psychology*, *30*, 461–480.
Uchida, Y., Norasakkunkit, V., & Kitayama, S. (2004). Cultural constructions of happiness: Theory and empirical evidence. *Journal of Happiness Studies*, *5*, 223–239.
Weisz, J. R., Rothbaum, F. M., & Blackburn, T. C. (1984). Standing out and standing in: The psychology of control in America and Japan. *American Psychologist*, *39*, 955–969.
Yamaguchi, S. (2001). Culture and control orientations. In D. Matsumoto (Ed.), *The handbook of culture and psychology* (pp. 223–242). New York: Oxford University Press.
Yang, K. (2000). Mono-cultural and cross-cultural indigenous approaches: The royal road to the development of a balanced global psychology. *Asian Journal of Social Psychology*, *3*, 241–263.

Chapter 8
Work: A Paradox in Flow Research

8.1 Work and Leisure: Two Separate Domains?

Work represents a fundamental human activity, aimed at providing resources that allow for the biocultural survival and reproduction of individuals and groups (see Chapter 2; Calegari & Massimini, 1978). Solutions to the universal problem of work organization and distribution among community members vary across societies, presenting an extensive gamut of economic systems regulating crucial aspects of productive life, such as means of production, access to work, and labor division. Variation is also found diachronically in a given population, reflecting cultural and technological development (i.e., cultural evolution) over time. For instance, the industrial revolution during the eighteenth and the nineteenth centuries marked the transition from previously manual labor and draft-animal-based economy to machine-based manufacturing.

Variations across societies are also found in relation to the amount of time devoted to work and leisure. While in some communities of hunter-gatherers, individuals spend only 3–5 h a day in productive tasks like providing food, shelter, clothing, and tools (Csikszentmihalyi, 1990), in others—such as traditional agricultural groups—work characterizes the bulk of people's daily life. What distinguishes societies even further is people's attitude toward the work–leisure division. In the western world, in particular, work has primarily become synonymous with duty, constraint, and boredom: People have to work to earn a living, whereas full self-actualization takes place in the free time, when one can be oneself, and engage in meaningful and creative activities. This vision is also reflected in the psychological literature on work that emphasizes the need for fostering workers' motivation and for countering the levels of stress and burnout associated with productive activities (Le Blanc, de Jonge, & Schaufeli, 2008; Schaufeli, Leiter, & Maslach, 2009). However, Parker (1997) has maintained that the relationship between work and leisure is not homogenous within a given society, as it primarily depends on people's occupations. He proposed three different patterns in the work–leisure relationship. The first pattern is labeled *extension*; it derives from the spill-over approach that posits mutual influences in terms of skill development and levels of satisfaction between different life areas. This pattern is typical of people involved in creative and

A. Delle Fave et al., *Psychological Selection and Optimal Experience Across Cultures*, Cross-Cultural Advancements in Positive Psychology 2,
DOI 10.1007/978-90-481-9876-4_8, © Springer Science+Business Media B.V. 2011

autonomy-supporting jobs, such as artists, scientists, and specialized professionals. The second pattern is *opposition*; it also originates from the spill-over approach and implies a contrast between work and leisure. It applies to people enrolled in risky and damaging jobs, who compensate through leisure for the frustrations and constraints of work. The third pattern is *separation*, according to which work and leisure are perceived as independent life domains having no mutual influences.

Indeed a key issue in work and leisure studies concerns the opportunities for self-expression and individual development provided in the two contexts (Delle Fave & Massimini, 2003). As will be shown in the Chapter 9, people may have a hard time deciding how to spend their free time; a great deal of it is generally spent in passive unstructured activities, such as watching TV, which may replenish the exhausted worker's energy but which certainly do not contribute to her personal growth. By contrast—and often contrary to people's common opinion—the work domain can offer meaningful occasions for proving one's worth, increasing one's competences, sustaining self-esteem, and ultimately contributing to a full life besides important life domains such as family and social relations (see Chapter 10; Delle Fave, 2009; Page & Vella-Brodrick, 2009). Attributing meaning to one's job sustains in-role performance and job flexibility in terms of willingness to change (van den Heuvel, Demerouti, Schreurs, Bakker, & Schaufeli, 2009). Additionally, Delle Fave, Brdar, Freire, Vella-Brodrick, and Wissing (2010) found that work ranked second among the meaningful things cited by participants from seven western countries (Australia, Croatia, Germany, Italy, Portugal, Spain, and South Africa), but only sixth among the domains related to the definition of happiness. Recently, Linley, Harrington, and Garcea (2010) dedicated an edited book to the ways people can find meaning and purpose in work settings, by giving coherence and direction to their activities, and by aligning organizations' strategies to support individuals' fulfillment and well-being.

In line with these results, studies have shown that work represents a privileged area for retrieving optimal experiences (Csikszentmihalyi & Lefevre, 1989; Lefevre, 1988). Following the same format we use in other chapters, we will present major findings obtained by flow researchers in the work domain, stressing the peculiarities of the work experience compared to leisure, and highlighting personal, organizational, as well as cultural factors associated with flow at work. Attention will also be paid to the potential of work in supporting individuals' psychological selection and well-being, by funneling psychic and material resources into pursuing professional fulfillment. To exemplify this potential, we will provide some findings obtained from musicians and teachers.

8.2 The Quality of Experience Associated with Work: A Persistent Paradox

Understanding the quality of experience associated with work is a crucial issue, considering that work accounts for a substantial portion of individuals' daily lives in most countries (Csikszentmihalyi, 1997). Thanks to ESM online investigation, researchers have repeatedly found that work is characterized by below-average scores of affect and motivation, and simultaneously by high cognitive investment, high current stakes in the task at hand, and long-term goals. This finding was observed across a variety of professions and tasks including white-collar workers, managers, assembly-line workers (Csikszentmihalyi & Lefevre, 1989; Haworth & Hill, 1992; Lefevre, 1988), high school teachers (Bassi, Coppa, Sartori, & Delle Fave, 2008a), and professional rescuers (Sartori, 2010; Sartori, Massimini, & Delle Fave, 2009). All participants constantly reported an experience of engagement, concentration, and clear goals while working, but they did not seem to find it particularly enjoyable or motivating. This experiential profile contrasts with the one associated with leisure activities such as sports and hobbies, which are characterized by high motivation, cognitive engagement, but by below-average goals and stakes in the activity. In addition, the same occupation presents a different experiential profile when it is performed to get payment or out of voluntary reasons. In an Italian study comparing professionals and volunteers engaged in the same rescuing activities, results showed that the former reported lower levels of excitement, freedom, and wish to do the activities than the latter (Sartori, 2010; Sartori et al., 2009).

These findings are not surprising, given the compulsory nature of work. Moreover, a similar experiential profile is reported by young people while studying at school (see Table 5.2), thus suggesting common experiential characteristics across compulsory productive activities. However, flow researchers were taken aback when they analyzed the quality of work experience reported by participants in situations of perceived match between high challenges and high skills. As theoretically hypothesized, respondents reported higher scores in all the cognitive, affective, and motivational dimensions of experience, than on average during work tasks. Nonetheless, the values of affect and intrinsic motivation were quite below their overall weekly average (Bassi, 2008; Csikszentmihalyi & Lefevre, 1989; Delle Fave & Massimini, 2005; Haworth & Hill, 1992; Lefevre, 1988; Rheinberg, Manig, Kliegel, Engeser, & Vollmeyer, 2007; Schallberger & Pfister, 2001). The same result was also obtained analyzing participants' flow opportunities at work with flow questionnaire (FQ; Chapter 4). In a study comparing the psychological features of optimal experience in productive activities, structured leisure, interactions, and media use across cultures, Delle Fave (2007a) showed that besides a stable cognitive core characterizing all flow activity categories, productive activities were associated with lower excitement and enjoyment as well as lower wish to do the activity (see Chapter 5). The findings illustrated in Chapter 7 partially confirmed this trend from a global cross-cultural perspective. This phenomenon was labeled *work paradox* (Csikszentmihalyi & Lefevre, 1989; Csikszentmihalyi, 1990, 1997; Hektner, Schmidt, & Csikszentmihalyi, 2007): Although work proved to offer opportunities for optimal experience, across studies participants consistently reported to wish to be doing something else. In the attempt to explain such paradox, Csikszentmihalyi and Lefevre (1989) proposed that the obligatory nature of work masks the positive experience it engenders. In other words, in deciding whether they wish to work or not, individuals judge their desires by social conventions rather than by the reality of their feelings. Haworth and Hill (1992) focused more closely on the motivational aspects involved in the work paradox. In particular, they distinguished between individuals' wanting or having to perform an activity (intrinsic vs. extrinsic motivation) and their wishing to be doing something else. In their study with white-collar workers, they found that those individuals who reported that they had to do the ongoing work activity (i.e., perceived the extrinsic nature of work) and simultaneously reported that they would not rather be doing something else scored higher on psychological well-being than individuals who reported wanting to do the activity but wishing to be doing something else. Rheinberg et al. (2007) tackled the work paradox from the goal perspective. In line with theoretical assumptions and empirical research, goals were found to be a crucial component of optimal experience both at work and during free time. However, goals also had a negative effect on perceived happiness, which could partially account for the work paradox.

All these potential explanations require future investigation in order to shed light on the work paradox. As shown in Chapter 5, a family of optimal experiences exists based on the characteristics of associated activities (Delle Fave & Massimini, 2005). Whether the findings pertaining to work represent a paradox, a domain-specific characteristic or job-specific features, studies have found that optimal experience is highly susceptible to contingent situations (see also Chapter 7). Using multilevel techniques among both students and workers, researchers have highlighted that most variance in flow is attributable to situational characteristics compared to dispositional factors (Bassi & Delle Fave, 2009; Fullargar & Kelloway, 2009; Schmidt, Shernoff, & Csikszentmihalyi, 2007). This can partially explain why empirical evidence confirmed that flow is not a monolithic experience and that flow-related productive activities can be associated with both autonomous and controlled motivation. It is the task of future research to highlight implications of these findings in terms of people's psychological selection, as well as in relation to individual and social well-being.

8.2.1 Optimal Experience in Work and Leisure Across Professions

Studies conducted through ESM with participants involved in a variety of professions have also found that work—relative to leisure—represents the most frequent opportunity for optimal experience during an ordinary week in daily life.

This was true of white- and blue-collar workers, managers, engineers, teachers, and rescuers (Bassi et al., 2008a; Csikszentmihalyi & Lefevre, 1989; Delle Fave & Massimini, 2005; Sartori et al., 2009). In the comparative study between professional and volunteer rescuers, for example, findings showed that professionals most frequently associated rescuing activities with optimal experience, while volunteers reported more relaxation and anxiety (Sartori, 2010; Sartori et al., 2009). ESM results also showed that the specific type of occupation affected the workers' perception of flow. During work, managers and engineers spent more time in flow than clerical and assembly-line workers (Lefevre, 1988). More specifically, among line managers, activities such as planning and problem solving and evaluation—but not brainstorming—were predictive of optimal experience (Nielsen & Cleal, 2010).

Table 8.1 Percentages of selected optimal activities across professions (and sample characteristics)

	Physicians ($N = 48$) %	Craftsmen ($N = 68$) %	White-collar workers ($N = 50$) %	Blue-collar workers ($N = 29$) %	Cashiers ($N = 55$) %
Work	39.6	57.6	30	38	16.4
Leisure	43.8	36.4	54	34.6	74.5
Studying	6.3	1.5	8	3.4	1.8
Interactions	4.2	1.5	2	10.3	1.8
Spiritual practice[a]	4.2	1.5	4	–	3.6
Introspection	2.1	1.5	2	10.3	1.8
Personal care	–	–	–	3.4	–
Group *N*	60	78	66	55	60
Age	28–69	14–77	20–53	21–56	21–64
Gender	M = 47; F = 13	M = 35; F = 43	M = 38; F =28	M = 51; F = 4	M = 12; F = 48
% of flow[b]	80	87.2	75.8	52.7	91.7

Note. Group *N* refers to the overall sample sizes.
[a]It includes yoga, meditation, and religious activities.
[b]It refers to the percentage of participants recognizing a flow activity in their lives.

Within our databank gathered through FQ, participants by and large quoted work and leisure tasks in almost equal percentages (see Chapter 7; Delle Fave, 2007a). However, differences across professions were detected. Table 8.1 illustrates the optimal activities selected by different Italian professionals: physicians (surgeons, anesthesiologists, and gynecologists), craftsmen (knitters, goldsmiths, tailors, carpenters), clerks, blue-collar workers, and cashiers (working at post offices, banks, supermarkets, or cinemas).

First of all, groups differed in the number of individuals recognizing optimal experiences in their lives, with percentages ranging between 52.7% among blue collars and 91.7% among cashiers. A second major distinction between groups regarded the percentages of work and leisure activities associated with flow (in the examined samples, leisure included hobbies such as reading, playing an instrument, dancing, and sports such as playing soccer, sailing, raising flowers). Leisure prevailed among cashiers and white collars, whereas work predominated among craftsmen. As for physicians, their optimal activities were almost equally distributed between work and leisure, with a slight predominance of leisure. Among blue collars, work prevailed over leisure. However, these workers also reported relatively high percentages of answers related to interactions and introspection, which, together with leisure, showed that work was not a dominant life domain in which they retrieved opportunities for optimal experience.

Here are some of the descriptions participants reported of their optimal experience at work

> [Work] is a great pleasure and a personal satisfaction, wishing that it can be of help to someone (Surgeon).

> [Work] is an activity that involves me mentally and physically. And it is also a pleasant way to earn a living (Goldsmith).
>
> [Work] is being alone with myself, being in the company of my work, doing something I love and that makes me feel good (Carpenter).
>
> [Work] is a way to best employ my knowledge and my experience in order to face all the different situations I am daily confronted with (Skilled blue collar).
>
> [Work] is an activity not only to get remuneration but also to put my skills to the test and to be useful to others (Cashier at post office).

Overall, answers stressed the potential of work as an opportunity for putting one's skills and competence into practice, thus deriving satisfaction, self-actualization, as well as helping other people in the case of professionals dealing with patients or customers. Across groups, in the few occasions in which the economic aspects of work were mentioned, these were a kind of pleasant side effect of doing an activity one enjoyed carrying out. However, data also clearly showed that not all jobs offered the same opportunities of optimal experience.

8.3 Individual Characteristics, Job Resources, and Cultures

Differences in the opportunities for optimal experience at work can be related to individual characteristics. In a study among secondary-school teachers, for instance, Salanova, Bakker, and Llorens (2006) found that self-efficacy beliefs facilitated work-related flow. Among employees from a large discount electronics and appliance retailer, Eisenberger, Jones, Stinglhamber, Shanock, and Randall (2005) showed that the perception of high challenges and high skills (flow) was related to high positive mood, task interest, and performance among achievement-oriented participants. Demerouti (2006) found a mediating effect of conscientiousness between optimal experience and performance among employees from a variety of companies. More recently, Mäkikangas, Bakker, Aunola, and Demerouti (2009) showed that the burnout dimension of exhaustion was an important predictor of optimal experience, with low levels of exhaustion predicting high levels of flow.

Another interesting difference was found in relation to gender. In a US sample, Larson and Richards (1994) showed that work generally represented a far more important life area for men than for women. Compared to women, men reported their most intense experiences at work, both the positive and the negative ones, suggesting that genders may have different cognitive styles at work that result in differences in subjective experience. This finding is further substantiated by Koh (2005) who reported that, among men, affect was more negative at work than at home, whereas women reported comparable levels of affect at home and in the workplace. In an ESM longitudinal study with primiparous couples (see Chapter 10), Delle Fave and Massimini (2004a) showed that women were much more focused on child-related activities than their husbands who, in their turn, more frequently reported their optimal experiences at work.

Personal differences also play a role in the motivational area, in particular affecting the reasons why people chose their profession. The evaluation of this aspect

Table 8.2 Percentage distribution of job motivation across professions

	Physicians ($N = 57$) %	Craftsmen ($N = 73$) %	White-collar workers ($N = 66$) %	Blue-collar workers ($N = 55$) %	Cashiers ($N = 60$) %
Material needs	13.9	31.5	31	34.7	59
Status	2.8	–	–	–	–
Income	–	–	15.6	16.7	8.4
Personal choice/interest	70.8	42.7	37.9	37.1	8.4
Previous studies	1.4	4.2	7.8	3.9	3.6
Family	1.4	13.6	4.9	3.9	3.6
Social relations	5.6	1	2.8	2.5	9.6
Working conditions	4.2	7.3	–	1.2	7.2
N answers	72	96	103	78	83

can shed light on the links between self-determination in starting one's career and the perception of optimal experience at work. Table 8.2 illustrates the job motivations that were provided by the groups of workers we introduced in Section 8.2.1. Participants were asked to answer the question in the life theme questionnaire: "Why did you choose your job?"

Results showed that cashiers—who reported a low percentage of flow in their occupation—quoted material pressures and needs (i.e., extrinsic motivation) as their most frequent reason for choosing their job. On the contrary, physicians primarily quoted personal choice (i.e., intrinsic motivation). For white collars, blue collars, and craftsmen, personal choice and material needs were mentioned in similar percentages. Income represented an additional relevant extrinsic motivation quoted by workers. As shown in Section 8.2, work as optimal activity can be associated with both intrinsic and extrinsic motivations. However, in particular among cashiers, predominance of extrinsic motivation may undermine the opportunities for optimal experience at work.

Besides personal characteristics, job resources were also investigated in relation to optimal experience at work. Once again, the answers provided by our participants concerning the most positive and negative situations they experienced at work will help better understand the crucial areas that can favor optimal experience at work.

As shown in Table 8.3, most professionals—physicians, white and blue collars, and cashiers—prominently quoted autonomy and positive relations among the most positive situations experienced at the workplace. By contrast, craftsmen rarely reported positive relations and, following autonomy, they referred to the perception of challenges. Among the negative situations, relations were the most frequent category reported by cashiers and blue collars, followed by work overload. Among white collars, these two categories accounted for equal percentages. For physicians and craftsmen, overload was by far the most frequent negative work situation.

Other studies investigated the role of job resources in favoring optimal experience through the Job Characteristic Model (JCM; Hackman & Oldham, 1980).

Table 8.3 Percentage distribution of positive and negative situations at work across professions

	Physicians %	Craftsmen %	White-collar workers %	Blue-collar workers %	Cashiers %
Positive situations					
Specific tasks	–	–	14	23.9	5.4
Challenge	25.4	42	22.1	12.7	10.7
Autonomy	35.4	49.4	31.4	30.1	31.5
Positive relations	36.2	8.6	31.4	28.5	47
Other	3.1	–	1.6	4.8	5.4
N answers	130	81	86	63	149
Negative situations					
Overload	45.7	45.6	35.3	29.1	24.7
Constraints	19.7	24.6	20.8	16.7	14.8
Negative relations	29.2	24.6	35.5	43.8	53.5
Other	4.7	5.3	8.6	10.4	7
N answers	127	57	82	48	142

The JCM identifies five main job characteristics influencing workers' attitudes and behavior: (1) skill variety—the degree to which the job requires different activities and skills to carry out the task; (2) autonomy—the extent to which the worker has independent discretion in determining the schedule and process of work; (3) task identity—the extent to which the job requires completion of a whole and identifiable piece of work; (4) task significance—the degree to which the job has a meaningful impact on other people; (5) feedback—the degree to which the worker is provided with information concerning how well she is performing. Job resources have motivational potential because they make employees' work meaningful, hold them responsible for work processes and outcomes, and provide them with information about the actual results of their work activities. Demerouti (2006) computed a motivating potential score (MPS) of a job, using an additive score for these job characteristics measured with the Job Diagnostic Survey (Hackman & Oldham, 1980). In her research with employees from various companies, she found that MPS was positively related with and predictive of flow at work. By analyzing single job characteristics among architects students engaged in studio work, Fullagar and Kelloway (2009) specifically found that skill variety and autonomy—but not task identity, task significance, and feedback—were significant predictors of flow. In a study conducted with music teachers, Bakker (2005) analyzed job resources such as social support and supervisory coaching, besides autonomy and feedback. He found that these variables had a positive relationship with the balance between challenges and skills, and that this balance, in turn, predicted participants' frequency of flow.

Additional job resources that proved to be associated with optimal experience were opportunities for professional development (Mäkikangas et al., 2009), innovation orientation, rules orientation (i.e., the extent to which the behavior of organizational members is regulated by formal norms and rules), and goals orientation (i.e., the extent to which activities and behaviors are oriented toward the attainment of previously established objectives) (Salanova et al., 2006). By contrast, applying ESM to line managers from a private accountancy firm and a public elder care organization, Nielsen and Cleal (2010) showed that the stable job characteristics of role clarity, influence (autonomy vs. control), and cognitive demands did not predict flow at work. Instead, differences emerged between organizations, with line managers in elder care experiencing flow more often than accountancy line managers.

All the findings we have thus far presented primarily regarded different professions and different tasks irrespective of the cultural origin of the participants. As a matter of fact, all studies were carried out in western countries including Italy, Denmark, Germany, the Netherlands, Spain, Switzerland, the United Kingdom, and the United States, which by and large share similar post-industrial service economies, work histories, and policies. Even though the western model is gradually spreading around the world, cultures can differ in the meaning and value they attribute to work. As shown in the introduction, in western cultures work has primarily become synonymous with duty and constraints: It is a means to earn one's living which is firmly opposed to free time as a precious occasion to relax from work and to engage in activities that can be conducive to self-actualization. While data have partly disconfirmed such a dichotomous view by showing the potential of work as optimal activity and as source of personal fulfillment, they also detected the high frequency of leisure among the selected self-reported optimal activities.

As maintained by Parker (1997) and as empirically shown in Section 8.2.1, the relationship between work and leisure is not homogenous within a given society, as it primarily depends on people's occupations. However, in our cross-cultural analysis—which is extensively presented in Chapter 7—we also detected differences in the percentages of work and leisure that can be attributed to cultural diversity. These differences can be related to the conceptualization of work and leisure, as sustained by Csikszentmihalyi (1990). In some cultures, work is a fundamental part of daily living, which is not opposed to leisure. In our studies, we analyzed traditional cultures in Northern Italy undergoing modernization (Delle Fave & Massimini, 1988, 1991, 1996; Massimini, Delle Fave, & Borri Gaspardin, 1992). Participants comprised the "elderly generation" which was not contaminated by modernization pressures and lived of the fruits of their work as farmers, peasants, and craftsmen. Findings showed that traditional tasks such as tilling the land, knitting, raising the cattle, growing vegetables were the most pervasive optimal activities. These participants engaged in complex challenging activities that kept them closely related to their natural environment and contributed to their satisfaction and well-being. Traditional activities have been shown to account for the high frequency of work-related optimal experiences also among participants belonging to a variety of cultures, such as Gypsies, Navajos, and Indonesians (Delle Fave & Massimini, 2004b; Delle Fave, 1999; Delle Fave, Bassi, & Massimini, 2003; Chapter 7). These activities clearly differ according to the local cultural heritage, but they all seem to present common characteristics such as complexity and challenge. They also require dexterity, imply a definite visible outcome (a crop, an artifact such as a woolen sweater, a carved utensil), and are often transmitted by parents or relatives, thus maintaining a strong connection among family members. In these traditional communities, leisure is more rarely reported as a source of optimal experience because there is no such strong dichotomy between work and leisure. As suggested by Csikszentmihalyi (1997), international data seem to hint that a society begins to rely heavily on leisure—especially on passive leisure—only when it has become incapable of offering meaningful productive occupation to its members.

8.4 Flow at Work and Individuals' and Organizations' Well-Being

In the wake of the positive psychology movement, great emphasis is currently being placed on identifying the factors promoting well-being at work, and their potential contribution to individuals' overall levels of well-being and to organizations' functioning (Linley et al., 2010; Page & Vella-Brodrick, 2009). Bakker (2008) found a positive relationship between flow at work and job satisfaction. Studies also showed that retrieving optimal experience in work activities enhances positive mood as an outcome of eudaimonic processes (Eisenberger et al., 2005; Fullargar & Kelloway, 2009; Lefevre, 1988). In particular, Fullagar and Kelloway (2009) tested the causal direction of the relationship between flow and mood using the lagged measures of these variables gathered longitudinally with ESM. Results suggested that lagged flow was predictive of mood, but that lagged mood was not associated with later flow.

Other studies have highlighted the role of optimal experience in promoting workers' performance at different levels, including both in- and extra-role tasks. In-role performance refers to the officially required outcomes and behaviors that directly serve the goals of the organization; extra-role performance comprises discretionary behaviors that promote the effective functioning of an organization without necessarily having a direct influence on an employee's productivity. Demerouti (2006) found that flow predicted both kinds of performances among conscientious employees. From a different point of view, Eisenberger et al. (2005) found that achievement-oriented employees perceiving high skills and high challenges in their occupations more frequently engaged in organizational spontaneity, namely extra-role behaviors such as making constructive suggestions, enhancing one's own knowledge and skills in ways that can help the organization, protecting it from potential problems, and helping co-workers. Salanova and her colleagues (2006) identified an upward spiral between flow, and personal and organizational resources in a two-wave study with teachers: Not only did resources facilitate work-related flow; work-related flow in turn had a positive influence on building resources over time. Similar results were obtained by Mäkikangas et al. (2009) in a three-wave follow-up study with employees of an employment agency. Both the levels and the changes in job resources and flow were found to be positively associated; in particular, the greater the increase in job resources across the three measurements, the greater the increase in flow across the same time period and vice versa. These results attest to the dynamic nature of optimal experience through the perceived high challenges and high skills relation (as shown in Chapter 3), to its crucial role in growth in competence and complexity, and to its contribution to the organization's human capital.

Finding flow at work has also been shown to promote people's adaptation to new living conditions. In this respect, Delle Fave and Bassi (2009) analyzed a group of first-generation immigrants who moved to Italy from Africa, India, South America, and Eastern Europe. Findings showed that the occurrence of optimal experiences, the features of the associated activities, as well as participants' perceived current challenges and future goals were primarily connected to the life opportunities offered by the hosting country, along with participants' cultural distance and length of stay (see also Chapter 13). In general, however, having a complex and satisfactory occupation that matched personal work training and skills facilitated the retrieval of optimal experience in the hosting country, thus giving continuation to one's life theme or planning it anew in a different country. Unfortunately, participants did not often find occupations suitable to their skills, and took up jobs that seldom provided them with flow occasions. This was the case of a group of Eastern European women who primarily found jobs as assistants to elderly people or as housemaids in Italian families, but who had worked as specialized professionals in their home countries (primarily as teachers) (Fianco, 2006). These participants reported work as their most frequent category of optimal experience at home, followed by reading. By contrast, in Italy, they mainly quoted social and family relations as predominant optimal activities.

Optimal experience at work can also have far-reaching implications at the social level, impacting on other people's survival and physical well-being. This phenomenon can primarily be seen among health professionals or teachers—so-called helping professionals—who, respectively, play a crucial role in promoting individuals' physical well-being, and in the transmission of culture to the future generations (Delle Fave & Massimini, 2003). Findings obtained from teachers will be discussed in detail in Section 8.5. As for health professionals, studies showed that the quality of experience they associated with their job influenced work performance, relationships with patients, and ultimately patients' well-being (Delle Fave, 2006). In particular, physicians' empathy and positive disposition toward patients fostered patients' satisfaction with consequently positive outcomes in the domains of both prevention and treatment (Majani, Pierobon, Giardini, & Callegari, 2000). Conversely, physicians reporting burnout symptoms were self-critical concerning their accomplishments, frequently perceiving suboptimal patient care practices (Shanafelt, Bradley, Wipf, & Back, 2002). In a study conducted by Delle Fave and Massimini (2003) among surgeons, anesthesiologists, and gynecologists (see also Table 8.1), over one-third of the participants associated work with optimal experience, mainly referring to performing a surgical operation, doing research work, and interacting with patients. Participants reported personal choice and interest (i.e., intrinsic motivation) for choosing the medical profession (Table 8.2). Among the most positive work experience, they quoted autonomy and good relationships with colleagues and patients; among the most negative experiences they mentioned work overload and conflicts with colleagues (Table 8.3). Similar results were obtained among nurses and delivery assistants (Delle Fave, 1996): 26% of them named work as their most pervasive optimal activity and personal choice and interest as main reason for choosing their jobs (54% of the answers). These samples represent clear examples of the importance of associating flow with activities that do not only provide growth-conducive experiences to single individuals, but also contribute to the well-being of the community as a whole (Massimini & Delle Fave, 2000). Findings additionally stress the importance of promoting a good working environment in which overload and relational conflicts do not undermine professionals' as well as patients' well-being.

8.5 Work as Core of Psychological Selection

As work generally accounts for a large share of individuals' daily life, we welcome the finding that occupations can offer meaningful opportunities for optimal experiences. Work can be perceived as an important domain in which to invest one's competences and efforts, to experience personal rewards, and to pursue well-being. It usually represents one of the many aspects of daily life, alongside other meaningful domains such as family, relations, and leisure. However, it can also become the center of individuals' psychological selection, thus taking on a fundamental and pervasive role in one's life (Delle Fave & Massimini, 2005; Massimini & Delle Fave, 2000). In our databank of workers, we have observed that, when this happens, the pattern between work and leisure is characterized by extension (Parker, 1997), that is, by mutual influences in terms of skill development and levels of satisfaction between different life areas. In this concluding section, we will discuss work as core of psychological selection in two groups of participants: musicians and teachers. Musicians represent the case in which a typical leisure activity becomes a full-time profession, blurring the line between work and leisure. Teachers exemplify the case of individuals who have centered their psychological selection on cultural transmission, extending its influence to all life domains as well as to students' potential engagement in school activities.

8.5.1 Career Building: The Case of Musicians

To investigate the role of optimal experience in the construction of one's career and life theme, we collected data from a group of individuals attending or having attended musical schools and classes (Massimini & Delle Fave, 1995). Such training requires high personal investment, discipline, and the commitment to devote many hours to musical practice every day. Participants' main instruments were the piano (53.2%), strings (20.3%), and winds (12.7%). Information about their psychological selection was gathered through flow questionnaire and life theme questionnaire (see Chapter 4).

As shown in Table 8.4, all participants except one recognized the occurrence of flow in their daily lives, and associated with it three activities on average. The most frequent optimal domain was sports and hobbies, followed by studying, and media.

Table 8.4 Percentages of optimal activities among teachers and musicians (and sample characteristics)

	Teachers ($N = 327$) %	Musicians ($N = 229$) %
Work	53.2	6.1
Sports and hobbies	13.1	47.2
Reading	13.1	6.6
Media	3.7	10.4
Studying	7.3	13.5
Interactions	4.9	7.8
Spiritual practice[a]	3.1	0.9
Introspection	1.5	5.3
Personal care	–	2.2
Group *N*	184	97
Age	26–63	15–51
Gender	M = 35; F = 149	M = 55; F = 42
% of flow[b]	90.1	99

Note. N = number of reported activities; Group *N* refers to the overall sample sizes.
[a]It includes yoga and meditation.
[b]It refers to the percentage of participants recognizing a flow activity in their lives.

Across categories, music accounted for more than half of the reported activities (53.3%). It was cultivated through work, learning, reading, and the use of media. However, it was more frequently reported as leisure, with answers such as playing, composing, improvising in which no direct reference was made to either work or study. When asked to select the activity associated with the most pervasive optimal experience, 73% of the participants reported playing music, describing it as a way to externalize one's "inner representations" giving substance to contents, which cannot be expressed verbally

> Composing music is the possibility to pour out acoustic sensations and make them as real as possible (Woman, 24 years old).

> Playing the violin is an activity that makes my soul pour out something which couldn't come out in other activities (Woman, 19 years old).

Such intense self-expression requires discipline and hard work in order to learn and master the techniques that make playing possible

> Studying a piece of music means concentration, fractioning the piece into many parts, studying single parts with various time intervals (i.e. breaks to rest, but primarily to ponder on what I am doing). With time one can succeed in knowing and mastering the piece. The goal is to reach unity between me and the piece (Man, 18 years old).

> My hands, the score, the keys, the room do not exist anymore; only emotions within you exist and come to surface in the shape of sounds. You and music become one, because music is exactly what you are expressing. I am used to playing by heart, because this process is thus facilitated. I never look at my hands, only for specific passages. I don't look at anything. Maybe I look inside me ... I don't think of what I am doing ... It takes years and years of studying to gain the necessary technical skills so that hands will obtain the sonority you want (Woman, 22 years old).

Music was also described as an activity permeating all dimensions of one's life

> To me, studying means shutting myself up in a room, alone, to concentrate as much as I can, and the longer I can, my violin and me. My way of life is shaped by these activities: Studying music, listening to it, playing the violin and the piano make up all my day, not considering the hours I spend at school ... Playing and studying the violin are for me extremely important; I am not particularly ambitious, but I am sure that I will keep following this track in the future (Woman, 16 years old).

As described by participants, and as shown in various studies (Byrne, MacDonald, & Carlton, 2003; Csikszentmihalyi, 1988; Macdonald, Byrne, & Carlton, 2006), music represents an ideal activity in which to retrieve optimal experience as it can offer challenges of virtually unlimited complexity. These challenges, however, can be seized only if participants invest in it all their mental and physical resources. Indeed, the role of music as the core of psychological selection further emerged in the analysis of our participants' current challenges and future goals, reported in Table 8.5.

Among current challenges, participants primarily mentioned the categories of work, study, and personal growth. Again music was the main challenge across categories (45.6% of the answers)

> My main challenge has been and will always be, with absolute certainty, my concert activity. Without this certainty, I wouldn't be spurred to find a job, and it is thus of capital importance. For this, it is necessary to be true to myself and to have courage. To face this challenge, I have adopted studying methods which do not allow me to get distracted; in the future I will look for new and more practical studying techniques. In any case, it is important to deeply believe in what I do, feeling it as a categorical imperative (Man, 27 years old).

Among future goals, work prevailed, followed by family and study. Music accounted for 47.8% of all the answers across categories, highlighting its pervasiveness in the life theme

> I would like to teach music to others, and to spread it among the many, because I love it. It will take me all my life to reach this goal, since in music you NEVER stop learning; you need courage, passion, perseverance and resignation to follow this track. Try to imagine a world without music: you will understand by yourself. Music is a universal language, like love (Woman, 16 years old).

Table 8.5 Percentage distributions of current challenges and future goals among musicians

	Challenges	Goals
Free time	1.1	5
Work	33.7	43.8
Family	8.7	26.3
Personal growth	16.3	5.6
Studying	35.9	13
Health	2.2	–
Material goods	1.1	5.6
Social commitment	1.1	0.6
N answers	92	160

8.5.2 Teachers and Cultural Transmission: The Centrality of Relationships

Much research has been carried out on teachers' opportunities for optimal experiences at work, in light of the relevant role these professionals play in transmitting cultural information to students (Bakker, 2005; Bassi, 2008; Bassi, Fianco, Preziosa, Steca, & Delle Fave, 2008b; Delle Fave & Massimini, 2003; Morgan, 2005). As previously reported, finding flow while teaching has also been related to an upward spiral of personal and organizational resources that teachers can implement in their daily working tasks (Salanova et al., 2006).

Specifically, our research group has investigated various samples of primary- and secondary-school teachers coming from different Italian regions. All our studies repeatedly identified an extremely high frequency of optimal experience in working tasks among these professionals. In particular, in a pilot study with ESM we found that teachers associated their work activities with optimal experience in 40.1% of the weekly self-reports (Bassi et al., 2008a).

Data gathered with the flow questionnaire confirmed this evidence. For exemplification purposes, Table 8.4 illustrates the percentage distribution of optimal activities in a group of Italian teachers (Delle Fave, 2007b). As many as 90.1% of the participants retrieved optimal experience and, on average, they associated with it two activities each. Teaching accounted for more than half of the answers (53.2%), and 61.2% of the respondents selected it as the opportunity for the most pervasive optimal experiences. No other professional group studied with these instruments associated work with flow in such a high percentage (see data in Table 8.1 for comparison).

Here are some of the descriptions provided by participants

> Teaching is discussing with pupils, working with them at both the didactic and at the human levels (Woman, 56 years old).
>
> I have this experience when I am immersed in research or in my work; time goes by, the world keeps living, but I am 'outside of it'; by research I mean studying and broadening my knowledge by acquiring information and to connect it to previous experiences (Woman, 27 years old).
>
> To give students what I think is best (Woman, 50 years old).

Among optimal activities, besides work, teachers reported reading, other hobbies such as painting, drawing, and creative writing, followed by studying. All these findings point to the central role of the acquisition and exchange of information in participants' psychological selection and construction of a life theme. Besides work, teachers primarily devoted their attention to books, artistic hobbies, and studying. Their profession allowed them to cultivate activities that were sources of intellectual pleasure, and to transmit love for knowledge to their students.

To delve deeper into the teachers' experience at work, Table 8.6 reports the most positive and negative aspects the participants identified in their profession.

The majority of answers clustered in the category "relations" for both positive and negative aspects. Positive interactions primarily took place with students,

Table 8.6 Percentage distribution of positive and negative situations at work among teachers

Positive situations	%
Specific tasks	18.7
Challenge	5.7
Autonomy	4.9
Positive relations	62.6
with students	*42.3*
with colleagues	*8.9*
not specified	*11.4*
N answers	246
Negative situations	%
Pressures	17.9
Bureaucracy/constraints	17.9
Boredom/routine	5.8
Negative relations	57.4
with students	*13.5*
with colleagues	*38.6*
not specified	*5.3*
Other	1
N answers	207

whereas negative ones with colleagues. These data clearly stress the relational nature of the teaching profession, as well as teachers' commitment to education and knowledge transmission (Bassi, Lombardi, & Delle Fave, 2006; Delle Fave & Massimini, 2003). The importance attributed to relations, however, makes teachers more susceptible to the negative implications of possible conflicts with colleagues, as shown in a great number of studies investigating the causes of teachers' burnout (Guglielmi & Tatrow, 1998; Hakanen, Bakker, & Schaufeli, 2006).

Interesting results on teachers' psychological selection were further obtained administering the eudaimonic and hedonic happiness investigation (EHHI, Delle Fave et al., 2010) to a group of 185 teachers (159 women, 26 men, aged 29–64), employed at primary and secondary institutions (Bassi et al., 2008b). After family, participants quoted work among their most important goals, the meaningful things in their lives, and contrary to other investigated samples, also among the most frequent occasions of intense happiness. Additionally, results showed that participants who attached to work high levels of meaningfulness and happiness scored higher in life satisfaction than those participants who did not. Over and above data gathered with FQ and life theme questionnaire, these findings stress that eudaimonic and hedonic components are complementary aspects of happiness in teachers' experience at work, making their profession an enjoyable and engaging component of their lives.

As happens for other helping professionals, the well-being of teachers at work has far-reaching effects on students' concept assimilation, adjustment at school, and overall development. As will be reported in Chapter 11, Bakker (2005) found a positive relationship between teachers' and students' flow. He showed that optimal experience can cross over from teachers to their students on the basis of emotional contagion. Indeed, some of our teachers reported their own professors at school as important positive influences in their lives, as they played a crucial role in transmitting them love for knowledge, and shaping their choices

> [Among my positive life influences] my teachers, two in particular. The one teaching Italian who made me appreciate the pleasure of knowledge (and hence of studying); and the one of drawing who 'sensitized' me to art in its various expressions (Woman, 31 years old).

However, our simultaneous ESM assessment of students' and teachers' experience at school showed that teachers mostly report flow while teaching (40.1% of the self-reports), whereas students mostly report apathy while listening to classes and taking notes (24%), followed by arousal (19.4%) and optimal experience (16.2%) (Bassi et al., 2008a). As previously shown, autonomy plays an important role in fostering optimal experience, both among professionals, and among students. The observed experiential differences between teachers and youths can thus be related to varying degrees of perceived autonomy. Laudadío and colleagues (2009) explored this topic among university professors who were administered the optimal experience survey (see Chapter 4). The authors found that teaching styles had an impact on the retrieval of optimal experience. Professors with a so-called transitive or teacher-centered style reported more flow than professors with a participating/reflexive student-centered style. In particular, differences concerned the affective and cognitive dimensions of optimal experience. On the one hand, professors with a teacher-centered style reported clear-cut goals whose achievement could be easily verified, and could be source of positive affect and reward. On the other hand, professors with a student-centered style did not limit teaching to transmission of knowledge. This could make their achievement evaluation more difficult, thus negatively influencing the cognitive and affective dimensions of their experience during classes. According to the authors, these professors seemed to have given up the possibility of having a more gratifying experience in teaching for the sake of setting more ambitious goals to their students. However, no differences were found in the flow components of achievement and skills based on teaching style. This suggests that teachers, in spite of setting distinctive (teacher- or student-oriented) goals, globally reported feeling able to meet them.

8.6 Concluding Remarks

Findings in this chapter have shown that the association of optimal experience with work activities can contribute to individuals' well-being and performance. Considering, however, international economic crises as well as disparities and inequalities in work treatment and security, much still needs to be done to provide workers with meaningful opportunities for high concentration, engagement, and personal initiative. In particular, not all jobs provide workers with the same personal rewards we have, for example, found among musicians and teachers. The more individuals are alienated from the products of their work and engage in repetitive and simple tasks, the more they develop work-related disorders and illnesses that undermine their quality of life (Linley et al., 2010; Massimini & Delle Fave,

2000). It is the goal of the international community to pursue "full employment and decent work for all" (ILO 2009); likewise, it is the goal of all occupational psychologists and social workers to support people in identifying their privileged areas of skills in career choice and to orient them toward opportunities for complex experiences which can extend beyond the working sectors and contribute to their overall psychological and physical well-being.

References

Bakker, A. B. (2005). Flow among music teachers and their students: The crossover of peak experiences. *Journal of Vocational Behavior, 66*, 26–44.

Bakker, A. B. (2008). The work-related flow inventory: Construction and initial validation of the WOLF. *Journal of Vocational Behavior, 72*, 400–414.

Bassi, M. (2008). Optimal experience, motivational orientations and the work paradox among teachers. Paper presented at *4th European Conference on Positive Psychology*, Book of Abstracts, 59. Opatija, Croatia, 2–4 July.

Bassi, M., Coppa, R., Sartori, R., & Delle Fave, A. (2008a). Condividere benessere per educare al benessere: l'esperienza quotidiana di insegnanti e studenti [sharing well-being to educate about well-being: Daily experience of teachers and students]. In C. Guido G. Vernì (a cura di), *Educazione al benessere e nuova professionalità docente. Ricerca, profili, riflessioni* (pp. 19–66). Bari: Ufficio Scolastico Regionale Puglia.

Bassi, M., & Delle Fave, A. (2009). Self-determination and optimal experience at school: Joining perspectives. Paper presented at *1st International Positive Psychology Conference*, Book of Abstracts, 43. Philadelphia, US, 18–21 June.

Bassi, M., Fianco, A., Preziosa, A., Steca, P., & Delle Fave, A. (2008b). La psicologia positiva e lo studio del benessere e della felicità: Una ricerca pilota con un gruppo di insegnanti [positive psychhology and the study of well-being and happiness: A pilot study with a group of teachers]. In C. Guido & G. Vernì (a cura di), *Educazione al benessere e nuova professionalità docente. Ricerca, profili, riflessioni* (pp. 133–164). Bari: Ufficio Scolastico Regionale Puglia.

Bassi, M., Lombardi, M., & Delle Fave, A. (2006). La professione relazionale dell'insegnante [the teacher's relational profession]. In O. Albanese (Ed.), *Disabilità, integrazione e formazione degli insegnanti. Esperienze e riflessioni* (pp. 193–205). Bergamo: Junior.

Byrne, C., MacDonald, R., & Carlton, L. (2003). Assessing creativity in musical compositions: Flow as an assessment tool. *British Journal of Musical Education, 20*, 277–290.

Calegari, P., & Massimini, F. (1978). *Psicologia dell'artefatto normativo sociale* [Psychology of the social normative artifact]. Milano: Franco Angeli.

Csikszentmihalyi, M. (1988). Motivation and creativity: Toward a synthesis of structural and energistic approaches to cognition. *New Ideas in Psychology, 6*, 159–176.

Csikszentmihalyi, M. (1990). *Flow: The psychology of optimal experience*. New York: Harper & Row.

Csikszentmihalyi, M. (1997). *Finding flow: The psychology of engagement wit everyday life*. New York: Basic Books.

Csikszentmihalyi, M., & Lefevre, J. (1989). Optimal experience in work and leisure. *Journal of Personality and Social Psychology, 56*, 815–822.

Delle Fave, A. (1996). Flow e attività tradizionali femminili: La continuità nella selezione e ritenzione delle informazioni [flow and traditional female activities: Continuity in the selection and acquisition of information]. In F. Massimini, P. Inghilleri, & A. Delle Fave (Eds.), *La selezione psicologica umana – teoria e metodo d'analisi* (pp. 599–614). Milano: Coop. Libraria IULM.

Delle Fave, A. (1999). Individual development and bicultural identity: The navajo way. In A. Delle Fave and F. Meli (Eds.), *Modernization and cultural identity* (pp. 49–68). Milano: Edizioni dell'Arco.
Delle Fave, A. (2006). The impact of subjective experience on the quality of life. a central issue for health professionals. In M. Csikszentmihalyi & I. Csikszentmihalyi (Eds.), *A life worth living: Contributions to positive psychology* (pp. 165–181). New York: Oxford University Press.
Delle Fave, A. (2007a). Individual development and community empowerment: Suggestions from studies on optimal experience. In J. Haworth & G. Hart (Eds.), *Well-being: Individual, community, and societal perspectives* (pp. 41–56). London: Palgrave McMillan.
Delle Fave, A. (2007b). Ottimizzare l'esperienza di docenti e studenti. Teorie, ricerche, proposte [optimizing the experience of teachers and students. Theories, research, proposals]. In C. Cosimo & G. Vernì (Eds.), *Scuola attraente e cultural del benessere. La scuola che promuove salute* (pp. 27–70). Bari: Ufficio Scolastico Regionale Puglia.
Delle Fave, A. (2009). Optimal experience and meaning: Which relationship? *Psychological Topics, 18*, 285–302.
Delle Fave, A., & Bassi, M. (2009). Sharing optimal experiences and promoting good community life in a multicultural society. *Journal of Positive Psychology, 4*, 280–289.
Delle Fave, A., Bassi, M., & Massimini, F. (2003). Coping with boundaries: The quality of daily experience of Rom nomads in Europe. *Psychology and developing societies, 15*, 87–102.
Delle Fave, A., Brdar, I., Freire, T., Vella-Brodrick, D. A., & Wissing, M. P. (2010). The eudaimonic and hedonic components of happiness: Qualitative and quantitative findings. *Journal of Happiness Studies*, published online 4 May 2010.
Delle Fave, A., & Massimini, F. (1988). Modernization and the changing context of flow in work and leisure. In M. Csikszentmihalyi, & I. Csikszentmihalyi (Eds.), *Optimal experience: Psychological studies of flow in consciousness* (pp. 193–213). New York: Cambridge University Press.
Delle Fave, A., & Massimini, F. (1991). Modernization and the quality of daily experience in a southern Italy village. In N. Bleichrodt & P. J. D. Drenth (eds.), *Contemporary issues in cross-cultural psychology* (pp. 110–119). Amsterdam: Swets & Zeitlinger B.V.
Delle Fave, A., & Massimini, F. (1996). Modernizzazione e fruizione dei media: Dati su due comunità italiane [modernization and use of media: Data from two Italian communities]. *Ikon, 32*, 95–117.
Delle Fave, A., & Massimini, F. (2003). Optimal experience in work and leisure among teachers and physicians: Individual and bio-cultural implications. *Leisure Studies, 22*, 323–342.
Delle Fave, A., & Massimini, F. (2004a). Parenthood and the quality of experience in daily life: A longitudinal study. *Social Indicators Research, 67*, 75–106.
Delle Fave, A., & Massimini, F. (2004b). The cross-cultural investigation of optimal experience. *Ricerche di Psicologia, 27*, 79–102.
Delle Fave, A., & Massimini, F. (2005). The investigation of optimal experience and apathy: Developmental and psychosocial implications. *European Psychologist, 10*, 264–274.
Demerouti, E. (2006). Job characteristics, flow, and performance: The moderating role of conscientiousness. *Journal of Occupational Health Psychology, 11*, 266–280.
Eisenberger, R., Jones, J. R., Stinglhamber, F., Shanock, L., & Randall, A. T. (2005). Flow experiences at work: For high need achievers alone? *Journal of Organizational Behavior, 26*, 755–775.
Fianco, A. (2006). *Migrazione e qualità dell'esperienza: Uno studio con experience sampling method* [Migration and quality of experience: A study with experience sampling method]. Doctoral Dissertation, University of Milano.
Fullagar, C. J., & Kelloway, E. K. (2009). 'Flow' at work: An experience sampling approach. *Journal of Occupational Health Psychology, 82*, 595–615.
Guglielmi, R., & Tatrow, K. (1998). Occupational stress, burnout, and health in teachers: A methodological and theoretical analysis. *Review of Educational Research, 68*, 61–99.
Hackman, J. R., & Oldham, G. R. (1980). *Work redesign*. Reading, MA: Addison-Wesley.

Hakanen, J. J., Bakker, A. B., & Schaufeli, W. B. (2006). Burnout and work engagement among teachers. *Journal of School Psychology, 43*, 495–513.

Haworth, J., & Hill, S. (1992). Work, leisure and psychological well-being in a sample of young adults. *Journal of Community and Applied Social Psychology, 2*, 147–160.

Hektner, J. M., Schmidt, J., & Csikszentmihalyi, M. (2007). *Experience sampling method: Measuring the quality of everyday life*. Thousand Oaks, CA: Sage.

International Labour Office (ILO). (2009). *Guide to the new millennium development goals employment indicators: Including the full set of decent work indicators*. Geneva: ILO.

Koh, C. (2005). The everyday emotional experiences of husbands and wives. In B. Schneider & L. J. Waite (Eds.), Being together working apart: Dual-career families and the work-life balance (pp. 169–189). New York: Cambridge University Press.

Larson, R. W., & Richards, M. H. (1994). *Divergent realities: The emotional lives of mothers, fathers, and adolescents*. New York: Basic Books.

Laudadío, J., Tezón, M., & Mesurado, B. (2009). Estilos de enseñanza universitaria y su relación con la experiencia subjetiva de los profesores [university-teaching styles and their relations with the subjective experience of professors]. In M. C. Richaud & J. E. Moreno (Eds.), *Investigación en ciencias del comportamento* (pp. 423–432). Buenos Aires: Ciipme-Conicet.

Le Blanc, P., de Jonge, J., & Schaufeli, W. (2008). Job stress and occupational health. In N. Chmiel (Ed.), *An introduction to work and organizational psychology: A european perspective* (pp. 119–147). Malden, MA: Blackwell.

Lefevre, J. (1988). Flow and the quality of experience during work and leisure. In M. Csikszentmihalyi, & I. Csikszentmihalyi (Eds.), *Optimal experience: Psychological studies of flow in consciousness* (pp. 307–318). New York: Cambridge University Press.

Linley, P. A., Harrington, S., & Garcea, N. (2010). *Oxford handbook of positive psychology and work*. New York: Oxford University Press.

Macdonald, R., Byrne, C., & Carlton, L. (2006). Creativity and flow in musical composition: An empirical investigation. *Psychology of Music, 34*, 292–306.

Majani, G., Pierobon, A., Giardini, A., & Callegari, S. (2000). Satisfaction profile (Sat_P) in 732 patients: Focus on subjectivity in HRQoL assessment. *Psychology and Health, 15*, 409–422.

Massimini, F., & Delle Fave, A. (1995). Qualità dell'esperienza e coltivazione di attività musicali [quality of experience and cultivation of musical activities]. *Comunicazioni Scientifiche di Psicologia Generale, 14*, 157–180.

Massimini, F., & Delle Fave, A. (2000). Individual development in a bio-cultural perspective. *American Psychologist, 55*, 24–33.

Massimini, F., Delle Fave, A., & Borri Gaspardin, M. (1992). Televisione e qualità dell'esperienza soggettiva: l'integrazione tra dati qualitativi e qualitativi [television and quality of subjective experience: Integrating qualitative and quantitative data]. *Ikon, 24*, 5–29.

Morgan, S. J. (2005). *JobLAB: A study into the experience of teaching*. Crawley: CrossLight.

Mäkikangas, A., Bakker, A. B., Aunola, K., & Demerouti, E. (2010). Job resources and flow at work: Modeling the relationship via latent growth curve and mixture model methodology. *Journal of Occupational Health Psychology, 83*, 795–814.

Nielsen, K., & Cleal, B. (2010). Predicting flow at work: Investigating the activities and job characteristics that predict flow states at work. *Journal of Occupational Health Psychology, 15*, 180–190.

Page, K. M., & Vella-Brodrick, D. A. (2009). The 'what', 'why' and 'how' of employee well-being. *Social Indicators Research, 90*, 441–458.

Parker, S. (1997). Work and leisure futures: Trends and scenarios. In J. Haworth (Ed.), *Work, leisure, and well-being* (pp. 180–191). London: Routledge.

Rheinberg, F., Manig, Y., Kliegel, R., Engeser, S., & Vollmeyer, R. (2007). Flow bei der arbeit, doch glück in der freizeit. Zielausrichtung, flow und glückgefühle [flow during work but happiness during leisure time: Goals, flow experience and happiness]. *Zeitschrift für Arbeits- und Organisationspsychologie, 3*, 105–115.

Salanova, M., Bakker, A., & Llorens, S. (2006). Flow at work: Evidence for an upward spiral of personal and organizational resources. *Journal of Happiness Studies*, *7*, 1–22.
Sartori, R. D. G. (2010). Flow experience in rescuing: A comparison between professionals and volunteers. Paper presented at the *I International conference: The concept of flow: Toward a scientific integration*. Book of Abstract, 4. TU Braunschweig, Germany, February 26–28.
Sartori, R. D. G., Massimini, F., & Delle Fave, A. (2009). Well-being in rescuing activities among professionals and volunteers. Paper presented at *IX ISQOLS Conference "Quality of life studies: Measures and goals for the progress of societies"*, Book of Abstract, 190. Florence, Italy, July, 19–23.
Schallberger, U., & Pfister, R. (2001). Flow-erleben in arbeit und freizeit. Eine untersuchung zum "paradox der arbeit" mit der experience sampling method (ESM) [Flow experiences in work and leisure: An experience sampling study about the paradox of work]. *Zeitschrift für Arbeits- und Organisationspsychologie*, *45*, 176–187.
Schaufeli, W. B., Leiter, M., & Maslach, C. (2009). Burnout: 35 years of research and practice. *Career Development International*, *14*, 204–220.
Schmidt, J., Shernoff, D., & Csikszentmihalyi, M. (2007). Individual and situational factors related to the experience of flow in adolescence: A multilevel approach. In A. D. Ong & M. van Dulmen (Eds.), *The handbook of methods in positive psychology* (pp. 542–558). Oxford: Oxford University Press.
Shanafelt, T. D., Bradley, K. A., Wipf, J. E., & Back, A. (2002). Burnout and self-reported patient care in an internal medicine residency program. *Annals of Internal Medicine*, *136*, 358–367.
van den Heuvel, M., Demerouti, E., Schreurs, B. H. J., Bakker, A. B., & Schaufeli, W. B. (2009). Does meaning-making help during organizational change? development and validation of a new scale. *Career Development International*, *14*, 508–533.

Chapter 9
Free Time: An Opportunity for Growth, Recreation, or Stagnation

9.1 Conceptualizing Free Time

Free time is, by definition, time that is free from duties or responsibilities, that can be spent on one's own activities, or tasks that one enjoys. While the term does not refer to any specific activity—which primarily depends on individuals' choice—it is basically opposed to productive activities, such as work and studying, which are compulsory and apparently less enjoyable (see Chapter 8). Such a dichotomy between work and free time has primarily come about in western societies (Olivier, 2000), supplanting the Aristotelian idea of *scholé* as time devoted to *philosophia* or the love of wisdom (Dumazedier, 1999). However, with the unrelenting westernization of habits and daily time-budget around the world, this dichotomy has gradually spread in most countries, thus representing an international phenomenon.

Besides being complementary to work, free time includes a wide range of activities, such as playing sports, practicing hobbies, idling, volunteering, interacting, watching TV, and playing videogames. A great number of partly overlapping conceptualizations and models have been proposed to account for such variety of activities and for their contribution to individuals' development and well-being. Leisure activities can be divided into active and passive leisure, on the basis of individuals' level of activation and engagement in the task at hand (Csikszentmihalyi, 1990). Passive activities, such as watching TV, require low energy investment and are primarily related to relaxation; on the contraty, active tasks, such as sports and hobbies, imply high activation and personal engagement.

Another classification of leisure is based on formal activity features. Free time can be divided into structured and unstructured tasks. The former are characterized by a clear set of rules and procedures, which promote concentration, and effort toward meeting challenges and achieving goals. Structured activities include sports, games, arts, and hobbies that merge the enjoyment of leisure with engagement toward meeting a goal such as winning a match, producing a painting, or improving one's ability level (Kleiber, Larson, & Csikszentmihalyi, 1986). Other activities, such as socializing, watching television, reading, and listening to music, are defined as unstructured or relaxed leisure (Larson & Kleiber, 1993), and provide pleasure and fun without high demands.

A. Delle Fave et al., *Psychological Selection and Optimal Experience Across Cultures*, Cross-Cultural Advancements in Positive Psychology 2,
DOI 10.1007/978-90-481-9876-4_9,

Stebbins more recently proposed an overarching classification of free time (1997, 2001, 2007), dividing the activities into serious and casual leisure according to the constancy and duration of individuals' engagement in performing them. Serious leisure is the systematic pursuit of amateur, hobbyist, or volunteer activities that are sufficiently substantial, interesting, and fulfilling to foster participants' commitment in the long term through the acquisition of special skills, knowledge, and experience (Stebbins, 2007). By contrast, casual leisure activities are more hedonistic, immediately enjoyable and rewarding, relatively short-lived, and requiring little or no specialist training.

Both types of leisure have been analyzed in relation to individuals' well-being and development. On the one hand, casual leisure has been shown to bring about benefits such as buffering immediate stress or the impact of negative life events, and sustaining coping efforts (Hutchinson & Kleiber, 2005). On the other hand, the notion of serious leisure constitutes a significant theoretical advancement, as it acknowledges that leisure entails long-term commitment, that it can sometimes be frustrating and boring, but that participants can gain a deep sense of satisfaction and fulfillment from their perseverance and dedication to it (Dilley & Scraton, 2010).

Stebbins's distinction between serious and casual leisure calls forth the potentially constructive role of free time in personal growth, not just as opportunity for fun and relaxation, but also as engaged commitment. Leisure in its current meaning basically flourished in industrial western societies, partly as a consequence of the deep differentiation of work tasks and environment from private and social activities and spaces (Delle Fave & Massimini, 1988). Western cultures offer a range of various formal and informal activities in which to invest individuals' time away from productive duties. Moreover, the growing amount of free time connected to the increased automation of most daily activities raises the question of how to make use of it. The consumer attitude and the work-spend-work-spend mentality, typical of countries centered on work ethics, foster escapism in leisure and a passive lifestyle (Iso-Ahola, 1997). Children, adolescents, and adults spend a relevant portion of their free time in unstructured tasks, such as buying and consuming goods, watching TV, and idling (Larson & Verma, 1999). The associated quality of experience is prominently negative: People report leisure-related boredom and apathy, as well as lower physical and mental health (Delle Fave & Bassi, 2003; Iso-Ahola, 1997). Having nothing to do and not knowing how to engage one's time can be dysfunctional. Idling can be associated with loss of concentration and motivation; the mind begins to wander and can focus on problems that cause anxiety (Csikszentmihalyi, 1990). Serious leisure can counter such scenarios, and provide opportunities for optimal experience, as well as long-term commitment to meaningful activities.

In particular, Csikszentmihalyi's early works (1990; Csikszentmihalyi & Csikszentmihalyi, 1988) have underlined the preferential association of flow with games, sports, or artistic and literary forms. Subsequent works have broadened the scope of investigation, both including a wider range of activities and exploring free time across cultures. Analyzing all the findings obtained in as vast a field as leisure over more than three decades is beyond the scope of this chapter. We will focus on major findings concerning the most frequently reported free time activities, illustrating the quality of associated experience, and their potential as flow opportunities. We will subsequently outline the individual and cultural features associated with optimal experience in leisure, as well as the risks of disengagement and deviant behavior entailed in free time. In the concluding section, we will analyze the role of leisure activities in individuals' psychological selection.

9.2 The Quality of Experience of Leisure Activities

Both the amount of free time and the types of activities available to individuals present wide variations around the world, depending on a number of factors such as working policies, religious practices, social rules, cultural values, age, and gender. Some of these factors will be analyzed in the Section 9.3. Nevertheless, at the global level few pervasive leisure categories have been identified across societies: sports and hobbies, media use, and social interactions. Here we will primarily focus on the first two categories, as an entire chapter is devoted to interactions (see Chapter 10).

As shown above, sports and hobbies are broadly classified as active structured leisure, whereas media use comprises both active structured activities such as playing video games, and passive unstructured ones, like watching TV and listening to music. These characteristics (structure vs. lack of structure; high vs. low activation) are reflected in the average quality of experience participants around the world associate with leisure activities (Delle Fave & Massimini, 2005; Jackson & Csikszentmihalyi, 1999; Kubey & Csikszentmihalyi, 1990). For exemplification purposes, let us once again consider the data gathered through ESM in a group of 199 Italian adolescents, as illustrated in Chapter 5, Table 5.2. The table shows that, on average, sports and hobbies were associated with an extremely positive experiential profile, characterized by high concentration, control, involvement, wish to do the activity, freedom, and happiness. However, on average participants did not associate them with relevant stakes or goals. In general, these activities represented pleasurable and engaging occupations, unrelated to long-term planning. While watching TV, participants reported average affect and cognitive investment, high ease of concentration and wish to do the activity, as well as low involvement, stakes, and goals. These findings highlight a passive relaxing activity, neither particularly positive nor meaningful, but perceived as desirable.

Sports and hobbies and watching TV further diverge as opportunities for optimal experience. In our sample of Italian adolescents, the former were associated with flow (channel 2) by 43.8% of the participants, whereas the latter by 24.4% of them. Optimal experience during both typologies of leisure activities was characterized by significantly positive values of most dimensions of the experience. However, at the motivational level, perceived stakes and goals scored above average for sports and hobbies, and around-average for watching TV.

Table 9.1 Percentages of selected optimal activities in the categories "sports and hobbies" and "watching TV" across cultures

	Sports and hobbies (%)	Watching TV (%)
Argentinian youths ($N = 801$)[a]	23.1	10 (80)
Chadian medical students ($N = 15$)	20	–
Indonesian adults ($N = 62$)	19.4	1.6 (1)
Iranian adults ($N = 26$)	3.8	7.7 (2)
Italian medical students ($N = 14$)	50	7.1 (1)
Navajo college students ($N = 62$)	19.4	–
Nepali high school students ($N = 34$)	17.7	2.9 (1)
Rom adults ($N = 48$)	19.2	2.1 (1)
Southern Italian adults ($N = 50$)	26	2 (1)
Ugandan high school students ($N = 39$)	10.2	–
Walser adults ($N = 47$)	30.4	–

Note: N refers to the total number of participants reporting optimal activities in each sample. Numbers within parenthesis refer to the participants reporting watching TV as optimal activity.
[a]Mesurado (2009a)

Wide discrepancies in percentages of optimal experience between the two leisure categories were also obtained in other ESM studies with Italian college students and adults, Nepalese teenagers (Delle Fave & Massimini, 2005), as well as American teenagers and adults (Csikszentmihalyi & Larson, 1984; Csikszentmihalyi & LeFevre, 1989; LeFevre 1988; Shernoff & Vandell, 2007).

Differences were also observed in cross-cultural studies using flow questionnaire (Delle Fave, 2007; Chapter 7): Hobbies and sports were reported as privileged flow opportunities by over one-third of the participants across cultures, while watching TV was selected by an irrelevant percentage of individuals. Table 9.1 reports some striking cross-cultural findings (Bassi, Coppa, & Delle Fave, 2008; Cavallo, Lombardi, & Stokart, 2006; Delle Fave & Massimini, 2004; Delle Fave, 1999).

Across cultures, very few participants, if any, reported watching TV as a pervasive optimal activity. Argentina was the only exception, with 10% of the participants (Mesurado, 2009a). This difference may be related to the young age (9–15 years) of the South American sample, compared to the other ones (see Section 9.3). By contrast, sports and hobbies were mentioned by a larger share of respondents, with variations across groups: Italian college students reported the highest percentage, whereas Iranian adults reported the lowest.

These differences are further corroborated by the distribution of the two leisure categories across the EFM channels detected in most studies conducted with ESM. In all the analyzed samples (Bassi & Delle Fave, 2004; Csikszentmihalyi & LeFevre, 1989; Delle Fave & Bassi, 2003; Delle Fave & Massimini, 2005), sports and hobbies are more frequently associated with channel 2, whereas watching TV primarily falls into channel 4 (relaxation) and 6 (apathy). In our group of adolescents, sports and hobbies are associated with flow in 22.4% of the self-reports, with relaxation in 14.6%, and with apathy in 8.1%. By contrast, the distribution of watching TV amounts to 7.5% for flow, 21.8% for relaxation, and 22.5% for apathy.

These findings raise important questions: What kind of activities do people report among sports and hobbies? What are the main characteristics of these activities, besides structure and engagement promotion? How frequently do participants watch television? Does the associated experience characterize also other medium-based activities such as playing video games, navigating in Internet, or listening to music?

9.2.1 Sports and Hobbies as Opportunities for Serious Leisure

An incredibly rich literature has been gathered on optimal experience in sports and hobbies, among both amateurs and professionals. Since the focus of our chapter is free time and not full-time professional engagement in sport or creative activities, we only focus on amateurs.[1] Some studies have targeted specific sports such as soccer (García, Cervelló, Jimenez, Iglesias, & Santos-Rosa, 2005), golf (Catley & Duda, 1997), marathon (Schüler & Brunner, 2009), swimming (Kowal & Fortier, 1999), outdoor recreation such as hiking, horseback riding, and fishing (Decloe, Kaczynski, & Havitz, 2009; Vittersø, Vorkinn, & Vistad, 2001; Whitmore & Borrie, 2005), rock climbing (Bassi & Delle Fave, 2010; Csikszentmihalyi, 1975; Delle Fave, Bassi, & Massimini, 2003a), and hobbies like theater acting (Martin & Cutler, 2002), playing music (Byrne, MacDonald, & Carlton, 2003; MacDonald, Byrne, & Carlton, 2006; Massimini & Delle Fave, 1995), rock dancing, playing chess (Csikszentmihalyi, 1975), and skateboarding (Seifert & Hedderson, 2010). Through flow questionnaire in which respondents were free to report the activities associated with optimal experience, and by means of ESM online assessment, an even longer list of free time activities has been collected across cultures, including a variety of traditional culture-specific hobbies like knitting or handicraft and, to a limited extent, volunteering in associations involved in humanitarian activities (Delle Fave & Massimini, 2004; Delle Fave, 2007).

As shown above, all these activities share similar characteristics: They have structure and require personal engagement, two features that favor their association with optimal experience. Structure implies clear rules and feedback (Chapters 3 and 5). Personal engagement reflects individuals' motivation. Studies on structured leisure conducted from the perspective of self-determination theory (SDT) have repeatedly stressed the relationship of sports, exercise, and hobbies with intrinsic motivation (Hagger & Chatzisarantis, 2007; Larson, 2000). In Section 9.2, we showed that optimal experience in sports and hobbies among Italian adolescents monitored with ESM was characterized by above-average levels of freedom and wish to do the activity (Table 5.2; Delle Fave & Bassi, 2000, 2003; Delle Fave & Massimini, 2005). Similar results were obtained with ESM among US adults (Csikszentmihalyi & LeFevre, 1989), and with FQ in various other cultures (Delle Fave & Massimini, 2004; Delle Fave, 2007).

---

[1] Readers interested in professionals can consult, among others, the extensive work done by Susan Jackson and her colleagues (Jackson & Csikszentmihalyi, 1999; Jackson & Kimiecik, 2008; Jackson & Roberts, 1992; Jackson et al., 2001). Some information is also provided in Chapter 8.

However, research has also shown that both intrinsic motivation and self-determined extrinsic motivation are positively related to flow. Kowal and Fortier (1999) obtained this result among swimmers, and further found a positive relation between flow and perception of autonomy, competence, and relatedness. González-Cutre, Sicilia, Moreno, and Fernández-Balboa (2009) found a positive correlation between dispositional flow and intrinsic and identified motivations among young people practicing individual and group sports. Martin and Cutler (2002) detected that theater actors rated acting as an intense optimal experience, and this condition was associated with both intrinsic and extrinsic reasons to perform. In a study among retired adults, Mannell, Zuzanek, and Larson (1988) showed that both intrinsically and extrinsically motivated freely chosen activities were associated with flow. However, the extrinsically motivated ones produced more intense optimal experiences than the intrinsically motivated ones. The authors interpreted this result by considering freely chosen extrinsically motivated activities as serious leisure (Stebbins, 2007), requiring more effort and commitment than "pure leisure" (e.g., freely chosen intrinsically motivated tasks). In other words, those activities that are freely chosen and for which there are also extrinsic reasons for participation could require more perseverance and long-term dedication, and could bring about a deeper sense of fulfillment through the development of skills and knowledge over time. This view is congruent with the eudaimonic perspective in positive psychology, particularly if extrinsic reasons are related to the well-being of other people and communities. More research attention is required to shed light on this interpretation.

9.2.2 The Television Paradox and Media Use

All studies focusing on watching TV have shown that this activity is rarely associated with optimal experience across age and cultures (Table 9.1; Bassi & Delle Fave, 2004; Delle Fave & Bassi, 2000, 2003; Delle Fave & Massimini, 1994; Kubey & Csikszentmihalyi, 1990, 2002). The few occasions in which viewing is associated with flow is when individuals report watching an interesting or stimulating movie or sport matches (Delle Fave & Massimini, 1994). These occasions are often reported in the presence of other people, thus making them primarily social activities (Larson & Kubey, 1983; Larson, 1995). Only in a group of Italian blind people did we find "watching" TV as a predominant flow activity: Participants described it as a means of keeping into contact with the wider world and to retrieve information and keep oneself updated (see Chapter 14; Delle Fave & Maletto, 1992; Massimini, Delle Fave, & Borri Gaspardin, 1992).

The analysis of ESM data with the EFM has pointed out that, at best, watching TV is associated with relaxation, but it is often characterized by apathy. In light of these findings, the high frequency of free time people—and primarily youths—devote to watching TV, mostly reporting the wish to do the activity, seems like a paradox (Flammer & Schaffner, 2003; Hektner, Schmidt, & Csikszentmihalyi, 2007; Larson & Verma, 1999). Viewing can partly be explained by the fact that television captures the individuals' attention irrespective of its content and long-term relevance for personal development (Kubey & Csikszentmihalyi, 2002), by triggering the orienting response, or people's instinctive visual or auditory reaction to any sudden or novel stimulus. The orienting response, however, does not account for the sometimes long hours spent in front of the TV set. Delle Fave and Massimini (1994) have proposed an explanation based on the analysis of the quality of experience perceived while watching TV on average, in association with channel 2 (optimal experience) and with channel 6 (apathy, i.e., the worst experiential condition characterized by below-average challenges and skills). In samples of Italian adolescents, they found that, under all the three conditions, watching TV was never associated with an extremely negative experience. Although it represents a passive entertainment not connected to relevant goals or stakes, and evoking no active personal engagement, it is freely sought after, provides relaxation and perceived control of the situation. Watching TV seems therefore to exert a sort of *parachute effect* preventing attention and consciousness from falling into the disruption and pervasive disengagement of apathy. At the same time, due to the lack of goals and engagement associated with it, TV does not help step out of apathy and head toward more complex and challenging opportunities for action. Therefore, watching TV does not represent a long-term source of development; rather, it primarily serves as a time filler and a passive entertainment (Massimini et al., 1992).

Besides watching TV, individuals daily engage in other medium-based activities, such as listening to music, navigating in Internet, chatting, and playing video games. ESM studies showed that listening to music is a passive activity like watching TV, and it presents a similar experiential profile characterized by above-average wish to do the activity, and by below-average values of goals and stakes (Larson & Kubey, 1983). However, listening to music is more frequently associated with optimal experience than watching TV, especially among youth (e.g., 14.2% vs. 7.5% in our sample of adolescents). Music—in terms of both sound and lyrics—can be more involving and challenging for developing individuals, and represent a mode of self-expression, tension release, and autonomy from adults.

Both the TV set and the radio (or CD player/stereo) are gradually being supplanted by the computer, especially among youth (Mannell, Kaczynski, & Aronson, 2005). The major difference between these media is that most computer-related activities require participants' active engagement (interactivity), both physically in executing the operations on the keyboard, and cognitively in following instructions or information on the screen. Activities such as navigating in Internet, chatting, and playing video games are also endowed with structure: Well-defined procedures are required to use a specific software, and rules and goals are associated with its content (the mediated message). Moreover, these activities offer challenges in which to invest one's ability (Mathwick & Rigdon, 2004; Sherry, 2004): To play a computer game, an individual first has to master keyword commands and then learn the rules of the game. Studies have shown that the average experience associated with computer-mediated activities is similar to the one associated with sports and hobbies (Bassi & Delle Fave, 2004). In addition, these activities represent opportunities for optimal experience (Chang & Wang, 2008; Chen, 2006; Chen, Wigand, & Nilan, 2000; Skadberg & Kimmel, 2004). Especially computer games are associated with flow among children, adolescents, and young adults (Bassi & Delle Fave, 2004; Mesurado, 2009b; Voiskounsky, Mitina, & Avetisova, 2004). The appeal of video games results predominantly from the challenges of solving the puzzle presented in the game (Sherry, 2004). Not only do players get immediate clear feedback about the performed activity; but they can also adjust the level of challenge to equal their skills, thus preventing boredom and favoring skills improvement and engagement over time.

9.3 Individual Characteristics, Cultural Features, and Optimal Experience in Leisure

One of the most pervasive individual differences found in the leisure domain is related to gender (Csikszentmihalyi & Larson, 1984; Hektner et al., 2007; Pavón and Moreno 2008). Differences start to emerge in early childhood and are present at all ages. Studies have repeatedly shown that females primarily devote free time to interactions and to hobbies; whereas males spend more time in sport activities, games, and watching TV. The more gender roles are separated within a society, the greater is the difference in free time allocation and preferences, especially when social restrictions limit the participation of women in leisure pursuits outside the home (Verma & Larson, 2003). Gender differences are also subject to change in time: In an ESM study with two groups of Italian adolescents sampled in 1986 and in 2000, Bassi and Delle Fave (2004) showed that among boys, leisure activities related to new technologies (primarily computer games) became by far the most frequent free time activity in 2000, substituting and not just accompanying more traditional sports and hobbies that were reported in 1986. These differences in free time activities are consistent with the opportunities for optimal experience prominently reported by genders: Girls report flow primarily during interactions and hobbies, and boys in sports, games, and Internet use (Bassi & Delle Fave, 2004; Delle Fave & Bassi, 2003; Mannell et al., 2005). However, no significant gender difference can be detected in the associated experiential profile.

Across age groups, differences have been identified in the percentage of time devoted to leisure (Hektner et al., 2007). They are primarily due to age-related variations in the partition of daily time-budget between work and free time. However, when asked to report their most pervasive optimal experiences, youth and adults in western countries report leisure activities in similar percentages (Bassi & Delle Fave, 2004; Csikszentmihalyi & LeFevre, 1989; Delle Fave & Massimini, 1996, 2003; Delle Fave, 1999), whereas in non-western cultures youth tend to more frequently report leisure, and adults to report work (Delle Fave & Massimini, 1988, 1991, 1996; Massimini et al., 1992). The type of reported activity seems to be related not only to respondents' all-time preferences—i.e., activities they have cultivated throughout the years—but also to their physical and cognitive abilities, with a reduction in active sports among older male adults in favor of serious hobbies or voluntary work (Mannell et al., 1988).

When sports are associated with optimal experience, individuals report the perception of meaningful goals and stakes in the task at hand (Table 6.2). Researchers investigated whether individuals' goal orientations (task and ego involvement) could predict the association of sports with optimal experience. In particular, Csikszentmihalyi (1990) argued that optimal experience should be associated with task involvement and mastery-oriented focus; he maintained that "when beating the opponent takes precedence in the mind over performing as well as possible, enjoyment tends to disappear. Competition is enjoyable only when it is a means to perfect one's skills; when it becomes an end in itself, it ceases to be fun" (p. 50). In a series of studies among young people involved in physical activities, both dispositional flow and achievement goal orientations were measured (Cervelló, Moreno, Alonso, & Iglesias, 2006; Moreno, Alonso, Martínez, Cervelló, & Ruiz, 2008). Results showed that optimal experience correlated positively with both ego and task orientations, and that both orientations were significant predictors of flow in physical activities. The authors of these studies did not bring forward any explanation for this unexpected finding. In line with our reasoning on goals and meaning (Section 5.3.1, Chapter 5, this volume), we can tentatively suggest that what counts most in favoring flow in leisure activities is individuals' tendency to perceive meaningful goals, be they task or ego related. However, more studies are needed to shed light on these findings and their implications in terms of individuals' well-being and sport performance.

Beside the individual differences we have presented, various cultural and contextual peculiarities can influence the occurrence and cultivation of optimal experience in the leisure domain (Delle Fave & Massimini, 1996; Massimini & Delle Fave, 2000; Massimini et al., 1992; Massimini, Inghilleri, & Delle Fave, 1996). From a broad perspective, individuals retrieve optimal experience in leisure activities offered by the cultures they belong to, thus contributing to replicate their memes and, at the same time, finding occasions of well-being and growth. However, processes such as modernization and encounters between different cultures—be they peaceful or characterized by imposition and domination—can create gaps in the cultural transmission of traditional leisure activities, thus potentially causing a hiatus between generations, on the one hand, and loss of traditional activities, on the other hand. Our cross-cultural analysis of leisure time highlighted different scenarios. Among Rom gypsies living in Italy, for example, young people were concerned with family and social interactions, just like their parents (Chapter 10). They were not interested in the modern leisure opportunities they could easily find outside the camp. By contrast, they reported optimal experiences in traditional Rom activities such as playing music, singing, dancing, and playing cards (Delle Fave, Bassi, & Massimini, 2003b). One participant described playing music in the following way

> I learned how to play guitar when I was very young ... I play all the time: in my shanty, on the grass, and during festivities and parties ... Sometimes I play the whole day, without eating or resting. But I feel very good, my heart is filled with great joy (30-year-old man).

On the opposite, a generational gap was detected among cultures undergoing modernization (Delle Fave & Massimini, 1988, 1991, 1996; Massimini et al., 1992).

This phenomenon was observed across three generations among members of Walser and Occitan communities living in the alpine areas of north-west Italy, and among people from a rural area in southern Italy, living on agriculture and sheep farming. Elderly and middle aged participants primarily quoted traditional work tasks as optimal activities (tilling the fields, knitting, raising the cattle, taking care of the vegetables). Leisure was reported less frequently, and in association with traditional outdoor recreation, such as walking in nature, alpine skiing, dancing. These participants had maintained a close relation with their natural environment, which was reflected in their choice of optimal activities. By contrast, young generations had embraced modernization: They reported watching TV in their free time, and they primarily found flow in activities such as ice-skating, reading, riding the bike, going to the disco. Some individuals—predominantly belonging to the middle generation—reported bicultural strategies in their leisure-time activities: They found flow in both traditional and modernized occupations, quoting side by side playing the accordion and riding the motorbike.

Among the Navajos (Delle Fave, 1999), whose traditional culture is threatened by western models, similar differences were detected between adolescents attending public schools and members of the Diné college, an institution aimed at promoting biculturalism among Navajo youth (further details are provided in Chapters 7 and 13). Adolescents mostly associated flow with western sports such as football, basketball, or jogging. Members of the Diné College quoted traditional Navajo practices such as hunting, fishing, and wandering in the countryside, besides western sports

> I experience flow in bowhunting. When I hunt, I become one with nature, that's my native side ... it starts when I am on a fresh track of recent passing of deer, or a sight of a good buck, and the beginning of the stalk ... the one thought that there was a challenge and I met that challenge and overcame it, the fear, the excitement, but most of all knowing that you can do it ... all this keeps the feeling going on (19-year-old man).

The family as well as the school environment play an important role in the regulation of available free time among youth, and in the transmission of leisure activities, be they traditional or modernized (Hektner, 2001; Larson, 2000; Rathunde, 2001; Verma & Larson, 2003). For example, in Asian cultures, adolescent life—including leisure—is enmeshed with the family. By virtue of the traditional suspicion about idle time, Korean and Japanese teenagers spend large amounts of their waking hours in school-related activities, and their free time in school extracurricular activities (Lee, 2003; Nishino & Larson, 2003). By contrast, US adolescents have large amounts of unregulated free time, running the risk of doing nothing, watching TV, or looking for excitement in deviant activities (Larson, 2000). Both family and school are therefore crucial in promoting positive development by providing youth with structured meaningful activities in which to invest personal skills and to find opportunities for optimal experience (Dworkin, Larson, & Hansen, 2003; Schmidt, 2003; Shernoff & Vandell, 2007).

9.4 Free Time and Well-Being: What You Do and How Long You Do It

As mentioned at the beginning of this chapter, free time can offer various activity opportunities that promote well-being, both at the individual level by fostering physical and mental health, and at the social level by contributing to community cohesion and other people's well-being (e.g., through volunteer activities) (Csikszentmihalyi, 1990; Massimini & Delle Fave, 2000; Stebbins, 2007). In particular, all these activities can promote well-being through their association with optimal experience (Delle Fave, 2009; Delle Fave and Fava, in press). For instance, regular physical activity is known to reduce the risk of developing diseases such as diabetes, heart disorders, colon cancer, and feelings of depression and anxiety, while promoting positive mood and affect, subjective and psychological well-being, and self-esteem (Mutrie & Faulkner, 2002). If an individual finds flow in sports and exercise, she will derive short-term satisfaction from investing personal skills in meaningful challenges; she is also likely to incorporate them in her life style, and to show commitment in cultivating them over time. In addition, finding flow in competitive sports has been shown to have a positive relationship with performance, both directly (Jackson & Roberts, 1992; Jackson, Thomas, Marsh, & Smethurst, 2001; Stavrou, Jackson, Zervas, & Karteroliotis, 2007) and indirectly by fostering pre-race training behavior (Schüler & Brunner, 2009). A significant correlation was also found between optimal experience and quality of composition among music students, in terms of levels of creativity evaluated by music specialists (Byrne et al., 2003; MacDonald et al., 2006). Ethnographic observation of skateboarders also attested to the relation between flow and peak performance (Seifert & Hedderson, 2010), with observers reporting participants' perseverance and more intense training in the face of unsuccessful stunts.

As shown in Chapter 3, in spite of its implications in development and in the positive quality of life, flow presents an amoral character (Csikszentmihalyi & Massimini, 1985; Csikszentmihalyi, 1990; Nakamura & Csikszentmihalyi, 2009). Individuals tend to pursue and reproduce flow activities whether they have, or not, positive consequences for the individual or for society. This is particularly the case of leisure time, in which people are freer from social constraints. In this respect, research has identified two major risks: (a) associating flow with deviant or illegal activities; (b) spending too much time in flow-related activities, which could have a negative impact on health.

Concerning the first risk, studies have found that optimal experience was associated with activities such as graffiti spraying (Rheinberg & Manig, 2003), and computer hacking (Voiskounsky & Smyslova, 2003). These activities are clearly harmful to the individual who could be inflicted severe punishment, and to the community, which could be violated in its environmental and information capital. The second risk is more subtle in that it is not necessarily related to deviant activities; these are harmful in their own right, irrespective of the amount of time one invests in it. Studies on flow and electronic media activities among youth have proved the displacement hypothesis, i.e., they have shown that associating optimal experience with computer and video games or Internet use can divert time from physically active leisure, social participation, and thus lead to withdrawn sedentary lives (Kubey & Csikszentmihalyi, 2002; Mannell et al., 2005). While this risk is also run by youth associating flow with solitary intellectual hobbies like reading, much concern among psychologists and educators is raised by the increasing amount of time youth spend in front of the computer, possibly by virtue of the association of computer activities with optimal experience.

Some studies have obtained empirical support to the hypothesis that flow could lead to addiction in activities such as playing video and computer games (Chou & Ting, 2003; Sherry, 2004), and big wave surfing (Partington, Partington, & Olivier, 2009). Another study, however, showed that flow was negatively correlated with addictive inclination in adolescents playing online games (Wan & Chiou, 2006). Moreover, optimal experience was not a significant predictor of players' subsequent addictive inclination, and addicts' flow state was significantly less intense than non-addicts'. Given this conflicting evidence, more research is needed to distinguish the contribution of optimal experience from that of personality factors or mental conditions in the development of addiction.

9.5 Leisure and Psychological Selection

As shown throughout this chapter, free time presents multiple facets. It can provide occasions for relaxation and casual leisure. It can be a curse if we do not know how to use it: We may end up in apathy or search for thrilling dangerous activities to fill in the void. It can offer flow opportunities in activities such as playing video games that are not growth conducive, but that can be challenging and rewarding in specific stages of life such as adolescence. It can also provide opportunities for serious leisure that individuals cultivate in time as privileged focus of their psychological selection. In some instances, activities can become so meaningful and pervasive that they can turn into regular occupations, as in the cases of professional athletes (Jackson & Csikszentmihalyi, 1999) or musicians (see Chapter 8; Massimini & Delle Fave, 1995). In most instances, however, they remain "restricted" to free time enriching life with satisfaction and fulfillment. This is the topic of the concluding section, in which we present findings on rock climbers (Bassi & Delle Fave, 2010; Delle Fave et al., 2003a) and amateur athletes (Delle Fave & Massimini, 1999) who have selected specific leisure activities in which to invest their time and energy over time.

9.5.1 The Experience of Rock Climbing and Mountaineering

Rock climbing is a recreational activity that presents structural components of real or perceived danger, in which the participants have to cope with an uncertain

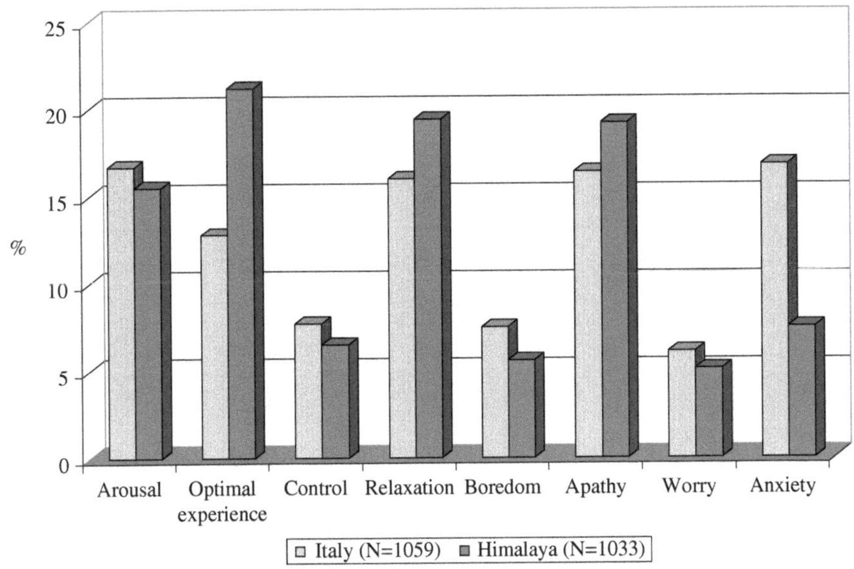

Fig. 9.1 Channel percentage distribution in Italy and in the Himalaya ($N = N$ self-reports)

outcome by means of personal skills and resources (Ewert & Hollenhorst, 1997). A number of studies have investigated the reasons why individuals should expose their lives to extreme dangers on the mountains by calling into question personality traits such as sensation seeking (Aşçi, Demirhan, & Dinç, 2007; Egan & Stelmack, 2003). Besides personality characteristics, however, we hypothesized that the quality of associated experience while climbing in the mountains could play an important motivational role (Delle Fave et al., 2003a). To test our hypothesis, we monitored six Italian climbers with ESM for one and a half months during an expedition on Thalay Sagar (6,904 m), one of the most difficult peaks in the Indian Himalaya. We also explored their daily life at home through an ESM session performed after the expedition. Our participants included skilful amateur climbers, who had their own profession at home: Four were skilled workers (carpenter, mason, blue collar, and photographer), one was researcher at the university, and one was a dentist. Results showed that, far from pursuing thrilling experiences such as arousal (channel 1 in the EFM; Fig. 4.1), climbers mostly reported optimal experience, characterized by a balance between high challenges and high skills. Flow was the most frequent experience during the expedition in general (Fig. 9.1), and it largely prevailed during camp and climbing activities (Fig. 9.2).

The expedition presented structural characteristics that allowed for flow onset. Above all, it offered meaningful outcomes—ultimately including personal survival—contingent upon the skills of the participants (Ewert, 1994). In addition, the analysis of participants' risk assessment highlighted no significant deviations from average across situations, showing that risk played a minor role in the overall climbing experience. This result was further substantiated by the low frequency

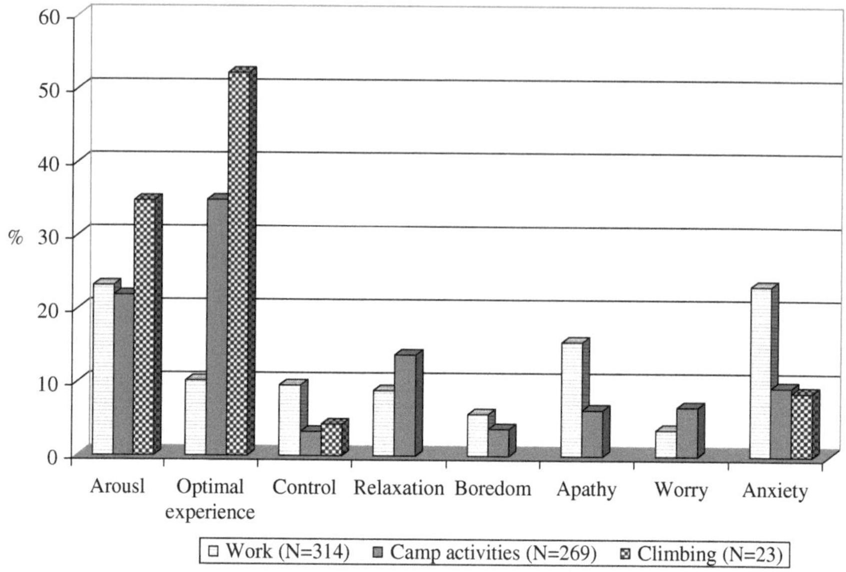

Fig. 9.2 Percentage distribution of work, and camp/climbing activities in the channels of the EFM ($N = N$ self-reports)

of anxiety (channel 8; Fig. 9.1) reported during the expedition. Any activity can potentially be risky, when the individual does not possess adequate skills to face the challenge. Over time climbers had undergone extensive training to sharpen their skills, so that they could identify risk associated, say, with bad weather conditions or poor physical shape, and avoid to put their lives in danger by going beyond personal capabilities (Csikszentmihalyi, 1975). In particular, anxiety control is functional to climbers' survival: If a climber is not able to master anxiety, she can lose control of the situation, fall into a crevice, or be unable to fully exploit her physical potential (Robinson, 1985).

Participants were also followed with ESM for 1 month during their daily life in Italy (Bassi, 1998). Ironically for the sedentary reader, climbers did not report the same control on daily environmental challenges that they had in the Himalaya. Data analysis with the EFM showed that participants mostly reported an imbalance between high challenges and moderate or low skills (arousal and anxiety, respectively; Fig. 9.1). In particular, during their daily life they reported twice as much anxiety as in the seemingly more dangerous Himalaya. Anxiety and arousal, with equal percentages, were prominent during work (Fig. 9.2). Last but not least, participants reported optimal experience much less frequently during their daily life, both in general and during work.

These findings point to the trend these climbers are pursuing in their psychological selection. Some of the participants lived in mountain areas so that they could spend as much time climbing as possible when they were off work. Other participants lived in metropolitan areas, but few hours away from the Alps. Climbing was the most rewarding activity in their lives, and they cultivated it beyond and above all the other daily duties, including work. With the passing of time, they had accumulated great skills and capabilities in climbing that made them feel more comfortable and competent on the roof of the world than in their daily life in Italy. For all of them, climbing played a crucial role in psychological selection, providing meaning to their life and opportunities for personal growth and development.

9.5.2 Track-and-Field: Amateurs and Professionals

In our exploration of psychological selection and leisure activities, we were also interested in comparing athletes who chose sport as a profession with those who performed it at the amateur level (Delle Fave & Massimini, 1999). We administered flow questionnaire and life theme questionnaire to a group of 100 track-and-field athletes (marathon, walking, and running), 58 professionals (aged 15–35), and 42 amateurs (aged 15–55). The former were primarily high-school or university students who were paid by their sport association and who trained between 1 and 3 h a day; the latter had a job that had nothing to do with their sport, and trained once or twice a week.

The majority of participants (98%) reported optimal experience in their lives, with professionals quoting 2.5 activities on average, and amateurs 1.5. As illustrated in Fig. 9.3, sport was by far the most frequent category for both groups.

In the category sport, professionals primarily quoted activities related to track and field (79%): training, competitions, jogging, or specific techniques; in 21%

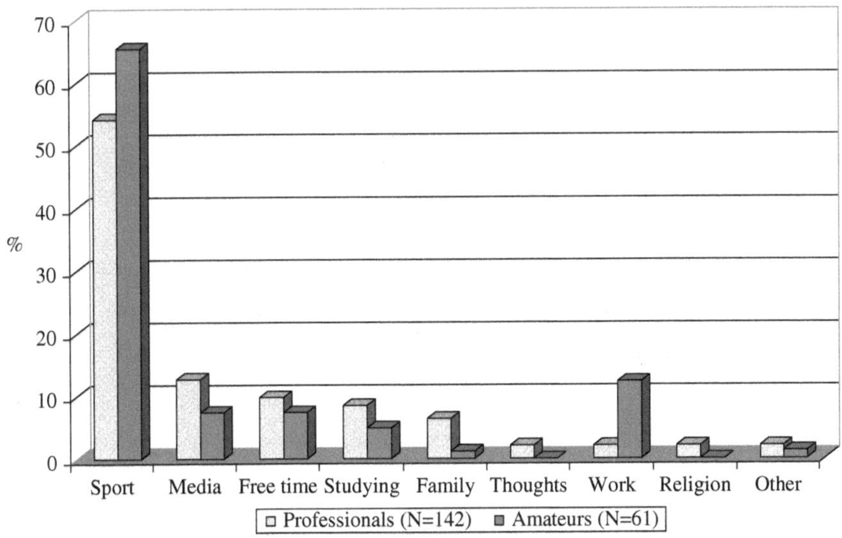

Fig. 9.3 Percentage distribution of flow activities among professional and amateur athletes (N = N answers)

Table 9.2 Percentage distributions of current challenges and future goals among athletes

	Challenges		Goals	
	Professionals (N = 52)	Amateurs (N = 40)	Professionals (N = 52)	Amateurs (N = 40)
Sport	28.8	2.1	21.1	8.1
Work	12.3	29.3	23.4	19.3
Family	9.6	29.3	23.4	29
Personal growth	8.2	2.7	12.8	11.3
Studying	37	10.1	10.6	3.2
Health	–	–	6.4	4.9
Material goods	–	1.8	14.9	17.7
Other	4.1	5.7	6.4	6.5
N answers	73	47	109	62

of their answers, they also described other sports such as tennis, swimming, and climbing. Among amateurs, by contrast, track and field accounted for only 48% of the category sport. Analyzing what participants meant for the sport activities they associated with optimal experience, another difference emerged between professionals and amateurs. For professionals, sport was an occasion for concentration, psychophysical coordination and peak performance. It required investment of time and energy in view of long-term objectives

> [It means] succeeding in isolating myself to such an extent that I can get the highest degree of concentration, thus proving unique feelings and sensations (23-year-old woman)
>
> A competition in which to prove to others and to myself my worth and the physical and psychic abilities that I can put into a run in a bunch of seconds (18-year-old man).

For amateurs sport took on different meanings, which had to do with recreation and socialization

> It helps release the tension I have built up during the day (54-year-old man)
>
> [It means] running, participating in competitions, but above all staying with other people, exchange ideas and opinions (42-year-old man).

These differences between professionals and amateurs were also observed in the analysis of participants' current challenges and future goals (Table 9.2).

For professionals, sport was the second most frequent current challenge, and it ranked third among the future goals. Amateurs rarely quoted sport among both challenges and goals, with other life domains being more important in the construction of their life theme.

These results show that for both amateurs and professionals sport activities were the primary source of optimal experience. Thanks to the rewarding experience associated with practice, participants cultivated these activities, gain increasing skills and competences, and sustain their effort and commitment in the face of difficulties and failures. However, sport activities played different roles in participants' psychological selection. For professionals, sport was a central focus of their life theme, both as current challenge and as future goal; for amateur, it had a marginal position compared to work, family, or material goods (such as buying one's own house). It was, however, a gratifying component of their lives, worth pursuing over time, providing them opportunities for socialization, and promoting a healthy lifestyle.

References

Aşçi, F. H., Demirhan, G., & Dinç, S. (2007). Psychological profile of Turkish rock climbers: An examination of climbing experience and route difficulty. *Perceptual and Motor Skills, 104*, 892–900.

Bassi, M. (1998). *L'interazione tra challenges e skills e le fluttuazioni dello stato esperienziale: Ricerca sul campo in condizioni estreme* [The challenges and skills interaction and experience fluctuation: Field research in extreme conditions]. Doctoral Dissertation, Università degli Studi di Milano, Italy.

Bassi, M., Coppa, R., & Delle Fave, A. (2008). Studiare medicina per condividere benessere: Una ricerca transculturale in ciad e in italia [studying medicine to share well-being: A cross-cultural research in Chad and Italy]. *Psicologia della Salute, 1*, 93–107.

Bassi, M., & Delle Fave, A. (2004). Adolescence and the changing context of optimal experience in time: Italy 1986–2000. *Journal of Happiness Studies, 5*, 155–179.

Bassi, M., & Delle Fave, A. (2010). Impact of extreme weather conditions on high-altitude climbers' goals and quality of experience. *Journal of Leisure Research, 42*, 469–488.

Byrne, C., MacDonald, R., & Carlton, L. (2003). Assessing creativity in musical compositions: Flow as an assessment tool. *British Journal of Musical Education, 20*, 277–290.

Catley, D., & Duda, J. L. (1997). Psychological antecedents of the frequency and intensity of flow in golfers. *International Journal of Sport Psychology, 28*, 309–322.

Cavallo, M., Lombardi, M., & Stokart, Z. (2006). Complessità e sviluppo di opportunità: Esperienza ottimale e selezione psicologica in un gruppo di adolescenti nepalesi [complexity and development of opportunities: Optimal experience and psychological selection in a group of Nepali adolescents]. *Passaggi, 11*, 77–100.

Cervelló, E. M., Moreno, J. A., Alonso, N., & Iglesias, D. (2006). Goal orientations, motivational climate and dispositional flow of high school students engaging in extracurricular involvement in physical activity. *Perceptual and Motor Skills, 102*, 887–892.

Chang, H., & Wang, I. (2008). An investigation of user communication behavior in computer mediated environments. *Computers in Human Behavior, 24*, 2336–2356.

Chen, H. (2006). Flow on the net-detecting web users' positive affects and their flow states. *Computers in Human Behavior, 22*, 221–233.

Chen, H., Wigand, R. T., & Nilan, M. S. (2000). Exploring web users' optimal flow experiences. *Information Technology & People, 13*, 263–281.

Chou, T., & Ting, C. (2003). The role of flow experience in cyber-game addiction. *Cyber Psychology, 6*, 663–675.

Csikszentmihalyi, M. (1975/2000). *Beyond boredom and anxiety*. San Francisco: Jossey Bass.

Csikszentmihalyi, M. (1990). *Flow: The psychology of optimal experience*. New York: Harper & Row.

Csikszentmihalyi, M., & Csikszentmihalyi, I. (Eds.) (1988). *Optimal experience: Psychological studies of flow in consciousness*. New York: Cambridge University Press.

Csikszentmihalyi, M., & Larson, R. W. (1984). *Being adolescents: Conflict and growth in teenage years*. New York: Basic Books.

Csikszentmihalyi, M., & LeFevre, J. (1989). Optimal experience in work and leisure. *Journal of Personality and Social Psychology, 56*, 815–822.

Csikszentmihalyi, M., & Massimini, F. (1985). On the psychological selection of bio-cultural information. *New Ideas in Psychology, 3*, 115–138.

Decloe, M., Kaczynski, A., & Havitz, M. (2009). Social participation, flow and situational involvement in recreational physical activity. *Journal of Leisure Research*, *41*, 73–90.

Delle Fave, A. (1999). Individual development and bicultural identity: The Navajo way. In A. Delle Fave and F. Meli (Eds.), *Modernization and cultural identity* (pp. 49–68). Milano: Edizioni dell'Arco.

Delle Fave, A. (2007). Individual development and community empowerment: Suggestions from studies on optimal experience. In J. Haworth & G. Hart (Eds.), *Well-being: Individual, community, and societal perspectives* (pp. 41–56). London: Palgrave McMillan.

Delle Fave, A., & Bassi, M. (2000). The quality of experience in adolescents' daily life: Developmental perspectives. *Genetic, Social, and General Psychology Monographs*, *126*, 347–367.

Delle Fave, A., & Bassi, M. (2003). Italian adolescents and leisure: The role of engagement and optimal experience. In S. Verma & R. Larson (Eds.), *Examining adolescent leisure time across cultures: Developmental opportunities and risks. New directions in child and adolescent development* (pp. 79–93). San Francisco: Jossey-Bass.

Delle Fave, A., Bassi, M., & Massimini, F. (2003a). Quality of experience and risk perception in high-altitude rock climbing. *Journal of Applied Sport Psychology*, *15*, 82–99.

Delle Fave, A., Bassi, M., & Massimini, F. (2003b). Coping with boundaries: The quality of daily experience of Rom nomads in Europe. *Psychology and developing societies*, *15*, 87–102.

Delle Fave, A., & Fava, G. A. (in press). Positive psychotherapy and social change. In R. Biswas-Diener (Ed.), *Positive psychology as social change*. Dordrecht, NL: Springer.

Delle Fave, A., & Maletto, C. (1992). Processi di attenzione e qualità dell'esperienza soggettiva nei non vedenti [attentional processes and quality of subjective experience in blind people]. In D. Galati (Ed.), *La psicologia dei non vedenti. Processi cognitivi, affettivi e strategie adattative* (pp. 321–353). Milano: Franco Angeli.

Delle Fave, A., & Massimini, F. (1988). Modernization and the changing context of flow in work and leisure. In M. Csikszentmihalyi, & I. Csikszentmihalyi (Eds.), *Optimal experience: Psychological studies of flow in consciousness* (pp. 193–213). New York: Cambridge University Press.

Delle Fave, A., & Massimini, F. (1991). Modernization and the quality of daily experience in a southern Italy village. In N. Bleichrodt & P. J. D. Drenth (eds.), *Contemporary issues in cross-cultural psychology* (pp. 110–119). Amsterdam: Swets & Zeitlinger B.V.

Delle Fave, A., & Massimini, F. (1994). Frequenza della fruizione televisiva quotidiana e qualità dell'esperienza [daily frequency of TV watching and quality of experience]. *Ikon*, *28*, 11–39.

Delle Fave, A., & Massimini, F. (1996). Modernizzazione e fruizione dei media: Dati su due comunità italiane [modernization and use of media: Data from two Italian communities]. *Ikon*, *32*, 95–117.

Delle Fave, A., & Massimini, F. (1999). Flow and sport in atleti agonisti e amatori [Flow and sport in professional and amateur athletes]. Atti del *1° Convegno Nazionale Flow e peak experience: Discipline a confronto* (pp. 49–57). Milano: Psicosport.

Delle Fave, A., & Massimini, F. (2003). Optimal experience in work and leisure among teachers and physicians: Individual and bio-cultural implications. *Leisure Studies*, *22*, 323–342.

Delle Fave, A., & Massimini, F. (2004). The cross-cultural investigation of optimal experience. *Ricerche di Psicologia*, *27*, 79–102.

Delle Fave, A., & Massimini, F. (2005). The investigation of optimal experience and apathy: Developmental and psychosocial implications. *European Psychologist*, *10*, 264–274.

Delle Fave, A. (2009). Optimal experience and meaning: which relationship? *Psychological Topics. Special issue on positive psychology*, *18*, 285–302.

Dilley, R. E., & Scraton, S. J. (2010). Women, climbing and serious leisure. *Leisure Studies*, *29*, 125–141.

Dumazedier, J. (1999). Importance cachée de la croissance du temps libre dans la métamorphose de la civilisation [hidden importance of the increase of free time in the metamorphosis of civilization]. *Society and Leisure*, *22*, 313–322.

Dworkin, J. B., Larson, R. W., & Hansen, D. (2003). Adolescents' accounts of growth experiences in youth activities. *Journal of Youth and Adolescence, 32*, 17–26.

Egan, S., & Stelmack, R. (2003). A personality profile of mount everest climbers. *Personality and Individual Differences, 34*, 1491–1494.

Ewert, A. W. (1994). Playing the edge: Motivation and risk taking in a high-altitude wildernesslike environment. *Environment & Behavior, 26*(1), 3–24.

Ewert, A. W., & Hollenhorst, S. J. (1997). Adventure recreation and its implications for wilderness. *International Journal of Wilderness, 3*, 21–26.

Flammer, A., & Schaffner, B. (2003). Adolescent leisure across European nations. In S. Verma & R. Larson (Eds.), *Examining adolescent leisure time across cultures: Developmental opportunities and risks. New directions in child and adolescent development* (pp. 65–77). San Francisco: Jossey-Bass.

García, T., Cervelló, E., Jimenez, R., Iglesias, D., & Santos-Rosa, F. (2005). Predictive variables related to goal involvement in soccer payers and the relationship between goal involvement, flow state and competition satisfaction. *Revista de Psicología del Deporte, 14*, 21–42.

González-Cutre, D., Sicilia, A., Moreno, J. A., & Fernández-Balboa, J. M. (2009). Disponsitional flow in physical education: Relationships with motivational climate, social goals, and perceived competence. *Journal of Teaching in Physical Education, 28*, 422–440.

Hagger, M. S., & Chatzisarantis, K. L. (Eds.) (2007). *Intrinsic motivation and self-determination in exercise and sport*. Champaign, IL: Human Kynetics.

Hektner, J. M. (2001). Family, school, and community predictors of adolescent growth conducive experiences: Global and specific approaches. *Applied Developmental Science, 5*, 172–183.

Hektner, J. M., Schmidt, J., & Csikszentmihalyi, M. (2007). *Experience sampling method: Measuring the quality of everyday life*. Thousand Oaks, CA: Sage.

Hutchinson, S. L., & Kleiber, D. (2005). Gifts of the ordinary: Casual leisure's contributions to health and well-being. *World Leisure Journal, 47*, 2–16.

Iso-Ahola, S. E. (1997). A psychological analysis of leisure and health. In J. T. Haworth (Ed.), *Work, leisure, and well-being* (pp. 131–144). London: Routledge.

Jackson, S. A., & Csikszentmihalyi, M. (1999). *Flow in sports: The keys to optimal experiences and performances*. Champaign, IL: Human Kinetics.

Jackson, S. A., & Kimiecik, J. C. (2008). The flow perspective of optimal experience in sport and physical activity. In T. H. Horn (Ed.), *Advances in sport psychology* (3rd ed., pp. 377–399). Champaign, IL: Human Kinetics.

Jackson, S. A., & Roberts, G. C. (1992). Positive performance states of athletes: Toward a conceptual understanding of peak performance. *Sport Psychologist, 6*, 156–171.

Jackson, S. A., Thomas, P. R., Marsh, H. W., & Smethurst, C. J. (2001). Relationships between flow, self-concept, psychological skills, and performance. *Journal of Applied Sport Psychology, 13*, 129–153.

Kleiber, D., Larson, R. W., & Csikszentmihalyi, M. (1986). The experience of leisure in adolescence. *Journal of Leisure Research, 18*, 169–176.

Kowal, J., & Fortier, M. S. (1999). Motivational determinants of flow: Contributions from self-determination theory. *Journal of Social Psychology, 139*, 355–368.

Kubey, R., & Csikszentmihalyi, M. (1990). *Television and the quality of life: How viewing shapes everyday experience*. Hillsdale, NJ: Erlbaum.

Kubey, R., & Csikszentmihalyi, M. (2002). Television addiction is no mere metaphor. *Scientific American, 286*, 62–68.

Larson, R. W. (1995). Secrets in the bedroom: Adolescents' private use of media. *Journal of Youth and Adolescence, 24*, 535–550.

Larson, R. W. (2000). Toward a psychology of positive youth development. *American Psychologist, 55*, 170–183.

Larson, R. W., & Kleiber, D. (1993). Daily experience of adolescents. In P. Tolan, and B. Cohler (Eds.), *Handbook of clinical research and practice with adolescents* (pp. 125–145). New York: Wiley.

Larson, R. W., & Kubey, R. (1983). Television and music: Contrasting media in adolescent life. *Youth & Society, 15*, 13–31.

Larson, R. W., & Verma, S. (1999). How children and adolescents spend time across the world: Work, play and developmental opportunities. *Psychological Bulletin, 25*, 701–736.

Lee, M. (2003). Korean adolescents' "examination hell" and their use of free time. In S. Verma & R. Larson (Eds.), *Examining adolescent leisure time across cultures: Developmental opportunities and risks. New directions in child and adolescent development* (pp. 9–21). San Francisco: Jossey-Bass.

Lefevre, J. (1988). Flow and the quality of experience during work and leisure. In M. Csikszentmihalyi, & I. Csikszentmihalyi (Eds.), *Optimal experience: Psychological studies of flow in consciousness* (pp. 307–318). New York: Cambridge University Press.

MacDonald, R., Byrne, C., & Carlton, L. (2006). Creativity and flow in musical composition: An empirical investigation. *Psychology of Music, 34*, 292–306.

Mannell, R. C., Kaczynski, A. T., & Aronson, R. M. (2005). Adolescent participation and flow in physically active leisure and electronic media activities: Testing the displacement hypothesis. *Society and Leisure, 28*, 653–675.

Mannell, R. C., Zuzanek, J., & Larson, R. (1988). Leisure states and "flow" experiences: Testing perceived freedom and intrinsic motivation hypothesis. *Journal of Leisure Research, 20*, 289–304.

Martin, J. J., & Cutler, K. (2002). An exploratory study of flow and motivation in theater actors. *Journal of Applied Sport Psychology, 14*, 344–352.

Massimini, F., & Delle Fave, A. (1995). Qualità dell'esperienza e coltivazione di attività musicali [quality of experience and cultivation of musical activities]. *Comunicazioni Scientifiche di Psicologia Generale, 14*, 157–180.

Massimini, F., & Delle Fave, A. (2000). Individual development in a bio-cultural perspective. *American Psychologist, 55*, 24–33.

Massimini, F., Delle Fave, A., & Borri Gaspardin, M. (1992). Televisione e qualità dell'esperienza soggettiva: L'integrazione tra dati qualitativi e qualitativi [television and quality of subjective experience: Integrating qualitative and quantitative data]. *Ikon, 24*, 5–29.

Massimini, F., Inghilleri, P., Delle Fave, A. (Eds.) (1996). *La selezione psicologica umana – teoria e metodo d'analisi* [Human psychological selection – Theory and method of analysis]. Milano: Coop. Libraria IULM.

Mathwick, C., & Rigdon, E. (2004). Play, flow, and the online search experience. *Journal of Consumer Research, 31*, 324–332.

Mesurado, B. (2009a). Actividad estructurada vs. Actividad desestructurada, realizadas en solitario vs. En compañia de otros y la experiencia óptima [structured activities vs. Unstructured activities, performed alone vs. With others and optimal experience]. *Anales de psicología, 25*, 308–315.

Mesurado, B. (2009b). La experiencia de flow en niños y adolescentes en el uso de la informática [optimal experience in children's and adolescents' use of informatics]. In M. C. Richaud and J. E. Moreno (Eds.), *Investigación en ciencias del comportamiento: Avances iberoamericanos* (pp. 219–230). Buenos Aires: Ed. CIIPME – Conicet.

Moreno, J. A., Alonso, N., Martínez, C., Cervelló, E., & Ruiz, L. M. (2008). Motivation, disciplined behaviour, equal treatment and dispositional flow in physical education students. *Journal of International Social Research, 1*, 446–466.

Mutrie, N., & Faulkner, G. (2002). Physical activity: Positive psychology in motion. In P. A. Linley and S. Joseph (Eds.), *Positive psychology in practice* (pp. 146–163). New York: Wiley.

Nakamura, J., & Csikszentmihalyi, M. (2009). Flow theory and research. In S. J. Lopez & C. R. Snyder (Eds.), *Handbook of positive psychology* (pp. 195–206). New York: Oxford University Press.

Nishino, H. J., & Larson, R. W. (2003). Japanese adolescents' free time: Juku, bukatsu, and government efforts to create more meaningful leisure. In S. Verma & R. Larson (Eds.), *Examining adolescent leisure time across cultures: Developmental opportunities and risks. New directions in child and adolescent development* (pp. 23–35). San Francisco: Jossey-Bass.

Olivier, G. G. F. (2000). Le ludique dans la formation sociale de l'homme: Une théorie critique du loisir [playfulness in the social formation of man: A critical theory of leisure]. *Society and Leisure, 23*, 21–39.
Partington, S., Partington, E., & Olivier, S. (2009). The dark side of flow: A qualitative study of dependence in big wave surfing. *Sport Psychologist, 23*, 179–185.
Pávon, A., & Moreno, J. A. (2008). Actitud de los universitarios ante la prática físico-deportiva: Diferencias por géneros [university students' attitute to physical exercise and sport: Gender differences]. *Revista de Psicología del Deporte, 17*, 7–23.
Rathunde, K. (2001). Family context and the development of undivided interest: A longitudinal study of family support and challenge and adolescents' quality of experience. *Applied Developmental Science, 5*, 158–171.
Rheinberg, F., & Manig, Y. (2003). Was macht spaß am graffiti-sprayen? Eine induktive anreizanalyse [what's entertaining about graffiti spraying? An inductive analysis on incentives]. *Report Psychologie, 28*, 222–234.
Robinson, D. W. (1985). Stress seeking: Selected behavioral characteristics of elite rock climbers. *Journal of Sport Psychology, 7*, 400–404.
Schmidt, J. (2003). Correlates of reduced misconduct among adolescents facing adversity. *Journal of Youth and Adolescence, 32*, 439–452.
Schüler, J., & Brunner, S. (2009). The rewarding effect of flow experience on performance in a marathon race. *Psychology of Sport and Exercise, 10*, 168–174.
Seifert, T., & Hedderson, C. (2010). Intrinsic motivation and flow in skateboarding: An ethnographic study. *Journal of Happiness Studies, 11*, 277–292.
Shernoff, D., & Vandell, D. L. (2007). Engagement in after-school program activities: Quality of experience from the perspective of participants. *Journal of Youth and Adolescence, 36*, 891–903.
Sherry, J. L. (2004). Flow and media enjoyment. *Communication Theory, 14*, 328–347.
Skadberg, Y. X., & Kimmel, J. R. (2004). Visitors' flow experience while browsing a web site: Its measurement, contributing factors and consequences. *Computers in Human Behavior, 20*, 403–422.
Stavrou, N. A., Jackson, S. A., Zervas, Y., & Karteroliotis, K. (2007). Flow experience and athletes' performance with reference to t eorthogonal model of flow. *Sport Psychologist, 21*, 438–457.
Stebbins, R. A. (1997). Serious leisure and well-being. In J. T. Haworth (Ed.), *Work, leisure, and well-being* (pp. 117–130). London: Routledge.
Stebbins, R. A. (2001). *New directions in the theory and research of serious leisure*. Lewiston, NY: The Edwin Mellen.
Stebbins, R. A. (2007). *Serious leisure: A perspective for our time*. London: Transaction Publishers.
Verma, S., & Larson, R. W. (Eds.) (2003). *Examining adolescent leisure time across cultures: Developmental opportunities and risks. New directions in child and adolescent development*. San Francisco: Jossey-Bass.
Vittersø, J., Vorkinn, M., & Vistad, O. D. (2001). Congruence between recreational model and actual behavior. A prerequisite for optimal experiences? *Journal of Leisure Research, 33*, 137–159.
Voiskounsky, A. E., Mitina, O. V., & Avetisova, A. A. (2004). Playing online games: Flow experience. *PsychNology Journal, 3*, 259–281.
Voiskounsky, A. E., & Smyslova, O. V. (2003). Flow-based model of computer hackers' motivation. *Cyber Psychology, 6*, 171–180.
Wan, C. S., & Chiou, W. B. (2006). Psychological motives and online games addiction: A test of flow theory and humanistic needs theory for Taiwanese adolescents. *Cyber Psychology & Behavior, 9*, 317–324.
Whitmore, J. G., & Borrie, W. T. (2005). Exploring the usefulness of the dispositional flow scale for outdoor recreation activities. In J. G. Peden and R. M. Schuster (Eds.), *Proceedings of the 2005 northeastern recreation research symposium* (pp. 371–378). Newtown Square, PA: Forest Service, Northeastern Research Station.

Chapter 10
Relationships: Safe Harbor for Flow Explorers

10.1 Introduction

The identity formation of human beings as social animals has deep roots in the quality of relationships. Moreover, as outlined in Chapter 2, human adaptation is only partially a biological matter: Individuals have also to develop a cultural fitness, a key resource to cope with environmental challenges. No other species requires such a long period of education to acquire the pool of information necessary to behave adaptively within the complexity of the cultural networks developed by human societies. In this perspective, the direction and complexity of the individual developmental path are strongly influenced by social models and interaction patterns.

From birth until old age, relationships play a crucial role in meeting basic needs that range from personal care to affiliation (Pöhlman, 2001), as well as age-specific requirements such as identity formation in adolescence (Schwartz & Pantin, 2006) and autonomy support during old age (Wiggins, Higgs, Hyde, & Blane, 2004). Relationships contribute to personal growth and individual self-actualization by providing trust, self-esteem, and support (An & Cooney, 2006; Burleson, Kunkel, Samter, & Werking, 1996; Myers, 2000; Noller, 2005). Ryff's model of psychological well-being includes positive relations as one of its six dimensions (Ryff & Keyes, 1995). Much effort is required to maintain constant relationships with relatives and friends in time. However, individuals who succeed in building solid and harmonious relationships benefit from emotional closeness, companionship, and social identity support (Sherman, Lansford, & Volling, 2006; Weisz & Wood, 2005). In particular, close social networks influence the selection, initiation, and maintenance of new relationships (MacDonald & Ross, 1999; Parks, 2007), as clearly showed in cross-cultural studies (Lalonde, Hynie, Pannu, & Tatla, 2004; Zhang & Kline, 2009).

In this chapter, we will specifically discuss the role of family and close relationships in influencing the quality of experience in daily life, in promoting optimal experience, and in orienting resource investment in present challenges and future goals. Empirically, evidence will be provided through findings derived from previous studies, and through the analysis of data coming from the cross-cultural sample we are using as a general database throughout this book (see Chapter 7).

A. Delle Fave et al., *Psychological Selection and Optimal Experience Across Cultures*, Cross-Cultural Advancements in Positive Psychology 2,
DOI 10.1007/978-90-481-9876-4_10, © Springer Science+Business Media B.V. 2011

10.2 Family Relationships and Well-Being

From a biocultural perspective, Super and Harkness (1986) analyzed family as one of the key components of the developmental niche, which comprises the set of factors influencing individual growth and behavior: the natural and cultural daily environment, the culturally based child-rearing practices, and the psychology and behavior of the caretakers. A growing body of studies shows that family is a powerful mediator of cultural rules and norms, especially as concerns personal relationships (Reis, Collins, & Berscheid, 2000). Child-rearing practices and the socialization patterns and values transmitted within families have been investigated across cultures, showing their connection with the individualistic or collectivistic value orientation of the society (Baer, Curtis, Grabb, & Johnston, 1996; Low, 1989; Wang & Tamis-Lemonda, 2003).

Among the prominent scholars of families in the cross-cultural perspective, Cigdem Kagitçibasi highlighted the role of family as a system situated within a cultural and social structural context. Within the developmental niche, parents set socialization goals for their children which are adequate to the cultural environment they will live in. Children usually internalize basic expectations and attitudes concerning social behavior through interactions with caregivers (Sroufe & Fleeson, 1986), and later on experiment and apply these relational patterns to different social contexts. Following the distinction between independent and interdependent self-construals (Markus & Kitayama, 1991) as orientations characterizing individualistic and collectivistic cultures respectively, Kagitçibasi identified three prototypical family interaction patterns in child-rearing practice: the traditional, collectivistic pattern of emotional and instrumental interdependence among family members; the individualistic model, typical of western cultures, fostering child independence; and a dialectical synthesis of the two models, the autonomous relatedness pattern, in which the promotion of children's autonomy and agency coexists with the psychological interdependence and relatedness among family members (Kagitçibasi, 1996). This approach allowed to overcome the rigid distinction between individualistic and collectivistic cultures, especially as concerns family relationships. Cross-cultural studies showed that, especially in the last decades, the modernization trend favored the prominence of the psychological interdependence pattern within non-western families (Kagitçibasi, 2005; Keller et al., 2006; Oyserman, Kemmelmeier, & Coon, 2002). This pattern supports both individual and family well-being thanks to the promotion of autonomy and relatedness, two of the basic psychological needs endorsed by self-determination theory (Ryan & Deci, 2000).

Alongside biological features and cultural norms, parenthood requires an experiential adjustment to new environmental challenges. Subjective experience and individual life history play an important role in parental behavior. Studies on imprinting, attachment, and Internal Working Models showed that early relationships have evolutionary consequences at the biocultural level. Missing or poor caretaking during infancy generates highly maladaptive consequences during adolescence and adulthood, in terms of self-identity, social behavior, and parenting

(Bowlby, 1969, 1988; De Wolff & van Ijzendoorn, 1997; Main and Goldwyn 1984; Freedman & Gorman, 1993). The classical experiments by Harlow and Harlow (1965) clearly highlighted the consequences of inadequate caretaking among non-human primates; as concerns humans, a non-organic "failure to thrive" syndrome was identified among infants whose mothers suffered deprivation of reliable relationships during childhood (Benoit, Zeanah, & Barton, 1989). The quality of home environment and of the care infants receive proved to be related to their affect and temperament in several studies, and across countries (Luster, Boger, & Hannan, 1993; Pierrehumbert et al., 2009; Seifer, Schiller, Sameroff, Resnick, & Riordan, 1996).

At the individual level, another important dimension promoting children's harmonious growth across cultures is parents' perceived self-efficacy (Bandura, 1997). Parental self-efficacy (PSE) represents the beliefs that parents hold in their capacity to influence their children's behavior and the environment in order to promote children's successful development (Ardelt & Eccles, 2001). Efficacious parents are more likely to adopt adequate parenting strategies, thus promoting their children's success in the social and academic domains (Bogenschneider, Small, & Tsay, 1997; Jones & Prinz, 2005; Shumow & Lomax, 2002; Xiang, McBride, & Bruene, 2003). In addition, across cultures PSE has proved to promote children's self-regulation and to prevent them from the risk of engaging in deviant activities (Cote et al., 2009; Hill & Bush, 2001; Izzo, Weiss, Shanahan, & Rodriguez-Brown, 2000; Murry & Brody, 1999). PSE also promotes positive family relationships through parental responsiveness (Gondoli & Silverberg, 1997) and open communication (Bogenschneider et al., 1997).

Studies on optimal experience have highlighted that a supportive and challenging environment at home is crucial for children's psychosocial adaptation. Parents providing their children with the right balance between support and challenge keep them in the zone of proximal development (Vygotsky 1978), wherein the growth of mastery and self-efficacy are more likely to take place (Rathunde, 2001). Family interactions and activities can provide opportunities for skill building and growth experiences vis-à-vis long-term developmental goals (Hektner, 2001). The influence of parents' support and challenge on children's moods and goals, as well as parental role in orienting children's investment of skills and resources in optimal activities is evident throughout childhood and adolescence (Rathunde, 2001). Positive interactions with parents may set a standard by which children attempt to forge important peer relationships (Brown, Mounts, Lamborn, & Steinberg, 1993; Rathunde, 1997).

10.2.1 Parenting: Biology, Culture, and Subjective Experience

The evolutionary approach highlighted the role of mate selection, pair bonding, and parental behavior in enhancing offspring's biological chances to survive and reproduce (Buss et al., 1990; Daly, 1990; Lampert, 1997; Tooby & Cosmides, 1996; Trivers, 1972). More recently, scholars are increasingly focusing on the combined influence of biology and culture in orienting individual and social behavior (see Chapter 2).

Biological constraints on couple and parenting roles at the gender level are unquestionable (Buss, 1989): pregnancy, delivery, and breast-feeding are women's domain (MacCormack & Strathern, 1980). Gender differences have been investigated in hormonal profile during pregnancy and after child birth. In particular, the levels of prolactin, the hormone stimulating lactogenesis, rise during pregnancy and fall within few weeks after child birth in females. Prolactin seems to facilitate maternal behavior in rats (Bridges, DiBiase, Loundes, & Doherty, 1985), but its influence on humans is not yet clearly understood. Other clinical findings suggest that adaptive maternal behavior is associated with female hormonal "readiness": Teenage girls run higher medical risks during pregnancy and show poor performance in being mothers (Montagu, 1981; Warren & Shortle, 1990). As concerns fathers, current knowledge on the physiological changes associated with child birth is still incomplete. Again, there is evidence of higher prolactin levels in nurturing nonhuman male primates (Dixson & George, 1982), but no clear results have been obtained yet from humans. More attention is also being paid to *couvade* syndrome, a complex set of physical and psychosomatic symptoms reported by a significant proportion of men in industrialized societies during their partner's pregnancy and delivery (Lipkin & Lamb, 1982; Teichman & Lahav, 1987; Trethowan & Conlon, 1965). The term *couvade* comes from anthropological literature, and it originally referred to rituals performed by fathers in some preindustrial cultures shortly before and after child birth (Malinowski, 1927; Munroe, Munroe, & Whiting, 1981). Its role in humans has been investigated from different perspectives, as a pattern of physiological changes mediating paternal responsiveness (Elwood & Mason, 1994), or as a consequence of men's cultural and psychological involvement in fatherhood (Bogren, 1983; Clinton, 1985; Yogman, 1990). The biological modifications associated with pregnancy and parenthood can explain cross-cultural recurring reproductive and parental behaviors (Manning & Chamberlain, 1991; Salk, 1960), as well as the gender difference in time and energy allocation on offspring (Hrdy, 1981; Towsend et al., 1995). However, genetically transmitted traits constantly interact with the natural environment, which places survival and reproduction constraints on the individual behavior (Kaplan & Hill, 1992). Moreover, epigenetic and cultural inheritance substantially affect development, as discussed in Chapter 2 (Jablonka & Lamb, 2005).

Current cross-cultural research is a valuable tool to analyze reproductive behavior and child-rearing patterns among human groups. It allowed for detecting differences between societies that in several cases can be only partially referred to differences in natural environment (Mealey & Mackey, 1990). As concerns reproductive behavior, the negative population growth curve of most European countries is just one of the numerous cases of divergent genetic and cultural fitness reported in recent years. Although the amount of material family resources could ensure the survival and reproduction of several descendants, parents tend to concentrate their investment on only one or two children, who will have more opportunities to learn, and to exploit cultural resources. Researchers have also analyzed the impact of childbirth on modern family life. Modernization has brought remarkable changes in gender roles in most western cultures, influencing family structure and parents' involvement to such an extent that it has been referred to as the second demographic transition (Buss, Shackelford, Kirkpatrick, & Larsen, 2001; Lesthaeghe, 1992). One of the main features of the modern family is the diversification of women's daily roles, in addition to the traditional domestic ones (Chafetz & Hagan, 1996; Hoffman & Youngblade, 1999). Nevertheless, traditional gender differences persist in the effect of parenthood on work: In comparison with childless women, mothers devote a lower amount of hours to paid work, while for men fatherhood is associated with a higher work effort (Kaufman & Uhlenberg, 2000). Changes were instead detected in the organization of housework and in childcare: Men's contribution has almost doubled in the last three decades (Bryant & Wang, 1990; Cooksey & Fondell, 1996; Gerson, 1993; Meyer and Garasky 1993), while women's one has strongly decreased (Bianchi, Milkie, Sayer, & Robinson, 2000; Lamb, 1987). However, studies conducted in various western countries show that father's involvement in parenting activities is generally lower than mothers' (Bryant & Zick, 1996; Clarke-Stewart, 1980; Drew, Emerek, & Mahon, 1998; Gottfried, Gottfried, & Bathurst, 1995; Rexroat & Shehan, 1987; Zick & Bryant, 1996), even when children grow older and both parents—at least in dual-income families—devote to work a considerable amount of their time (Drew, 1998; McBride & Rane, 1998). Culturally sanctioned gender roles, economic constraints, and employment policies strongly influence the male's active engagement as nurturer (Yogman, 1990).

Alongside biological features and cultural norms, parenthood implies a radical overhaul of individuals' hierarchy of values, and a redistribution of the limited psychic resources in the daily life. Several studies investigated behavioral changes and psychological adjustment of new parents (Belsky, 1985; Coffman, Levitt, & Brown, 1994; Fiese, Hooker, Kotary, & Schwagler, 1993; Kach & McGhee, 1982; Ruble, Fleming, Hackel, & Stangor, 1988; Tomlinson, 1987). In particular, the quality of caregiving is related to parents' psychological health. Personal enjoyment and satisfaction in the relationship with the child—and with the spouse—play a crucial role in the quality of parental care (Simons, Beanman, Conger, & Chao, 1993). As described in Chapter 3, within and beyond the constraints biology and culture place on humans, the long-term process of psychological selection is directed step by step by subjective evaluations of the environmental requests and challenges during daily life. In order to investigate these issues we run a pilot study with ESM among five primiparous Italian women and their husbands during and after pregnancy (Delle Fave & Massimini, 2004). The couples took part to 8 ESM sessions, four before delivery (10th, 20th, 30th, and 35th week of pregnancy) and four after child birth (3rd and 7th week, 3rd and 6th month). Results highlighted some of the biological, cultural, and individual factors influencing the development of parental role.

Across self-reports, parenthood was described as a complex and demanding situation. Both mothers and fathers prominently associated child care with the perception of high challenges and engagement, positive mood and intrinsic motivation. Over 70% of ESM self-reports referring to parenting were comprised in channels 1, 2, and 8 of the EFM model, all characterized by the perception of above-average challenges (see Chapter 5 for details on the model). Both parents perceived child related activities as significantly more engaging, challenging, and relevant for their life goals, in comparison with the rest of daily situations. Moreover, optimal experience in parenting was characterized by the highest values of all psychological variables, if compared with the other daily activities. Some gender differences emerged in the parents' time-budget: fathers spent a much lower amount of time with their children than mothers did. Considering that the data were gathered within 6 months after child birth, biological constraints connected with breast-feeding, and cultural factors such as gender roles and provisions for maternity leave could explain this difference (Delle Fave & Massimini, 2000). Gender differences also emerged in the activities parents performed with the child, and in the quality of related experience. Fathers prominently played and interacted with the newborn, and reported significantly high values of mood and intrinsic reward. Mothers attended a variety of parenting tasks, and perceived significantly low levels of confidence and personal skills.

The association of optimal experience with child care can be considered a good starting point for child development. Moving from Vygotsky's approach, several researchers have stressed the influence of family context on individual development (Bruner, 1990; Rogoff, 1990). An enjoyable environment at home and a constructive parent–child relationship greatly support both children and family well-being (Crnic, Greenberg, Ragozin, Robinson, & Basham, 1983; Sacco & Murray, 1997; Wenk, Hardesty, Morgan, & Blair, 1994). More specifically, as stated by Rathunde (1989) and Csikszentmihalyi and Rathunde (1991), parents who perceive engagement, involvement, and intrinsic motivation in the daily opportunities for action—child care, but also work, leisure, and social interactions—are more likely to encourage their children's search for challenges and commitment to skill cultivation. In the perspective of self-determination theory (Deci & Ryan, 2000), such a family context fosters internalization of motives, promoting children's competence and autonomy, on one hand, and relatedness, on the other hand. The difficulties reported by the mothers in coping with their new role can be related to three major aspects: the lack of experience of primiparous mothers (Boukydis & Burgess, 1982; Fleming, 1990); the proportionally longer time devoted to parenting compared with fathers, which entails all minor and major difficulties involved in daily child caring; the relative isolation of postmodern nuclear families, in which mothers are totally in charge of the newborn. On the other hand, the enjoyment and intrinsic reward reported by fathers in the interaction with the child is consistent with other studies: For example, Yogman (1990) describes fathers' behavior as more playful, stimulating, and arousing than mothers'. Since males are not traditionally socialized to become caretakers, wives' constant presence and prominent role enable them to engage in the exciting and motivating aspects of child care, whereas mothers seem more responsive to the psychological burden and responsibility entailed in daily parenting activities.

In terms of psychological selection, the association of a positive and challenging experience with parenting enhances the probability that the parents will preferentially select and cultivate child-related activities in the future. This is an important premise, because the building of a constructive and well-balanced family relationship is based not just on the amount of time mothers and fathers spend in child care, but on the quality of the interaction, primarily related to the subjective experience (Bonney, Kelley, & Levant, 1999). The perceived importance of child birth is a prerequisite for adequate investment of attention on child care and education. From a biocultural perspective, it will ultimately facilitate the cross-generational transmission of those behavioral instructions the child will need to fit the biocultural environment. For the participants in our study, the relevance of parenthood was not limited to the present time, but it was also projected into the future as their main goal. This entails a strong and long-term commitment to develop the complex behavioral and social skills related to parenthood. The outcome will directly influence child growth, as shown by extensive research studies investigating the consequences of early family interactions on child and adult behavior (Bretherton & Waters, 1985; Crowell & Feldman, 1991; Hinde & Stevenson-Hinde, 1988; van Ijendoorn, 1992).

Within this approach further studies should be performed in order to shed light on cross-cultural differences in the daily quality of experience of new parents. Some data among pregnant South American immigrant women were recently gathered in our research group (Stokart, 2010), but the work is still in progress.

10.2.2 Adolescents and Family: Constraints and Opportunities

Across cultures, adolescents rate their parents as important landmarks in their lives, as sources of emotional and material support as well as providers of opportunities for development and identity building (Branje, van Aken, & van Lieshout, 2002; Collins, 1990; Helsen, Vollenbergh, & Meeus, 2000; Lanz, Iafrate, Marta, & Rosnati, 1999; McHale, Crouter, & Whiteman, 2003). The prolonged and strong ties with the family of origin that characterize humans can be related to neoteny at the biological level, and to the complex adaptation pressures imposed by increasingly articulated cultural systems on individual behavior. In particular, the lengthening of the formal education phase spreading in most countries implies the forced dependence of adolescents of both genders from their parents, requiring some kind of mutual adjustment (Bonifazi, Menniti, Misiti, & Palomba, 1999; Shulman & Ben-Artzi, 2003; Smetana, 1995; van Wel, Linssen, & Abma, 2000). Parents have to cope with teenagers' growing autonomy and exploration needs arising from biological maturation, psychological development, and cultural expectations. In their turn, adolescents have to find a balance between the attraction toward extra-family challenges and the need for family support. They often adopt disengagement and distance from family intimacy, rules, and values as strategies to achieve individual autonomy, while living in daily close contact with their parents (Collins, 1995; Larson, Richards, Moneta, Holmbeck, & Duckett, 1996; Searight, Thomas, Manley, & Ketterson, 1995; Wigfield, Eccles, & Pintrich, 1996).

The urge to autonomy along with the storm and stress characterizing adolescence can lead to family conflicts and misconduct (Santrock, 1997). The family itself can be the source of adolescents' malaise. Delinquency, drug abuse, academic difficulties are just some of the problems associated with a "depriving environment" in which family violence and neglect play a central role (Levesque, 2001). Similarly, cross-cultural research has provided compelling evidence of the influence of perceived parental rejection–acceptance on psychological adjustment and the development of deviant behaviors during adolescence and adulthood (Kim & Rohner, 2003; Rohner & Britner, 2002).

From an opposite perspective, researchers are increasingly paying attention to the role of family in promoting optimal development (Seligman & Csikszentmihalyi, 2000). The study of well-functioning and satisfied families can highlight interaction patterns and processes that may be applied to problematic families (Rich, 2003). Several studies have focused on adolescents' relations with parents and siblings, particularly referring to attachment and intimacy (Bowlby, 1982; Buist, Dekovic, Meeus, & Van Aken, 2002; Zavattini, Tambelli, Volpi, Chiarolanza, & Macone, 2002). The strong and secure relationship with the family, and with parents in particular, seems to play a fundamental role in the lives of adolescents, and it proves to be of lasting importance during young adulthood (van Wel et al., 2000). In particular, a secure attachment pattern can foster a prominent allocation of attention on extra-family opportunities and relationships during adolescence (Cobb, 1996; Delle Fave & Bassi, 2003; Larose & Boivin, 1998; Mounts, 2002).

At the cross-cultural level, a growing number of studies investigated the impact on adolescents' well-being of culturally valued models of family relationship (Dwairy & Achoui, 2006). For example, Chinese-American youth high in filial piety (respect and devotion to parents, subordination of one's own interests to family needs and requirements; Ho, 1996) were less prone to smoking and drug abuse (Juang & Nguyen, 2009). Similar findings were obtained among Latino adolescents scoring high in familism, which implies a strong family connection at both the emotional and instrumental levels (Gil, Wagner, & Vega, 2000). The previously cited approach developed by Kagitçibasi (2005), based on the distinction among different socialization patterns, allows for interpreting differences in child rearing from both the developmental and cultural perspectives.

One crucial aspect of family relationships is represented by the quality of experience associated with daily interactions. As adolescents spend a limited amount of time with their parents, shared situations become substantial opportunities for them to exchange ideas, receive suggestions, and also play an active role in family matters. In particular, optimal experience in family interactions plays a key role for both parents and children, increasing the enjoyment and the intrinsic reward derived from their relationship (Rathunde, 1997). Moreover, besides family interactions, parents retrieving optimal experiences in other domains of their lives can facilitate and encourage their children's capacity to derive optimal experiences from opportunities for action outside the family circle, such as at school and in learning tasks, by supporting their self-regulation and self-efficacy beliefs (Rathunde, 2001; Steca, Bassi, Caprara, & Delle Fave, 2010). Consistent with this approach are the findings gathered from the perspective of self-determination theory (Ryan & Deci, 2000), showing that teenagers' rejection of their schools' values is related to the undermining of intrinsic motivation. Children who have more fully internalized the regulation for positive school-related behaviors are those who feel securely connected to, and cared for by, their parents and teachers (Ryan, Stiller, & Lynch, 1994).

Research has also highlighted the preferential socialization with the same-sex parent in adolescence (Gecas & Seff, 1990; McHale et al., 2003). Mother–daughter relationships are more intense (Peters, 1994) and females perceive greater intimacy with the mothers than males (Field, Lang, Yando, & Bendell, 1995). This phenomenon, widely spread in all human communities, as pointed out in anthropological research (Schlegel, 1977), can be related to Gilligan's seminal work (Gilligan, 1982) showing that females devote a large amount of attention to personal relationships, and in self-descriptions they emphasize their role in relation to others. Other researchers have pointed out a stronger female orientation toward intimacy and self-disclosure (Fallon & Bowles, 1997; Paterson, Field, & Pryor, 1994; Searight et al., 1995); girls seem to be more inclined toward other-directed activities and behavior (Bruno, 1996; Ma & Huebner, 2008). However, preferential socialization with the same-sex parent can also be related to the cultural transmission of gender roles: Parents' interactions are characterized by the emphasis on separation with sons and on closeness with daughters (Leaper et al., 1989; Shulman & Ben-Artzi, 2003).

Studies conducted with ESM among Italian adolescents (Bassi & Delle Fave, 2004, 2006; Delle Fave, Bassi, & Massimini, 2002) confirmed theoretical assumptions and previous research evidence. Globally, adolescents associated to family interaction an experience of free and pleasant relaxation: Both boys and girls perceived average mood values, significantly low levels of engagement, high confidence and intrinsic motivation. Time with the family was devoted to passive leisure (watching TV) and maintenance activities. Optimal experience was mostly associated with socializing (talking, conversation, discussions).

These results are consistent with the findings obtained in ESM studies conducted among US adolescents (Larson et al., 1996) and among Indian teenagers (Larson & Verma, 1999). A relaxing family context counterbalances the high mandatory engagement in studying activities, and the exciting peer meetings. As Simmons and Blyth stated (1987), a stable family environment provides an "arena of comfort" which helps adolescents cope with external challenges, and fulfill their need for asserting personal identity (Damon & Hart, 1988) and individuation from parents (Allen, Hauser, Bell, & O'Connor, 1994; Belsky, Steinberg, & Draper, 1991; McElhaney, Porter, Thompson, & Allen, 2008).

The different amount of time Italian adolescents sampled through ESM reported spending with each parent was consistent with the results obtained in other studies (Amato, 1994; Buist et al., 2002; Kerns & Stevens, 1996; Lanz et al., 1999; Larson et al., 1996; Rosnati, 1996). The mother was more present and available than the father, and both daughters and sons spent a larger amount of time with her. However, girls reported being with their mothers more frequently than boys, prominently spent this shared time socializing, and reported flow as the most frequent experience. In contrast, boys most frequently associated the time spent with their mothers with the experience of apathy. Boys did not spend more time with their fathers than girls, nor did they talk more with him. Interestingly enough, the most frequent activity they reported while with their fathers was watching TV. However, despite the limited amount of shared time and the kind of activities performed, apparently poor in communication and interaction opportunities, boys reported a remarkably positive experience with their fathers, especially as concerned mood and intrinsic motivation.

Social roles in postindustrial societies are far from being rigidly and uniquely determined by gender and family expectations. Most participants in the ESM studies conducted in the US and Italy had not yet identified their main interests in study or work, and their future was still to be defined (Rosnati, 1996). This process requires energy investment in and attention focus on the cultural opportunities offered by the society, in order to discern which ones best suit individual attitudes and goals (Csikszentmihalyi, Rathunde, & Whalen, 1993; Delle Fave & Bassi, 2000). This process also allows the individual to practice personal skills in various domains, and to discover new sources of rewarding, positive, and complex experiences (Massimini & Delle Fave, 2000). From this perspective, family both provides a safe harbor and a microcosm in which parents can encourage children's attention investment into meaningful activities and relationships (Rathunde, 1989). Adolescents in the Italian sample associated family talking and socializing with positive and gratifying experiences: This is an important premise for open communication and information exchange, one of the fundamental and most enriching activities adolescents and their parents can share.

At the cross-cultural level, an investigation with ESM conducted among Nepalese high school students living in Kathmandu confirmed the role of family as a context of relaxation, positive mood, and intrinsic motivation (Delle Fave & Massimini, 2005; Delle Fave et al., 2003a). However, Nepalese adolescents mostly devoted the time spent with family to domestic work and to the care for younger siblings (Stokart, Cavallo, Fianco, & Lombardi, 2007). In traditional societies, the involvement of children in family work activities is part of the cultural education strategy (Goodnow, 1988; Nsamenang, 1992). The involvement of children in work shows great variations, according to the economic needs of the family, the features of the natural and cultural environment, the local opportunities for work, and the gender, age, and school attendance of the child. Recent surveys of the International Labour Organisation (ILO) estimated that some 250 millions of children aged between 5 and 14 work (see Chapter 15 for a more detailed analysis of the issue). However, in many cases their active contribution to family welfare involves activities that neither hamper their development, nor prevent them from going to school. On the opposite, performing domestic chores, and taking care of siblings or of other children in the family can promote individual responsibility and gratification (Whiting & Edwards, 1988).

The relationship between parental efficacy beliefs and children's optimal experience was recently investigated in another study with Italian adolescents (Steca et al., 2010). Results showed that children of high PSE parents were more engaged and motivated in learning and perceived higher levels of happiness and freedom during family and peer interactions than adolescents with low PSE parents. In addition, adolescents with high PSE parents reported a significantly higher percentage of optimal experiences. Considering the role of flow in the process of competence development and long-term goal pursuit (Massimini & Delle Fave, 2000; Chapter 3), these results suggested that adolescents with high PSE parents lived in a supportive and challenging environment, rich in growth experiences (Rathunde, 2001), sustaining their cognitive investment in learning activities, and happiness in social relations. In addition, they perceived more autonomy in both productive activities and relationships, including family interactions.

10.2.3 Sibling Relations: A Case Study on Twins

Sibling relationships represent the most enduring of all family bonds (Sherman et al., 2006; Stewart, Verbrugge, & Beilfuss, 1998). They tend to peak during childhood, when children live with parents, and wane during adulthood, when individuals' attention is primarily devoted to their own partners and family (Buhrmester & Furman, 1990). In old age, especially sisters maintain their relationship, sharing memories and support (Lee, Mancini, & Maxwell, 1990).

Within sibling relationships, twin bonds show some peculiarities. The most distinctive aspect of the twin couple is that it constitutes a unit from birth (Valente Torre, 1998). In their families, the dyadic parent–child interaction is actually a triadic condition, in which the twin children form the basic dyad (Robin, Josse, & Tourette, 1988). In particular monozygotic (MZ) twins share a very intense relationship, often characterized by social closure and affective self-sufficiency, especially in female pairs (Penninkilampi-Kerola, Moilanen, & Kaprio, 2005; Thorpe & Gardner, 2005).

Psychological research primarily focused on the impact of genetic and sociocultural factors on their personality and behavior (Boomsma, Busjahn, & Peltonen, 2002; Pike & Atzaba-Poria, 2003; Plomin, Reiss, Hetherington, & Howe, 1994). Negative consequences of twinship on psychological development were identified, such as language delays due to social closure (Thorpe, 2006), exclusive within-couple linguistic expressions (Zani, Carelli, Benelli, & Cicognani, 1991; Zazzo, 1960/2005), and shared habitual gestures and facial expressions. Moreover, the physical identity of MZ twins may hamper the process of identification–separation which is essential for identity formation (Akerman & Suurvee, 2003). Parents often amplify twins' identical appearance, dressing and combing their children in the same way.

In spite of the physical resemblance, Zazzo (1984) identified a strong differentiation process at the psychological level, the so-called paradox of twins. In their daily interaction with the environment, twins invest their attention and resources in diversified opportunities and activities, thus growing as unique individuals (Plomin & Daniels, 1987). However, at the same time they develop a couple identity consisting of complementary roles which favor the dyad cohesion (Zazzo, 1984). In particular, one of the twins takes care of "public relations" with other people, while the other one becomes responsible for the couple, acting as its guide and guardian. Researchers have labeled these complementary roles as the Minister of Foreign Affairs and the Minister of Domestic Affairs, respectively (von Bracken, 1934).

A longitudinal study with an MZ twin couple of young women, followed for 1 year through 12 ESM samplings (one per month), allowed us to shed light on the daily unfolding of this dyadic relationship and of the pair's psychological selection patterns (Bassi & Delle Fave, 2009). In order to detect similarities and differences in the experience associated by twins to shared contexts and situations, their beeper schedules were synchronized. The two members of the couple, conventionally named Paola and Chiara, showed similarities in both productive and leisure domains: They attended the same university courses and shared the same part-time job. Convergence was also detected in their daily social contexts: They lived with their parents and spent over one third of their time together, prominently at home, and performing typical family routine activities, such as maintenance, interactions, watching TV, reading magazines and books, and studying. Both members of the couple spent far more time with their co-twin than with friends.

The uniqueness of the twin bond further emerged in the participants' patterns of daily experience fluctuation (assessed through the Experience Fluctuation Model described in Chapter 5), and in the activities associated with optimal experience. Results showed a strong psychological juxtaposition within the dyad, confirming Zazzo's paradox of twins. In particular, when the twins were together, Paola reported low-challenge and high-challenge experiences in similar percentages, whereas Chiara primarily reported low-challenge experiences. For Paola, the most frequent experience while being with the co-twin was boredom, followed by arousal and optimal experience, while apathy prevailed for Chiara, followed by control and boredom.

As concerns opportunities for optimal experiences together, both participants prominently reported reading, studying, and miscellaneous tasks. Although performed in the presence of the co-twin, these typically individual tasks do not require interaction. However, a crucial difference emerged in the couple: Interaction with the twin accounted for the 25% of the opportunities for optimal experience reported by Paola, while Chiara never quoted it. This confirms that living in the same environment does not mean sharing the same experiences (Plomin & Daniels, 1987), nor does genetic identity imply the development of identical personalities. In this MZ twin couple each member achieved her personal differentiation. Although they shared academic and leisure interests, they differed in the daily appraisal of their relationship. Results identified the twins' complementary roles described by Zazzo (1984): Paola played the role of the minister of domestic affairs, being the guardian of the couple, while Chiara, as the minister of foreign affairs, was more projected outward. More generally, this study confirmed the potential of ESM in detecting unique individual features in the daily unfolding of psychological selection, and its usefulness in shedding light on the psychological features of dyadic interaction patterns.

10.3 Friendship Construction Through Shared Experiences

The primary quality of friendship is individual choice (Dunn, Slomkowski, & Beardsall, 1994; Sherman, de Vries, & Lansford, 2000). Same-sex aggregation among peers already appears during childhood (Schneider, 2000), and cross-cultural studies showed its substantial independence on gender roles and social norms (Maccoby, 1998; Munroe and Romney 2006). During adolescence, interactions with peers and friends acquire increasing relevance (Brown, 2004; Larson & Richards, 1994; Richards, Crowe, Larson, & Swarr, 1998). They provide sense of belonging through sharing problems and interests (Csikszentmihalyi & Larson, 1984), opportunities to enact competences acquired from family (Shulman, Seiffge-Krenke, Levy-Shiff, Fabian, & Rotenberg, 1995), and emotional and instrumental support (Heatherington, 1983). Girls usually invest more resources and energies in relationships than boys; they also report higher levels of intimacy and tackle more personal matters during conversation (Oxley, Dzindolet, & Miller, 2002; Thomas & Daubman, 2001).

Peer "crowds" —groups by which a teenager's reputation and status among peers are demarcated—emerge during adolescence (Brown, 1990). While norms of some crowds correspond closely to conventional adult values and expectations, helping members to move easily through adult-controlled institutions (Brown et al., 1993), others can endorse deviant lifestyles and behaviors. This is why family and peers have traditionally been considered two opposing magnets attracting youth to different developmental trajectories (Csikszentmihalyi & Larson, 1984; Shulman et al., 1995). However, affiliation with a crowd normally reflects preexistent choices and developmental trajectories of teenagers (Brown & Huang, 1995). Hence, group affiliation does not necessarily contrast family influence, nor necessarily brings about deviant behavior (Dekovic, Engels, Shirai, de Kort, & Anker, 2002; Field, Diego, & Sanders, 2002). After having internalized basic expectations and attitudes concerning social partners' behavior through relationships with caregivers (Sroufe & Fleeson, 1986), teenagers and youth tend to test them in different social contexts.

Literature has focused on criteria for friend selection (Burleson, 2003). Children are primarily attracted to peers having similar social skill levels, and pairs of friends have similar levels of skills related to the expression and management of emotional states (Burleson, 1994). Together they build a unique form of attachment that provides a safe haven during adolescence (Markiewicz, Lawford, Doyle, & Haggart, 2006).

Similarities also emerge in deviant behavior (Bagwell & Coie, 2004): Nonaggressive boys and their friends show greater positive engagement and reciprocity in their interactions compared with aggressive boys and their friends, who provide more enticement for rule violations and engage in more rule-breaking behaviors. Within an evolutionary framework, preference for similarity is explained by the distinctive role of shared interests and mutual knowledge in the pursuit of common goals through joint activity (Cole & Teboul, 2004).

Long-lasting and elective friendships typically flourish during adolescence, and undergo major changes through the subsequent stages of life, such as transition to college (Oswald & Clark, 2003). Best friendship is primarily established within same-gender dyads (Thomas & Daubman, 2001), who show striking similitude in attitudes, behaviors, values, and beliefs (Johnson, 1989; Sprecher, 1998). In addition, best friends resemble each other in ego identity and personality characteristics (Akers, Jones, & Coyl, 1998; Rubin, Wojslawowicz, Rose-Krasnor, Booth-LaForce, & Burgess, 2006). Best friendships are characterized by intimacy, loyalty, commitment, trust, and altruism which promote exclusive collaboration and support (Cole & Bradac, 1996; Tooby & Cosmides, 1996).

ESM studies conducted among adolescents in the United States (Csikszentmihalyi and Larson 1984; Csikszentmihalyi et al., 1993), Italy, and Nepal, (Delle Fave et al., 2002, 2003a) showed that being with friends had a positive impact on mood and intrinsic motivation, both dimensions scoring the highest compared with the other contexts. At the same time, adolescents reported average levels of engagement and confidence. The average level of engagement suggests that the company of friends provides fun and excitement, but does not require the investment of high cognitive resources: For example, while with friends Italian adolescents scored significantly low in concentration, but significantly high in alertness and activation. Flow and relaxation were the most frequent experiences they associated with peer interactions. Nepalese adolescents reported average levels of cognitive, emotional, and motivational variables during peer interactions (Delle Fave et al., 2003a), and a more homogeneous distribution of their answers across the various experiences identified by the EFM.

Some deeper insight in the daily experience of friendship was provided by a longitudinal study in which two young women, best friends, were followed over 1 year by means of 12 monthly ESM sessions (Bassi & Delle Fave, 2009). Since we were interested in comparing their experience in shared contexts and situations, their beeper schedules were synchronized. Individuals in the couple showed similarities in both productive and leisure domains: They had chosen to attend the same university course and were jointly working on the same dissertation topic. Convergence was also detected in daily time-budget. Both lived with their parents and siblings, who represented their most frequent social context. Their time together was mostly spent at one's or the other's house, and to a smaller extent at university, and in public places. Interactions were by far their main shared activity, accounting for 63% of the time they spent together.

The two friends reported striking similarities in their experience fluctuation together and in the activities associated with optimal experience. Both primarily reported high-challenge experiences in their daily life, with optimal experience being the most frequent one. In addition, both participants prominently associated shared activities with optimal experience. Quite interestingly, they were so much on the same wavelength that they reported synchronous optimal experiences while interacting.

These findings highlighted some specificities of the dyadic friendship relation: intentional choice and similarity. More specifically, results were consistent with the evolutionary theoretical framework on close relations, holding that similarity represents a key element in the pursuit of common goals through joint activity. The two participants in the study had been friends since high school, sharing adolescence turmoil, and managing to remain friends in young adulthood, by virtue of a special bond based on shared psychological selection patterns, vocational choices, and interests. They spent time together talking and thus strengthening communication and contact within the dyad. The cultivation of their relationship provided them with gratification and shared opportunities for optimal experience.

Considering that friendships are exposed to change with time, according to events and priorities intervening in subsequent stages of life, scientific research could gain further insight into human relationships by planning extensive longitudinal studies in this domain.

10.4 Relationships Across Cultures: Daily Experiences and Lifelong Perspectives

The analysis of the findings obtained from the cross-cultural adult sample described in Chapter 7 can provide further hints on the role of relationships—and in particular of family ties—in daily experience and in the long-term perspective. As reported in Chapter 7, interactions accounted for about 10% of the activities associated with optimal experience, and they were selected by 77 participants (10.5% of the total sample, equally distributed between western and non-western cultures) as opportunities for pervasive optimal experiences. The majority of answers within both the global list of optimal activities and among selected ones referred to family and couple relationships (69%) and to a lesser extent to socialization with friends and significant others. The psychological features of optimal experience during interactions were extremely positive, with most variables reaching their highest values across domains (See Table 7.1).

Additional information was obtained through flow questionnaire, since each participant was asked to rate the average experience associated with three daily domains: being with family, work, and being alone. Table 10.1 shows the experience

Table 10.1 The average quality of experience associated with the main daily contexts in western and non-western cultures

	Productive activities (W = 509, NW = 333)		Being with family (W = 506, NW = 307)		Being alone (W = 498, NW = 319)	
Variables	W *M (sd)*	NW *M (sd)*	NW *M (sd)*	NW *M (sd)*	W *M (sd)*	NW *M (sd)*
Involvement	5.3 (1.8)	5.5 (2.2)	5.2 (1.8)	5.8 (2.2)	3.7 (2.2)	3.0 (2.7)
Clear feedback	6.4 (1.6)	5.6 (2.1)	6.4 (1.6)	5.6 (2.1)	5.3 (2.2)	3.2 (2.5)
Intrinsic motivation	5.0 (2.7)	5.0 (2.7)	6.1 (2.2)	6.2 (2.2)	4.1 (2.4)	2.9 (2.7)
Excitement	6.1 (1.8)	5.6 (2.3)	6.5 (1.6)	6.8 (1.7)	4.9 (2.4)	3.7 (3.0)
Ease of concentration	5.0 (2.4)	4.7 (2.6)	5.6 (2.1)	5.9 (2.2)	5.6 (2.2)	3.7 (2.7)
Unselfconsciousness	3.5 (2.7)	4.2 (2.5)	3.9 (2.5)	5.0 (2.5)	4.8 (2.6)	3.3 (2.8)
Enjoyment	5.6 (2.1)	5.6 (2.5)	5.4 (2.0)	5.9 (2.0)	3.9 (2.2)	3.0 (2.7)
Concentration	5.2 (2.1)	5.0 (2.3)	4.3 (2.1)	5.8 (1.8)	2.0 (2.3)	3.3 (2.6)
Relaxation	4.9 (2.2)	5.1 (2.5)	5.5 (2.1)	5.9 (2.4)	5.8 (2.1)	4.5 (3.0)
Clear goals	6.6 (1.6)	6.0 (2.0)	5.9 (1.9)	6.1 (2.1)	5.3 (2.1)	3.9 (2.7)
Control of situation	5.9 (1.8)	5.7 (2.3)	5.5 (1.9)	5.8 (2.0)	5.7 (2.2)	4.2 (2.8)
Challenges	5.6 (2.0)	5.1 (2.4)	5.7 (1.9)	5.1 (2.3)	4.0 (2.3)	2.5 (2.4)
Skills	6.2 (1.5)	5.3 (2.0)	5.8 (1.5)	5.6 (2.0)	5.1 (2.0)	3.3 (2.6)

described by western and non-western participants during work, family interactions, and while alone. A paired t-test procedure was used to detect differences between the experience in family, at work, and in solitude within the two groups.

Among participants from western cultures, no difference between family and work experiences was found for the levels of involvement, enjoyment, and challenge. Family interactions were associated with significantly higher values than work, prominently as concerns motivational and emotional variables: intrinsic motivation ($t = 9.2, p < 0.0001$), excitement ($t = 3.9, p < 0.0001$), ease of concentration ($t = 4.6, p < 0.0001$), unselfconsciousness ($t = 3.2, p < 0.01$), and relaxation ($t = 5.6, p < 0.0001$). On the contrary, most cognitive variables scored significantly higher at work: clear feedback ($t = 2.7, p < 0.01$), concentration ($t = 7.5, p < 0.0001$), clear goals ($t = 7.3, p < 0.0001$), control of the situation ($t = 3.5, p < 0.001$), and skills ($t = 4.3, p < 0.0001$). The comparison between the experience with family and in solitude showed a more homogeneous trend. During family interactions, participants reported significantly higher values for the great majority of the variables: involvement ($t = 10.9, p < 0.0001$), clear feedback ($t = 7.4, p < 0.0001$), intrinsic motivation ($t = 14.3, p < 0.0001$), excitement ($t = 11.5, p < 0.0001$), enjoyment ($t = 10.7, p < 0.0001$), concentration ($t = 2.6, p < 0.05$), clear goals ($t = 5.6, p < 0.0001$), challenges ($t = 12.4, p < 0.0001$), and skills ($t = 7.5, p < 0.0001$). No difference was detected in the levels of ease of concentration and control of the situation. Solitude was associated with higher values of relaxation ($t = 2.3, p < 0.05$).

Findings from non western participants showed similar response profiles. The experience associated with the family context was more positive than work, especially as concerns the emotional and motivational variables: intrinsic motivation ($t = 3.9, p < 0.0001$), excitement ($t = 6.3, p < 0.0001$), ease of concentration ($t = 6.8, p < 0.0001$), unselfconsciousness ($t = 2.0, p < 0.05$), concentration ($t = 3.5, p < 0.001$), and relaxation ($t = 3.3, p < 0.001$). Most cognitive variables such as clear feedback, control of the situation, clear goals, challenges and skills did not differ significantly between the two situations. The comparison with solitude highlighted significantly higher values of most variables during family interactions: involvement ($t = 12.0, p < 0.0001$), clear feedback ($t = 10.4, p < 0.0001$), intrinsic motivation ($t = 13.5, p < 0.0001$), excitement ($t = 12.4, p < 0.0001$), ease of concentration ($t = 9.5, p < 0.0001$), unselfconsciousness ($t = 4.7, p < 0.0001$), enjoyment ($t = 13.2, p < 0.0001$), concentration ($t = 10.5, p < 0.0001$), relaxation ($t = 4.1, p < 0.0001$), clear goals ($t = 9.6, p < 0.0001$), control of the situation ($t = 6.4, p < 0.0001$), challenges ($t = 11.1, p < 0.0001$), and skills ($t = 10.4, p < 0.0001$).

Nonparametric Wilcoxon statistics highlighted cross-cultural similarities and differences in the quality of experience in the three contexts. As concerns work experience, no significant group difference emerged for involvement, intrinsic motivation, ease of concentration, enjoyment, concentration, clear goals, and control of the situation. Western participants reported significantly higher values of clear feedback ($Z = 5.3, p < 0.0001$), excitement ($Z = 3.0, p < 0.01$), clear goals ($Z = 3.5, p < 0.001$), challenges ($Z = 3.5, p < 0.001$), and skills ($Z = 6.9, p < 0.0001$), while non-western participants scored significantly higher for unselfconsciousness ($Z = 3.1$, $p < 0.01$) and relaxation ($Z = 2.1$, $p < 0.05$). With family, non-western participants reported significantly higher values for most variables: involvement ($Z = 4.7$, $p < 0.0001$), excitement ($Z = 3.6$, $p < 0.001$), ease of concentration ($Z = 2.4$, $p < 0.05$), unselfconsciousness ($Z = 5.4$, $p < 0.0001$), enjoyment ($Z = 4.0$, $p < 0.0001$), concentration ($Z = 9.7$, $p < 0.0001$), relaxation ($Z = 3.5$, $p < 0.001$), clear goals ($t = 2.3$, $p < 0.05$), and control of the situation ($Z = 2.7$, $p < 0.01$). Western participants scored instead higher for clear ideas ($Z = 3.2$, $p < 0.01$) and challenges ($Z = 3.5$, $p < 0.001$). An opposite trend was evident for solitude, in which western participants reported a substantially better experience: They scored significantly higher in involvement ($Z = 5.0$, $p < 0.0001$), clear feedback ($Z = 11.0$, $p < 0.0001$), intrinsic motivation ($Z = 6.5$, $p < 0.0001$), excitement ($Z = 5.6$, $p < 0.0001$), ease of concentration ($Z = 10.1$, $p < 0.0001$), unselfconsciousness ($Z = 6.6$, $p < 0.0001$), enjoyment ($Z = 5.4$, $p < 0.0001$), concentration ($Z = 3.7$, $p < 0.0001$), relaxation ($Z = 5.4$, $p < 0.0001$), clear goals ($t = 7.6$, $p < 0.01$), control of the situation ($Z = 7.0$, $p < 0.0001$), challenges ($Z = 8.3$, $p < 0.0001$), and skills ($Z = 9.5$, $p < 0.0001$).

These results raise some major considerations. First, the globally positive experiential features of daily family interactions are consistent with the findings obtained from other samples and discussed in the previous pages. For both western and non-western participants, the family context provides involvement, enjoyment, and intrinsic motivation, at the same time offering relaxation from the challenges and social evaluations of the work environment. It also supports well-being through the satisfaction of affiliation and relatedness needs (Oppedal, Roysamb, & Sam, 2004), missing in the condition of solitude. Second, family represents the most stable nucleus of continuity in individuals' life, as well as the prominent target of long-term resource investment. As shown in Chapter 7, family is the domain most frequently quoted across past, present, and future dimensions of the life history. Finally, the discrepancies between cultures in the daily experience associated with family interactions and solitude can be related to their individualistic versus collectivistic orientation. Non-western participants scored higher in family and lower in solitude than their western counterparts. Similar results were detected by Asakawa and Csikszentmihalyi (2000) in a study with ESM conducted with Asian-American and Caucasian-American adolescents. In both groups the levels of happiness improved in presence of other people, but the increase was more significant among Asian-American adolescents. In addition, when Asian-American participants were alone their levels of happiness were very low, as compared to their Caucasian-American counterparts. The interdependent conception of the self, typical of Asian cultures, can explain these findings (Markus & Kitayama, 1991; Chapter 7).

Across cultures, however, a certain amount of variability can be detected in the relevance attributed to relationships and aloneness. In the following pages we will provide two opposite examples of this variability, derived from two ancient and traditional societies.

10.4.1 Relationships as the Core of Gypsy Culture

Within the wide range of cross-cultural research on flow and psychological selection patterns, a study conducted in two Gypsy communities living in Italy detected an absolute peculiarity of this culture: the pervasive investment on family and social relationships both as opportunities of optimal experiences and as the core constituents of the long-term process of psychological selection (Delle Fave et al., 2003b).

Throughout the centuries, a nomadic lifestyle characterized Gypsies. They lived in relatively small groups, usually consisting in one extended family or genetically interrelated members. Moving from North-Western India to Persia and the Byzantine Empire, in the fifteenth century they reached Europe, giving rise to communities differing in language, area of immigration, and traditional occupations: Rom, Sinti, Manouches, Kale, Romanichel (Arlati, 1998; Bloch, 1934; Minorsky, 1982). They were renown as metal smiths, horse breeders, and musicians, as well as roundabout attendants, palmists, and fortune-tellers (Rasmussen, 1991).

Gypsies had developed their own oral traditions, rules, and norms, and they were traditionally impermeable to local laws, defying justice and unwilling to settle down in one area and to integrate into the local sedentary communities. Therefore, their relations with Europeans (called Gage, non-men, in Romany language) were often characterized by hostility. Gypsies were often prevented from traveling, banned from urban centers, and expelled from some countries. In Romania they were slaves until 1856 (de Vaux de Foletier, 1970). In Germany they suffered from segregation during the Nazi period, and extermination during World War II (Hancock, 1996; Rummel, 1992). In most European countries, prejudice and hostility against Gypsy minorities are still spread today (Adams, Okely, Morgan, & Smith, 1975; Zani & Kirchler, 1995). Presently, Rom are among the most impoverished cultural groups in Central and Eastern Europe (Unicef, 2005). Nearly 84% of Rom in Bulgaria, 88% in Romania, and 90% in Hungary live below the national poverty lines. Because of limited education, a low level of skills and discrimination in the labor market, in some settlements not a single person is regularly engaged in formal employment. Many children attend separate schools or are segregated when attending mainstream schools.

Despite these difficulties, Gypsy communities substantially managed to resist change (Arayici, 1998). Their culture was successfully transmitted through social learning, and their nomadic attitude survived the establishment of national boundaries. These aspects are still visible in the limited dimension of the communities, and in the avoidance of artifacts accumulation.

However, the modern social and legal systems adopted by the European countries during the last two centuries forced Gypsies to get a stable residency and a national citizenship in order to benefit from job opportunities, health services, and education programs. As a consequence, most groups accepted sedentary or semi-sedentary ways of life, often settling in camps located in the cities' outskirts, and living in caravans or shanties. While their traditional jobs and activities became obsolete with time, social cohesion and family ties are still very strong today, and represent the

Table 10.2 Percentage distribution of optimal activities, positive influences, present challenges, and future goals reported by gypsy participants

Categories	Optimal activities ($N = 48$)	Positive influences ($N = 59$)	Present challenges ($N = 60$)	Future goals ($N = 59$)
Family	32.4	70.8	40.5	40.3
Material goods	–	–	14.4	25.5
Personal growth	5.0	10.9	14.4	14.1
Work	27.5	–	14.4	8.7
Health, personal care	5.0	–	2.9	5.4
Social issues	–	0.8	7.7	2.7
Travels	7.5	7.3	–	1.3
Social relations	11.3	3.6	3.8	1.3
Leisure	11.3	0.8	1.9	0.7
School	–	5.8	–	–
Total percentage	100	100	100	100
N answers	80	137	104	149

Note: $N =$ number of participants.

biocultural core of Gypsy life. Extended families maintain strong ties even when scattered across different regions or countries, and marriages strengthen inter-family relationships and social cohesion.

This centrality of relationships was highlighted by the answers provided to flow questionnaire and life theme questionnaire by 28 men and 32 women living in suburban camps in Northern Italy, mostly migrated from the Balkans after the dissolution of ex-Yugoslavia (Delle Fave et al., 2003b).

Optimal experience was recognized by 48 participants (80%), while 12 respondents reported suffering and hardship due to death or imprisonment of relatives and to destitution. As shown in Table 10.2, the domain of family was prominent among flow activities, positive life influences, present challenges, and future goals. As an opportunity for optimal experience, it mostly comprised rearing children and grandchildren among both men and women, as testified by the words of a 19-year-old father: "I very much like to spend time with my little daughter, she is 10 months old and I go crazy for her because she is so beautiful! . . . I take her around and I do all I can for her."

The primary role of parents and grandparents in shaping the individuals' developmental niche and transmitting cultural information was strikingly evident among positive influences. As for present challenges and future goals, parenting and educating one's own children again predominated: In particular, participants emphasized their role in supporting children's development and self-actualization at work and in family, as well as in transmitting them moral rules and social values. Peaceful relations with the spouse and solid and trustful ties within the extended family were also quoted as challenges and goals. Gypsies' substantial investment on children's education partially explains their diffidence toward formal education. In a study promoted by the municipality of Milano to investigate the relationship between local Gypsy communities and Gage through the cultural network model, Gypsy parents highlighted that the role of schools should be to equip youth with notions and basic useful information, while only families are entitled to provide education and to transmit values and social norms (Delle Fave & Lombardi, 2000). Other studies have focused on the difficulties in introducing Rom pupils in western schools (Okely, 1997; Smith, 1997), mainly related to discipline and rule observance.

Work ranked second among flow activities, but it mostly comprised domestic tasks such as cooking, cleaning, repair works in the shanty (77.8% of the answers). Participants emphasized the importance of these activities for family well-being, as a 46-year-old woman clearly described: "... There are many people here, and there is always something to do... Large families are like that, if you love them you have to be very active and work all the time." Paid work accounted for only 22.3% of the answers in this category, and it referred to handicrafts and manual activities. Even among present challenges and future goals work did not result especially relevant. Most participants complained about the time and rule constraints characterizing modern jobs, setting freedom and independence as prerequisites to get optimal experience. Nevertheless, as detected in other studies (Delle Fave & Lombardi, 2000), vocational trainings have become increasingly attractive within European Rom communities in the last two decades. A growing number of adults are employed in stable jobs, and engagement in cooperative enterprises represents an interesting alternative to wage earning in industries or workshops. Anyway, due to the centrality of family in Rom communities, work is not valued at the individual level, but in terms of benefits for the group. An a 46-year-old man stated, "If you toil for someone else, then you get paid, but if you do it for yourself you don't get money but build a house, or a fence for the animals."

Among optimal activities, leisure comprised traditional Rom arts and entertainments, typically performed within a social context, such as playing music, singing, and dancing. Traveling was analyzed as a separate category, due to the traditional relevance of this activity, and the importance participants still attribute to visiting relatives in other regions or in other countries, mostly for family celebrations. Since sedentary lifestyle deeply restrained group mobility, traveling accounted for a low percentage of answers. As a 65-year-old man remarked, "My children travel less frequently than me, because they have their business here, but now life is different, I think that my grandchildren will even build a house for themselves!".

The importance of relationships in daily life was confirmed by participants' ratings of the average quality of experience in daily routine activities (Delle Fave et al., 2003b). While family interactions provided a globally positive experience, being alone was associated with significantly lower values of emotional, motivational, and cognitive dimensions. Unlike other cultures, which consider solitude as a context for autonomy, creativity, and self-expression (Larson, 1997), Rom people, since childhood, learn to avoid isolation as a threat against personal well-being and social integration. A 38-year-old man stated: "Only mad people are alone and talk to themselves." Another male participant explained: "When you are in trouble and

Table 10.3 Percentage distribution of selected optimal activities among Gypsy men and women

Categories	Women ($N = 26$)	Men ($N = 22$)
Family	46.2	22.7
Work	34.6	13.7
Free time	19.2	63.6
% of answers	100	100

nobody helps you and everyone kicks you out, then you are alone. But this happens only if you deserve it. If you do something very bad, for example if you kill or rape another Rom."

Some peculiar gender differences were detected in our study, which are consistent with the patriarchal organization of nomadic societies, and with the primary role of women as mothers and housewives. Table 10.3 shows the gender distribution of selected optimal activities. The broad category "free time" included leisure, socializing, personal care, and introspection. Almost half of the women reported the most pervasive optimal experience in child care and family interactions, followed by work, which prominently comprised domestic tasks. On the opposite, the majority of men selected free time activities (socializing, hobbies, resting, or idling). A significant gender difference was detected in this distribution ($\chi^2 = 9.9, p < 0.01$). We were also interested in assessing congruence of the Family domain across participants' answers to the flow questionnaire and the life theme questionnaire. Among the 48 participants who reported optimal experiences in their lives, ten (20.8%, including 9 women and 1 man) described family as an opportunity for flow, as well as a positive influence, a present challenge, and a future goal. A significant gender difference was detected ($\chi^2 = 6.5$, $p < 0.05$), since family was a recurrent component of the psychological selection pattern for 35% of the women in the group.

Finally, we did not find the generation gap characterizing most cultures undergoing modernization (Delle Fave & Massimini, 1988, 1991). Young people were concerned with family and community relations just like their parents. Modern leisure opportunities easily available outside the camps were not specifically attractive to them.

In sum, the psychological selection pattern of the participants was consistent with the collectivistic organization of their society. The development and preservation of harmony within the community was deemed more important than personal autonomy and achievements. Individuals reported to allocate most of their psychological and material resources in the pursuit of this shared aim.

10.4.2 Solitude Across Cultures and Among Navajos

In western countries, several studies showed that the amount of time spent alone increases from preadolescence to adolescence (Larson, 1997). Teenagers often intentionally look for retreat and isolation from family and social contexts. Time alone can be an opportunity to think about oneself, reflect on everyday events, rehearse acquired behaviors, and build personal identity; together with family, solitude can also buffer stress and social pressures (Larson & Lee, 1996). Studies conducted with ESM among US, Italian, and Nepalese adolescents showed that being alone was associated with significantly low values of mood and intrinsic motivation, but also with average or above-average levels of confidence (Cavallo, Lombardi, & Stokart, 2006; Delle Fave et al., 2002; Larson et al., 1996).

This experiential pattern held to be true of the cross-cultural adult sample described in the previous pages. For most participants across cultures being alone was associated with relaxation and control of the situation, but also with low enjoyment and engagement. The negative aspects of solitude were emphasized to a greater extent by non-western participants, who lived in societies organized around extended families, and characterized by collectivism and a strong social cohesion.

However, a peculiar response pattern was detected among Navajo participants, enrolled as students, teachers, and clerks at the Diné College in Tsaile (further details on this group are provided in Chapter 7 and Chapter 12). These participants associated optimal experience with the category "introspection" in 18.1% of their answers, more than double compared with the percentage reported by the global non-western sample, and three times the percentage reported by western participants. More specifically, 52% of the answers in this category referred to thinking and reflecting.

This result is related to a specific feature of the Navajo culture: the deep respect for the individual. Although group and family ties are the essential woof of Navajo society, the individual identity and freedom of the single person are considered core values, as highlighted by Navajo traditions and anthropological studies (Chisholm, 1995; Kluckhohn & Leighton, 1974). In addition, a nomadic and pastoralist traditional lifestyle, together with the dispersion of the homesites throughout wide spaces and prairies favor solitude and the attitude toward lonely reflections and meditation (Mishra, 2001). Children's raising practices are based on close physical contact and limited verbal interaction, as in most Eastern Asian regions (the original Navajo homeland). The Navajo attitude toward silence and quietness can be partially traced back to a biological trait shared with Sino-Mongolian populations, as research studies on newborns highlighted (Freedman, 1979).

Some quotations from Navajo participants can help highlight the features and function of this tendency toward solitude and reflection. A 36-year-old man stated: "I enjoy solitude frequently. It helps me think and rationalize more clearly." On the same wavelength, a 23-year-old woman reported: "There are times when I enjoy taking a walk or jogging alone just to help my concentration."

The quality of experience associated by Navajo participants with solitude (Table 10.4) further strengthened this evidence. Compared with the other non-western participants, Navajo reported significant higher values for most variables: intrinsic motivation ($Z = 3.2$, $p < 0.01$), excitement ($Z = 2.3$, $p < 0.05$), ease of concentration ($Z = 3.2$, $p < 0.01$), unselfconsciousness ($Z = 2.9$, $p < 0.01$), enjoyment ($Z = 3.9$, $p < 0.0001$), concentration ($Z = 3.4$, $p < 0.001$), relaxation ($Z = 3.5$, $p < 0.001$), clear goals ($Z = 2.0$, $p < 0.05$), challenges ($Z = 3.5$, $p < 0.001$), and skills

Table 10.4 The average quality of experience associated with solitude among Navajo participants

Variables	*M (sd)*
Involvement	3.4 (2.5)
Clear feedback	3.2 (2.6)
Intrinsic motivation	3.8 (2.6)
Excitement	4.4 (3.0)
Ease of concentration	4.6 (2.7)
Unselfconsciousness	4.2 (3.1)
Enjoyment	4.0 (2.6)
Concentration	4.3 (2.7)
Relaxation	5.7 (2.5)
Clear goals	4.4 (2.6)
Control of situation	4.7 (2.7)
Challenges	3.3 (2.4)
Skills	4.0 (2.6)

($Z = 2.6$, $p < 0.01$). No differences between the two groups were instead detected for involvement, clear feedback, and control of the situation.

In spite of this peculiarity, Navajos perceived the experience of solitude more negatively than western participants. They reported significantly lower values of several cognitive variables: clear feedback ($Z = 6.2$, $p < 0.0001$), ease of concentration ($Z = 3.0$, $p < 0.01$), clear goals ($Z = 2.6$, $p < 0.05$), control of the situation ($Z = 2.5$, $p < 0.05$), challenges ($Z = 2.3$, $p < 0.05$), and skills ($Z = 3.4$, $p < 0.001$). However, no group differences were detected in the ratings of the emotional and motivational dimensions: These findings confirmed the prominent role of solitude in promoting calmness and balance, rather than supporting cognitive engagement among Navajos.

10.5 Concluding Remarks

In summary, the findings gathered through different procedures and presented in this chapter allow for three major considerations.

The first one concerns the universally acknowledged pivotal role of relationships in providing the individual with emotional support, behavioral models, a context for developing both social competencies and personal identity, and opportunities for positive and rewarding states of consciousness. All the studies quoted in this chapter confirmed this role. From an opposite perspective, findings discussed in Chapter 15 in reference to child and adolescent maladjustment will highlight the negative developmental consequences of dysfunctional family and peer relations.

The second consideration concerns the occurrence of optimal experience during interactions. As discussed in Chapter 7 and in the previous pages, being with others does not necessarily provide flow per se. The quality of experience is primarily related to the kind of activities people perform when they are together. Interacting with one another is included among these activities, but it is not the only one, and it can be instrumental to other goals, such as performing a shared task.

ESM studies showed that for adolescents across cultures family represented a safe harbor and a warm and relaxing context, in which maintenance, unstructured leisure activities, and domestic work were prominent. The company of peers offered moments of thrill and excitement, but also situations of apathy and disengagement. Nevertheless, across cultures the daily relational context of adolescents resulted substantially positive at the experiential level; moreover, interactions with same-sex parent and with best friends emerged as opportunities for optimal experiences.

Similar findings were detected in the adult cross-cultural sample examined with flow questionnaire. Interactions were not prominently associated with flow, but when this happened, the experience described by the participants was characterized by the highest levels of positivity for all cognitive, motivational, and emotional variables. Moreover, across cultures the daily family context provided adult participants with a more positive experience than work and solitude.

The third and final consideration concerns the differences detected across cultures in the average daily experience associated with interactions and solitude. Collectivistic orientation (Triandis, 1999) and the prominence of interdependent self-construal (Markus & Kitayama, 1991) can play a major role in the more positive experience associated with family and in the more negative experience associated with solitude during daily life by non-western participants. However, each culture has its own peculiarities, and the tendency to generalize should not obscure them, as the examples of Navajo and Gypsies have shown.

References

Adams, B., Okely, J., Morgan, D., & Smith, D. (1975). Gypsies: current policies and practices. *Journal of Social Policy, 4*, 129–150.

Akerman, B. A., & Suurvee, E. (2003). The cognitive and identity development of twins at 16 years of age: A follow-up study with 32 twin pairs. *Twin Research, 6*, 328–333.

Akers, J., Jones, R., & Coyl, D. (1998). Adolescent friendship pairs: Similarities in identity status development, behaviors, attitudes, and intentions. *Journal of Adolescent Research, 13*, 178–201.

Allen, J., Hauser, S., Bell, K., & O'Connor, T. (1994). Longitudinal assessment of autonomy and relatedness in adolescent-family interactions as predictors of adolescent ego development and self-esteem. *Child Development, 65*, 179–194.

Amato, P. R. (1994). Father–child relations, mother–child relations, and offspring psychological well-being in early adulthood. *Journal of Marriage and the Family, 56*, 1031–1042.

An, J. S., & Cooney, T. M. (2006). Psychological well-being in mid to late life: the role of generativity development and parent-child relationships across the lifespan. *International Journal of Behavioral Development, 30*, 410–421.

Arayici, A. (1998). The gypsy minority in Europe—some considerations. *International Social Science Journal, 2*, 253–262.

Ardelt, M., & Eccles, J. S. (2001). Effects of mothers' parental efficacy beliefs and promotive parenting strategies on inner-city youth. *Journal of Family Issues, 22*, 944–972.

Arlati, A. (1998). Gli zingari in italia [Gypsies in Italy]. In Opera Nomadi Nazionale (Ed.), *Progettazioni sperimentali, verifiche, osservazioni sui corsi di formazione per mediatori culturali rom e sinti* (pp. 36–39). Milano: Cooperativa di Solidarità Sociale Romano Drom.

Asakawa, K., & Csikszentmihalyi, M. (2000). Feelings of connectedness and internalization of values in Asian American adolescents. *Journal of Youth and Adolescence, 29*, 121–145.

Baer, D., Curtis, J., Grabb, E., & Johnston, W. (1996). What values do adults prefer in children? A comparative analysis of survey evidence from fifteen countries. In C. Seligman, J. M. Olson, & M. P. Zanna (Eds.), *The psychology of values: The Ontario symposium* (Vol. 8, pp. 299–328). Mahwah, NJ: Lawrence Erlbaum.

Bagwell, C. L., & Coie, J. D. (2004). The best friendships of aggressive boys: Relationship quality, conflict management, and rule-breaking behavior. *Journal of Experimental Child Psychology, 88*, 5–24.

Bandura, A. (1997). *Self-efficacy: The exercise of control.* New York: Freeman.

Bassi, M., & Delle Fave, A. (2004). Adolescence and the changing context of optimal experience in time: Italy 1986–2000. *Journal of Happiness Studies, 5*, 155–179.

Bassi, M., & Delle Fave, A. (2006). The daily experience of Italian adolescents' in family interactions. Gender and developmental issues. In A. Delle Fave (Ed.), *Dimensions of well-being. Research and intervention* (pp. 172–190). Milano: FrancoAngeli.

Bassi, M., & Delle Fave, A. (2009). Daily experience and psychological selection in dyadic relationships: Monozygotic twins and best friends. In T. Freire (Ed.), *Understanding positive life. Research and practice in positive psychology* (pp. 65–84). Lisboa: Climepsi Editores.

Belsky, J. (1985). Experimenting with the family in the newborn period. *Child Development, 56*, 407–414.

Belsky, J., Steinberg, L., & Draper, P. (1991). Childhood experience, interpersonal development, and reproductive strategy: An evolutionary theory of socialization. *Child Development, 60*, 335–339.

Benoit, D., Zeanah, C. H., & Barton, M. L. (1989). Maternal attachment disturbances in failure to thrive. *Mental Health Journal, 10*, 185–202.

Bianchi, S. M., Milkie, M. A., Sayer, L. C., & Robinson, J. P. (2000). Is anyone doing the housework? Trends in the gender division of household labor. *Social Forces, 79*, 191–228.

Bloch, J. (1934). *L'indo-aryen, du veda aux temps modernes* [Indo-Aryan from the vedas to modern times]. Paris: Adrien-Maisonneuve.

Bogenschneider, K., Small, S. A., & Tsay, J. C. (1997). Child, parent, and contextual influences on perceived parenting competence among parents of adolescents. *Journal of Marriage & the Family, 59*, 345–362.

Bogren, L. Y. (1983). Couvade. *Acta Psychiatrica Scandinavica, 68*, 55–65.

Bonifazi, C., Menniti, A., Misiti, M., & Palomba, R. (1999). *Giovani che non lasciano il nido: Atteggiamenti, speranze, condizioni all'uscita da casa* [Youth who do not leave the nest: Attitudes, hopes, conditions for leaving home]. Roma: Istituto di Ricerche sulla Popolazione.

Bonney, J. F., Kelley, M. L., & Levant, R. F. (1999). A model of fathers' behavioral involvement in child care in dual-earner families. *Journal of Family Psychology, 13*, 401–415.

Boomsma, D., Busjahn, A., & Peltonen, L. (2002). Classical twin studies and beyond. *Nature Reviews/Genetics, 3*, 872–882.

Boukydis, C. F., & Burgess, R. L. (1982). Adult physiological response to infant cries: Effects of temperament of infant, parental status and gender. *Child Development, 53*, 1291–1298.

Bowlby, J. (1969). *Attachment and loss. Vol. 1. Attachment.* New York: Basic Books.

Bowlby, J. (1982). *Attachment and loss: Vol. 1, Attachment* (2nd ed.). New York: Basic Books.

Bowlby, J. (Ed.). (1988). *A Secure Base.* New York: Basic Books.

Branje, S., van Aken, M., & van Lieshout, C. (2002). Relational support in families with adolescents. *Journal of Family Psychology, 16*, 351–362.

Bretherton, I., & Waters, E. (Eds.). (1985). Growing points in attachment theory and research. *Monographs of the Society for Research in Child Development, 50*, 1–2.

Bridges, R. S., DiBiase, R., Loundes, D. D., & Doherty, P. C. (1985). Prolactin stimulation of maternal behavior in female rats. *Science, 227*, 782–784.

Brown, B. B. (1990). Peer groups and peer cultures. In S. S. Feldman & G. R. Elliott (Eds.), *At the threshold: The developing adolescent* (pp. 171–196). Cambridge, MA: Harvard University Press.

Brown, B. B. (2004). Adolescents' relationships with peers. In R. M. Lerner & L. Steinberg (Eds.), *Handbook of adolescent psychology* (pp. 364–394). New York: Wiley.

Brown, B. B., & Huang, B. (1995). Examining parenting practices in different peer contexts: Implications for adolescent trajectories. In L. J. Crockett & A. C. Crouter (Eds.), *Pathways through adolescence* (pp. 151–174). Mahwah, NJ: Lawrence Erlbaum Associates Inc.

Brown, B. B., Mounts, N., Lamborn, S. D., & Steinberg, L. (1993). Parenting practices and peer group affiliation. *Child Development, 64*, 467–482.

Bruner, J. S. (1990). *Acts of meaning*. Cambridge, MA: Harvard University Press.

Bruno, J. E. (1996). Time perceptions and time allocation preferences among adolescent boys and girls. *Adolescence, 31*, 109–126.

Bryant, W. K., & Wang, Y. (1990). Time together, time apart: an analysis of wives' solitary time and shared time with spouses. *Lifestyles: Family and Economic Issues, 11*, 89–119.

Bryant, W. K., & Zick, C. D. (1996). An examination of parent–child shared time. *Journal of Marriage and the Family, 58*, 227–237.

Buhrmester, D., & Furman, W. (1990). Perceptions of sibling relationships during middle childhood and adolescence. *Child Development, 61*, 1387–1398.

Buist, K., Dekovic, M., Meeus, W., & Van Aken, M. (2002). Developmental patterns in adolescent attachment to mother, father and sibling. *Journal of Youth and Adolescence, 31*, 167–176.

Burleson, B. R. (1994). Friendship and similarities in social-cognitive and communication abilities: Social skill bases of interpersonal attraction in childhood. *Personal Relationships, 1*, 371–389.

Burleson, B. R. (2003). The experience and effects of emotional support: What the study of cultural and gender differences can tell us about close relationships, emotion, and interpersonal communication. *Personal Relationships, 10*, 1–23.

Burleson, B. R., Kunkel, A. W., Samter, W., & Werking, K. J. (1996). Men's and women's evaluations of communication skills in personal relationships: When sex differences make a difference—and when they don't. *Journal of Social and Personal Relationships, 13*, 201–224.

Buss, D. (1989). Sex differences in human mate preferences: Evolutionary hypotheses tested in 37 cultures. *Behavioral and Brain Sciences, 12*, 1–49.

Buss, D. M., Abbott, M., Angleitner, A., Asherian, A., Biaggio, A., Blanco-Villasenor, A., et al. (1990). International preferences in selecting mates. A study of 37 cultures. *Journal of Cross-Cultural Psychology, 21*, 5–47.

Buss, D. M., Shackelford, T. K., Kirkpatrick, L. A., & Larsen, R. L. (2001). A half century of mate preferences: The cultural evolution of values. *Journal of Marriage and the Family, 63*, 491–503.

Cavallo, M., Lombardi, M., & Stokart, Z. (2006). Complessità e sviluppo di opportunità: Esperienza ottimale e selezione psicologica in un gruppo di adolescenti nepalesi [Complexity and opportunità development: Optimal experience and psychological selection among Nepalese adolescents]. *Passaggi. Rivista Italiana di Scienze Transculturali, 11*, 77–100.

Chafetz, J. S., & Hagan, J. (1996). The gender division of labor and family change in industrial societies: A theoretical accounting. *Journal of Comparative Family Studies, 27*, 187–219.

Chisholm, J. S. (1995). Learning 'respect for everything': Navajo images of development. In L. J. Crockett & A. C. Crouter (Eds.), *Pathways through adolescence* (pp. 138–151). Mahwah, NJ: Lawrence Erlbaum.

Clarke-Stewart, K. A. (1980). The fathers' contribution to children's cognitive and social development in early childhood. In F. A. Pedersen (Ed.), *The father-infant relationship: observational studies in a family setting* (pp. 111–146). New York: Holt, Rinehart and Winston.

Clinton, J. F. (1985). Couvade: Patterns, predictors, and nursing management. *Western Journal of Nursing Research, 7*, 221–243.

Cobb, C. T. H. (1996). Adolescent-parent attachments and family problem-solving styles. *Family Processes, 35*, 57–80.

Coffman, S., Levitt, M. J., & Brown, L. (1994). Effects of clarification of support expectations in prenatal couples. *Nursing Research, 43*, 111–116.

Cole, T., & Bradac, J. (1996). A lay theory of relational satisfaction with best friends. *Journal of Social and Personal Relationships, 13*, 57–83.

Cole, T., & Teboul, B. (2004). Non-zero-sum collaboration, reciprocity, and the preference for similarity: Developing an adaptive model of close relational functioning. *Personal Relationships, 11*, 135–160.

Collins, W. A. (1990). Parent–child relationship in the transition to adolescence: continuity and change in interaction, affect, and cognition. In R. Montemayor, G. Adams, & T. Gullotta (Eds.), *From childhood to adolescence: A transitional period? Advances in adolescent development: Vol. 2. The transition from childhood to adolescence* (pp. 85–106). Beverly Hills, CA: Sage.

Collins, W. A. (1995). Relationships and development: Family adaptation to individual change. In S. Shulman (Ed.), *Close relationship and socio-emotional development* (pp. 28–154). Norwood, NJ: Ablex Publishing Corporation.

Cooksey, E. C., & Fondell, M. M. (1996). Spending time with his kids: Effects of family structure on father's and children's lives. *Journal of Marriage and the Family, 58*, 693–707.

Cote, S. M., Boivin, M., Liu, X., Nagin, D. S., Zoccolillo, M., & Tremblay, R. E. (2009). Depression and anxiety symptoms: Onset, developmental course and risk factors during. *Journal of Child Psychology and Psychiatry, 50*, 1201–1208.

Crnic, K., Greenberg., M., Ragozin., A., Robinson, N., & Basham, R. (1983). Effects of stress and social support on mothers of premature and full-term infants. *Child Development, 54*, 209–217.

Crowell, J. A., & Feldman, S. S. (1991). Mothers' working models of attachment relationships and mother and child behavior during separation and reunion. *Developmental Psychology, 27*, 597–605.

Csikszentmihalyi, M., & Larson, R. (1984). *Being Adolescent*. New York: Basic Books.

Csikszentmihalyi, M., & Rathunde, K. (1991). Adolescent happiness and family interaction. In K. Pillmer & K. McCartney (Eds.), *Parent–Child Relations through Life* (pp. 143–161). Hillsdale, NJ: Erlbaum.

Csikszentmihalyi, M., Rathunde, K., & Whalen, S. (1993). *Talented Teenagers*. New York: Cambridge University Press.

Daly, M. (1990). Evolutionary theory and parental motives. In N. A. Krasnegor & R. S. Bridges (Eds.), *Mammalian Parenting* (pp. 25–39). Oxford: Oxford University Press.

Damon, W., & Hart, D. (1988). *Self-understanding in childhood and adolescence*. Cambridge, MA: Harvard University Press.

de Vaux de Foletier, F. (1970). *Mille ans d'historie des Tsiganes* [A thousand years of Gypsy history]. Paris: Librairie Arthème Fayard.

De Wolff, M. S., & van Ijzendoorn, M. (1997). Sensitivity and attachment: A meta-analysis on parental antecedents of infant attachment. *Child Development, 68*, 571–591.

Deci, E. L., & Ryan, R. M. (2000). Self-determination theory and the facilitation of intrinsic motivation, social development, and well-being. *American Psychologist, 55*, 68–78.

Dekovic, M., Engels, R. C. M. E., Shirai, T., de Kort, G., & Anker, A. L. (2002). The role of peer relations in adolescent development in two cultures. *Journal of Cross-Cultural Psychology, 33*, 577–595.

Delle Fave, A., & Bassi, M. (2000). The quality of experience in adolescents' daily life: Developmental perspectives. *Genetic, Social, and General Psychology Monographs, 126*, 347–367.

Delle Fave, A., & Bassi, M. (2003). Italian adolescents and leisure: The role of engagement and optimal experience. In S. Verma & R. W. Larson (Eds.), *Examining adolescent leisure time across cultures: Developmental opportunities and risks. New directions in child and adolescent development* (pp. 79–93). San Francisco: Jossey-Bass.

Delle Fave, A., Bassi, M., & Lombardi, M. (2003a). Adolescents' optimal experiences, psychological selection and life goals: Developmental implications. Paper presented at the *11th European Conference on Developmental Psychology,* Book of Abstracts, 283. Milano, August 27–31.

Delle Fave, A., Bassi, M., & Massimini, F. (2002). Quality of experience and daily social context of Italian adolescents. In A. L. Comunian & M. Gershenfeld (Eds.), *It's all about relationships* (pp. 159–172). Lengerich: Pabst Science Publishers.

Delle Fave, A., Bassi, M., & Massimini, F. (2003b). Coping with boundaries: The quality of daily experience of rom nomads in Europe. *Psychology and Developing Societies, 15*, 87–102.

Delle Fave, A., & Lombardi, M. (2000). *Rom e Gagè: una relazione interculturale* [Rom and Gage: An intercultural relation]. Milano: Comune di Milano.

Delle Fave, A., & Massimini, F. (1988). Modernization and changing contexts of flow in work and leisure. In M. Csikszentmihalyi & I. Csikszentmihalyi (Eds.), *Optimal experience. Psychological studies of flow in consciousness* (pp. 193–213). New York: Cambridge University Press.

Delle Fave, A., & Massimini, F. (1991). Modernization and the quality of daily experience in a southern Italy village. In N. Bleichrodt & P. J. D. Drenth (Eds.), *Contemporary issues in cross-cultural psychology* (pp. 110–119). Amsterdam: Swets & Zeitlinger B.V.

Delle Fave, A., & Massimini, F. (2000). Subjective experience and the building of parental roles in a biocultural perspective. In A. L. Comunian & U. P. Gielen (Eds.), *International perspectives in human development* (pp. 159–175). Lengerich: Pabst Science Publishers.

Delle Fave, A., & Massimini, F. (2004). Parenthood and the quality of experience in daily life: A longitudinal study. *Social Indicators Research, 67*, 75–106.

Delle Fave, A., & Massimini, F. (2005). The investigation of optimal experience and apathy: Developmental and psychosocial implications. *European Psychologist, 10*, 264–274.

Dixson, A. F., & George, L. (1982). Prolactin and parental behaviour in a male new world primate. *Nature, 295*, 551–553.

Drew, E. (1998). Changing family forms and the allocation of caring. In E. Drew, R. Emerek, & E. Mahon (Eds.), *Women, work and the family in Europe* (pp. 27–35). London: Routledge.

Drew, E., Emerek, R., & Mahon, E. (Eds.). (1998). *Women, work and the family in Europe*. London: Routledge.

Dunn, J., Slomkowski, C., & Beardsall, L. (1994). Sibling relationships from the preschool period through middle childhood and early adolescence. *Developmental Psychology, 30*, 315–324.

Dwairy, M., & Achoui, M. (2006). Introduction to three cross-regional research studies on parenting styles, individuation and mental health in Arab societies. *Special Section of the Journal of Cross-Cultural Psychology, 37*, 221–271.

Elwood, R. W., & Mason, C. (1994). The couvade and the onset of paternal care: A biological perspective. *Ethology and Sociobiology, 15*, 145–156.

Fallon, B. J., & Bowles, T. V. (1997). The effect of family structure and family functioning on adolescents' perceptions of intimate time spent with parents, siblings, and peers. *Journal of Youth and Adolescence, 26*, 25–43.

Field, T., Diego, M., & Sanders, C. (2002). Adolescents' parents and peer relationship. *Adolescence, 37*, 121–129.

Field, T., Lang, C., Yando, R., & Bendell, D. (1995). Adolescents' intimacy with parents and friends. *Adolescence, 30*, 133–140.

Fiese, B. H., Hooker, K. A., Kotary, L., & Schwagler, J. (1993). Family rituals in early stages of parenthood. *Journal of Marriage and the Family, 55*, 633–642.

Fleming, A. (1990). Hormonal and experiential correlates of maternal responsiveness in human mothers. In N. A. Krasnegor & R. S. Bridges (Eds.), *Mammalian Parenting* (pp. 184–208). Oxford: Oxford University Press.

Freedman, D. G. (1979). *Human Sociobiology*. New York: Academic Press.

Freedman, D. G., & Gorman, J. (1993). Attachment and the transmission of culture. An evolutionary perspective. *Journal of Social and Evolutionary Systems, 16*, 297–329.

Gecas, V., & Seff, M. (1990). Families and adolescents: A review of the 1980s. *Journal of Marriage and the Family, 48*, 37–46.

Gerson, K. (1993). *No man's land: Men's changing commitments to family and work*. New York: Basic Books.

Gil, A., Wagner, E., & Vega, W. (2000). Acculturation, familism and alcohol use among Latino adolescent males: Longitudinal relations. *Journal of Community Psychology, 28*, 443–458.

Gilligan, C. (1982). *In a different voice. Psychological theory and women's development.* Cambridge, MA: Harvard University Press.

Gondoli, D. M., & Silverberg, S. B. (1997). Maternal emotional distress and diminished responsiveness: The mediating role of parenting efficacy and parental perspective taking. *Developmental Psychology, 33*, 861–868.

Goodnow, J. J. (1988). Children's household work: Its nature and functions. *Psychological Bulletin, 103*, 5–26.

Gottfried, A. E., Gottfried, A. W., & Bathurst, K. (1995). Maternal and dual.-Earner employment status and parenting. In *Handbook of Parenting: Vol. 2. Biology and ecology of parenting* (pp. 139–160). Mahwah, NJ: Lawrence Erlbaum Ass.

Hancock, I. (1996). Responses to the Porrajmos : The Romani holocaust. In A. Rosenbaum (Ed.), *Is the Holocaust unique? Perspectives on comparative genocide* (pp. 39–64). Boulder, CO: Westview Press Inc.

Harlow, H. F., & Harlow, M. K. (1965). The affectional systems. In A. M. Schrier, H. F. Harlow, & F. Stollnitz (Eds.), *Behavior of Non-human primates* (pp. 287–334). New York: Academic Press.

Heatherington, E. M.(Ed.). (1983). *Handbook of child psychology: Socialization, personality and social development* (Vol. 4). New York: Wiley.

Hektner, J. (2001). Family, school, and community predictors of adolescent growth-conducive experiences: Global and specific approaches. *Applied Developmental Science, 5*, 172–183.

Helsen, M., Vollenbergh, W., & Meeus, W. (2000). Social support from parents and friends and emotional problems in adolescence. *Journal of Youth and Adolescence, 29*, 319–335.

Hill, N. E., & Bush, K. R. (2001). Relationships between parenting environment and children's mental health among African American and European American mothers and children. *Journal of Marriage and the Family, 63*, 954–966.

Hinde, R. A., & Stevenson-Hinde, J. (Eds.). (1988). *Relations within families.* Oxford: Oxford University Press.

Ho. (1996). Filial piety, authoritarian moralism, and cognitive conservatism in Chinese societies. *Genetic, Social and General Psychology Monographs, 120*, 347–365.

Hoffman, L. W., & Youngblade, L. M. (1999). *Mothers at work: Effects on children's well-being.* Cambridge: Cambridge University Press.

Hrdy, S. B. (1981). *The Woman that never evolved.* Cambridge, MA: Harvard University Press.

Izzo, C., Weiss, L., Shanahan, T., & Rodriguez-Brown, F. (2000). Parental self-efficacy and social support as predictors of parenting practices and children's socio-emotional adjustment in Mexican immigrant families. *Journal of Prevention & Intervention in the Community, 20*, 197–213.

Jablonka, E., & Lamb, M. J. (2005). *Evolution in Four Dimensions. Genetic, epigenetic, behavioural and symbolic variations in the history of life.* Cambridge, MA: MIT Press.

Johnson, M. A. (1989). Variables associated with friendship in adult population. *Journal of Social Psychology, 129*, 379–390.

Jones, T. L., & Prinz, R. J. (2005). Potential roles of parental self-efficacy in parent and child adjustment: A review. *Clinical Psychology Review, 25*, 341–363.

Juang, L. P., & Nguyen, H. H. (2009). Misconduct among Chinese American adolescents. The role of acculturation, family obligation, and autonomy expectations. *Journal of Cross-Cultural Psychology, 40*, 649–666.

Kach, J., & McGhee, P. (1982). Adjustment of early parenthood: The role of accuracy of preparenthood experiences. *Journal of Family Issues, 3*, 375–388.

Kagitcibasi, C. (1996). The autonomous-relational self: A new synthesis. *European Psychologist, 1*, 180–186.

Kagitcibasi, C. (2005). Autonomy and relatedness in cultural context: Implications for self and family. *Journal of Cross-Cultural Psychology, 36*, 403–422.

Kaplan, H., & Hill, K. (1992). The evolutionary ecology of food acquisition. In E. A. Smith & B. Winterhalder (Eds.), *Evolutionary Ecology* (pp. 167–201). Hawthorne, NY: Aldine-de Gruyter.

Kaufman, G., & Uhlenberg, P. (2000). The influence of parenthood on the work effort of married men and women. *Social Forces, 78*, 931–949.

Keller, H., Lamm, B., Abels, M., Yovsi, R., Borke, J., Jensen, H., et al. (2006). Cultural models, socialization goals and parenting ethnotheories. *Journal of Cross-Cultural Psychology, 37*, 155–172.

Kerns, K. A., & Stevens, A. C. (1996). Parent–child attachment in late adolescence: Links to social relations and personality. *Journal of Youth and Adolescence, 25*, 323–342.

Kim, S., & Rohner, R. P. (2003). Perceived parental acceptance and emotional empathy among university students in Korea. *Journal of Cross-Cultural Psychology, 34*, 723–735.

Kluckhohn, C., & Leighton, D. (1974). *The Navaho*. Cambridge, MA: Harvard University Press.

Lalonde, R. N., Hynie, M., Pannu, M., & Tatla, S. (2004). The role of culture in interpersonal relationships: Do second generation south Asian Canadians want a traditional partner? *Journal of Cross-Cultural Psychology, 35*, 503–524.

Lamb, M. E. (1987). The emergent American father. In M. E. Lamb (Ed.), *The father's role: Cross-cultural perspectives* (pp. 3–26). Hillsdale, NJ: Lawrence Erlbaum.

Lampert, A. (1997). *The evolution of love*. Berlin: Praeger Publishers.

Lanz, M., Iafrate, R., Marta, E., & Rosnati, R. (1999). Significant others: Italian adolescents' rankings compared with their parents'. *Psychological Reports, 84*, 459–466.

Larose, S., & Boivin, M. (1998). Attachment to parents, social support expectations, and socioemotional adjustment during the high school-college transition. *Journal for Research on Adolescence, 8*, 1–27.

Larson, R. W. (1997). The emergence of solitude as a constructive domain of experience in early adolescence. *Child Development, 68*, 80–93.

Larson, R. W., & Lee, M. (1996). The capacity to be alone as a stress buffer. *Journal of Social Psychology, 136*, 5–16.

Larson, R. W., & Richards, M. H. (1994). *Divergent Realities*. New York: Basic Books.

Larson, R. W., Richards, M. H., Moneta, G., Holmbeck, G., & Duckett, E. (1996). Changes in adolescents' daily interactions with their families from ages 10 to 18: Disengagement and transformation. *Developmental Psychology, 32*, 744–754.

Larson, R. W., & Verma, S. (1999). How children and adolescents spend time across the world: Work, play, and developmental opportunities. *Psychological Bulletin, 125*, 701–736.

Leaper, C., Hauser, S. T., Kremen, A., Powers, S. I., Jacobson, A. M., Noam, G. G., et al. (1989). Adolescent-parent interaction in relation to adolescents' gender and ego development pathway: a longitudinal study. *Journal of Early Adolescence, 9*, 335–361.

Lee, G. R., Mancini, J. A., & Maxwell, J. W. (1990). Sibling relationships in adulthood: Contact patterns and motivations. *Journal of Marriage and the Family, 52*, 431–440.

Lesthaeghe, R. (1992). The second demographic transition in western countries: An interpretation. Paper delivered at the *Seminar on Gender and Family Change in Industrial Countries, International Union for the Scientific Study of Population*, Rome, Italy.

Levesque, R. (2001). *Culture and family violence: Fostering change through human rights law*. Washington, DC: American Psychological Association.

Lipkin, M., Jr., & Lamb, G. S. (1982). The couvade syndrome: An epidemiologic study. *Annals of Internal Medicine, 96*, 509–511.

Low, B. S. (1989). Cross-cultural patterns in the training of children: An evolutionary perspective. *Journal of Comparative Psychology, 103*, 311–319.

Luster, T., Boger, R., & Hannan, K. (1993). Infant affect and home environment. *Journal of Marriage and the Family, 55*, 651–661.

Ma, C., & Huebner, S. (2008). Attachment relationship an adolescents' life satisfaction: Some relationships matter more to girls than boys. *Psychology in the Schools, 45*, 177–190.

Maccoby, E. (1998). *The two sexes: Growing up apart, coming together*. Cambridge, MA: Harvard University Press.

MacCormack, C., & Strathern, M. (Eds.). (1980). *Nature, Culture and Gender*. Cambridge: Cambridge University Press.
MacDonald, T. K., & Ross, M. (1999). Assessing the accuracy of predictions about dating relationships: How and why do lovers' predictions differ from those made by observers. *Personality and Social Psychology Bulletin, 25*, 1417–1429.
Main, M., & Goldwyn, R. (1984). Predicting rejection of her infants from mother's representation of her own experience: implications for the abused-abusing intergenerational cycle. *International Journal of Child Abuse and Neglect, 8*, 203–217.
Malinowski, B. (1927). *Sex and Repression in Savage Society*. London: Routledge.
Manning, J. T., & Chamberlain, A. T. (1991). Left-side cradling and brain lateralization. *Ethology and Sociobiology, 12*, 237–244.
Markiewicz, D., Lawford, H., Doyle, A. B., & Haggart, N. (2006). Developmental differences in adolescents' and young adults' use of mothers, fathers, best friends, and romantic partners to fulfil attachment needs. *Journal of Youth and Adolescence, 35*, 127–140.
Markus, R., & Kitayama, S. (1991). Culture and the self: Implications for cognition, emotion, and motivation. *Psychological Review, 98*, 224–253.
Massimini, F., & Delle Fave, A. (2000). Individual development in a bio-cultural perspective. *American Psychologist, 55*, 24–33.
McBride, B. A., & Rane, T. R. (1998). Parenting alliance as a predictor of father involvement: an exploratory study. *Family Relations, 47*, 229–236.
McElhaney, K., Porter, M., Thompson, L., & Allen, J. (2008). Apples and oranges: Divergent meanings of parents' and adolescents' perceptions of parental influence. *The Journal of Early Adolescence, 28*, 206–229.
McHale, S., Crouter, A., & Whiteman, S. (2003). The family contexts of gender development in childhood and adolescence. *Social Development, 21*, 125–148.
Mealey, L., & Mackey, W. (1990). Variation in offspring sex ratio in women of differing social status. *Ethology and Sociobiology, 11*, 83–95.
Meyer, D. R., & Garasky, S. (1993). Custodial fathers: Myths, realities, and child support policy. *Journal of Marriage and the Family, 55*, 73–89.
Minorsky, V. (1982). *Medieval Iran and its neighbours*. London: Variorum Reprints.
Mishra, R. C. (2001). Cognition across cultures. In D. Matsumoto (Ed.), *The Handbook of Culture and Psychology* (pp. 119–135). New York: Oxford University Press.
Montagu, A. (1981). The adolescent's unreadiness for pregnancy and motherhood. *Pediatric Annals, 10*, 497–511.
Mounts, N. (2002). Parental management of adolescent peer relationships in context: The role of parenting style. *Journal of Family Psychology, 16*, 58–89.
Munroe, R. L., & Kimball Romney, A. (2006). Gender and age differences in same-sex aggregation and social behaviour. *Journal of Cross-Cultural Psychology, 37*, 3–19.
Munroe, R. L., Munroe, R. H., & Whiting, J. W. M. (1981). Male sex role resolutions. In R. H. Munroe, R. L. Munroe, & B. B. Whiting (Eds.), *Handbook of Cross-Cultural Human Development* (pp. 611–632). New York: Garland.
Murry, V. M., & Brody, G. H. (1999). Self-regulation and self-worth of black children reared in economically stressed, rural, single mother-headed families. *Journal of Family Issues, 4*, 458–484.
Myers, D. G. (2000). The funds, friends and faith of happy people. *American Psychologist, 55*, 56–67.
Noller, P. (2005). Sibling relationships in adolescence: Learning and growing together. *Personal Relationships, 12*, 1–22.
Nsamenang, A. B. (1992). *Human development in cultural context: A third world perspective*. Newbury Park, CA: Sage.
Okely, J. (1997). Non-territorial culture as the rationale for the assimilation of gypsy children. *Childhood, 4*, 63–80.

Oppedal, B., Roysamb, E., & Sam, D. L. (2004). The effect of acculturation and social support on change in mental health among young immigrants. *International Journal of Behavioral Development, 28*, 481–494.

Oswald, D., & Clark, E. (2003). Best friends forever? High school best friendships and the transition to college. *Personal Relationships, 10*, 187–196.

Oxley, N., Dzindolet, M., & Miller, J. (2002). Sex differences in communication with close friends. Testing tannen's claims. *Psychological Reports, 91*, 537–544.

Oyserman, D., Kemmelmeier, M., & Coon, H. (2002). Rethinking individualism and collectivism: evaluation of theoretical assumptions and meta-analyses. *Psychological Bulletin, 128*, 97–110.

Parks, M. R. (2007). *Personal relationships and personal networks*. Mahwah, NJ: Lawrence Erlbaum.

Paterson, J., Field, J., & Pryor, J. (1994). Adolescents' perceptions of their attachment relationships with their mothers, fathers, and friends. *Journal of Youth and Adolescence, 23*, 579–600.

Penninkilampi-Kerola, V., Moilanen, I., & Kaprio, J. (2005). Co-twin dependence, social interactions, and academic achievement: A population-based study. *Journal of Social and Personal Relationships, 22*, 519–541.

Peters, J. F. (1994). Gender socialization of adolescents in the home: Research and discussion. *Adolescence, 29*, 913–934.

Pierrehumbert, B., Santelices, M. P., Ibanez, M., Alberdi, M., Ongari, B., Roskam, I., et al. (2009). Gender and attachment representations in the preschool years. Comparison between five countries. *Journal of Cross-Cultural Psychology, 40*, 543–566.

Pike, A., & Atzaba-Poria, N. (2003). Do sibling and friend relationships share the same temperamental origins? A twin study. *Journal of Child Psychology and Psychiatry, 44*, 598–611.

Plomin, R., & Daniels, D. (1987). Why are children in the same family so different from one another? *Behavioral and Brain Sciences, 10*, 1–16.

Plomin, R., Reiss, D., Hetherington, E. M., & Howe, G. (1994). Nature and nurture: Genetic influence on measures of the family environment. *Developmental Psychology, 30*, 32–43.

Pöhlman, K. (2001). Agency- and communion-orientation in life goals: Impacts on goal pursuit strategies and psychological well-being. In P. Schmuck & K. Sheldon (Eds.), *Life goals and well-being: Towards a positive psychology of human striving* (pp. 68–84). Ashland, OH: Hogrefe & Huber Publishers.

Rasmussen, L. V. (1991). Gypsy music in Yugoslavia: Inside the popular cultural tradition. *Journal of the Gypsy Lore Society, 1*, 127–139.

Rathunde, K. (1989). The context of optimal experience: An exploratory model of the family. *New Ideas in Psychology, 7*, 91–97.

Rathunde, K. (1997). Parent–adolescent interaction and optimal experience. *Journal of Youth and Adolescence, 26*, 669–689.

Rathunde, K. (2001). Family context and the development of undivided interest: A longitudinal study of family support and challenge and adolescents' quality of experience. *Applied developmental science, 5*, 158–171.

Reis, H. T., Collins, W. A., & Berscheid, E. (2000). The relationship context of human behavior and development. *Psychological Bulletin, 126*, 844–872.

Rexroat, C., & Shehan, C. (1987). The family life cycle and spouses' time in household. *Journal of Marriage and the Family, 49*, 737–750.

Rich, G. J. (2003). The positive psychology of youth and adolescence. *Journal of Youth and Adolescence, 32*, 1–3.

Richards, M. H., Crowe, P. A., Larson, R., & Swarr, A. (1998). Developmental patterns and gender differences in the experience of peer companionship during adolescence. *Child Development, 69*, 154–163.

Robin, M., Josse, D., & Tourette, C. (1988). Mother-twin interaction during early childhood. *Acta Geneticae Medicae et Gemellologiae, 37*, 151–159.

Rogoff, B. (1990). *Apprenticeship in thinking: Cognitive development in social context*. New York: Oxford University Press.

Rohner, R. P., & Britner, P. A. (2002). Worldwide mental health correlates of parental acceptance-rejection. Review of cross-cultural and intracultural evidence. *Cross-cultural Research, 36*, 16–47.

Rosnati, R. (1996). Comunicazione e supporto familiari e aspettative per il futuro in età adolescenziale [Communication and family support and future expectations in adolescence]. *Archivio di Psicologia, Neurologia e Psichiatria, 57*, 280–299.

Rubin, K. H., Wojslawowicz, J. C., Rose-Krasnor, L., Booth-LaForce, C., & Burgess, K. B. (2006). The best friendships of shy/withdrawn children: prevalence, stability, and relationship quality. *Journal of Abnormal Child Psychology, 34*, 143–157.

Ruble, D., Fleming, A., Hackel, L., & Stangor, C. (1988). Changes in the marital relationship during the transition to first-time motherhood: Effects of violated expectations concerning division of household labor. *Journal of Personality and Social Psychology, 55*, 78–87.

Rummel, R. J. (1992). *Democide: Nazi genocide and mass murder*. New Brunswick, NJ: Transaction Publishers.

Ryan, R. M., & Deci, E. L. (2000). Self-determination theory and the facilitation of intrinsic motivation, social development, and well-being. *American Psychologist, 55*, 68–78.

Ryan, R., Stiller, J., & Lynch, J. (1994). Representations of relationships to teachers, parents, and friends as predictors of academic motivation and self-esteem. *Journal of Early Adolescence, 14*, 226–249.

Ryff, C. D., & Keyes, C. L. M. (1995). The structure of psychological well-being revisited. *Journal of Personality and Social Psychology, 69*, 719–727.

Sacco, W. P., & Murray, D. W. (1997). Mother–child relationship satisfaction: The role of attributions and trait conceptions. *Journal of Social and Clinical Psychology, 16*, 24–42.

Salk, L. (1960). The effects of the normal heartbeat sound on the behaviour of the newborn infant: Implications for mental health. *World Mental Health, 12*, 168–175.

Santrock, J. (1997). *Life-span development* (6th ed.). Madison, WI: Brown & Benchmark.

Schlegel, A. (1977). *Sexual stratification*. New York: Academic Press.

Schneider, B. (2000). *Friend and enemies. Peer relations in childhood*. London: Arnold.

Schwartz, S. J., & Pantin, H. (2006). Identity development in adolescence and emerging adulthood: The interface of self, context, and culture. In A. P. Prescott (Ed.), *The concept of self in psychology* (pp. 45–85). Hauppauge, NY: Nova Science Publishers.

Searight, H. R., Thomas, S. L., Manley, C. M., & Ketterson, T. U. (1995). Self-disclosure in adolescents: A family systems perspective. In K. J. Rotenberg (Ed.), *Disclosure processes in children and adolescents* (pp. 204–225). New York: Cambridge University Press.

Seifer, R., Schiller, M., Sameroff, A. J., Resnick, S., & Riordan, K. (1996). Attachment, maternal sensitivity, and infant temperament during the first year of life. *Developmental Psychology, 32*, 12–25.

Seligman, M., & Csikszentmihalyi, M. (2000). Positive psychology: An introduction. *American Psychologist, 55*, 5–15.

Sherman, A. M., de Vries, B., & Lansford, J. E. (2000). Friendship in childhood and adulthood: Lessons across the life span. *International Journal of Aging and Human Development, 51*, 31–51.

Sherman, A. M., Lansford, J. E., & Volling, B. L. (2006). Sibling relationships and best friendships in young adulthood: Warmth, conflict, and well-being. *Personal Relationships, 13*, 151–165.

Shulman, S., & Ben-Artzi, E. (2003). Age-related differences in the transition from adolescence to adulthood and links with family relationships. *Journal of Adult Development, 10*, 217–226.

Shulman, S., Seiffge-Krenke, I., Levy-Shiff, R., Fabian, B., & Rotenberg, S. (1995). Peer group and family relationships in early adolescence. *International Journal of Psychology, 30*, 573–590.

Shumow, L., & Lomax, R. (2002). Parental self-efficacy: predictor of parenting behavior adolescent outcomes. *Parenting, Science and Practice, 2*, 127–150.

Simmons, R., & Blyth, D. A. (1987). *Moving into adolescence: The impact of pubertal change and school context*. New York: Aldine de Gruyter.

Simons, R. L., Beanman, J., Conger, R. D., & Chao, W. (1993). Childhood experience, conceptions of parenting, and attitudes of spouse as determinants of parental behavior. *Journal of Marriage and the Family, 55*, 91–106.
Smetana, J. G. (1995). Conflict and coordination in adolescent–parent relationships. In S. Shulman (Ed.), *Close relationship and socioemotional development* (pp. 155–184). Norwood, NJ: Ablex Publishing Corporation.
Smith, T. (1997). Recognising difference: The Romani "gypsy" child socialisation and education process. *British Journal of Sociology of Education, 18*, 243–256.
Sprecher, S. (1998). Insiders' perspectives on reasons for attraction to a close other. *Social Psychology Quarterly, 62*, 287–300.
Sroufe, L. A., & Fleeson, J. (1986). Attachment and the construction of relationships. In W. W. Hartup & Z. Rubin (Eds.), *Relationships and development* (pp. 51–77). Hillsdale, NJ: Lawrence Erlbaum Associates Inc.
Steca, P., Bassi, M., Caprara, G. V., & Delle Fave, A. (2010). Parents' self-efficacy beliefs and their children's psychosocial adaptation during adolescence. *Journal of Youth and Adolescence*, DOI 10.1007/s10964-010-9514-9.
Stewart, R., Verbrugge, K., & Beilfuss, M. (1998). Sibling relationships in early adulthood: A typology. *Personal Relationships, 5*, 59–74.
Stokart, Z. C. (2010). *Gravidanza, maternità e progetto migratorio: l'esperienza quotidiana di donne sudamericane in Italia* [Pregnancy, motherhood, and migration project: The daily experience of South-American women in Italy]. Unpublished PhD dissertation, University of Milano.
Stokart, Z. C., Cavallo, M., Fianco, A., & Lombardi, M. (2007). Esperienza ottimale e identità femminile: uno studio transculturale su tre gruppi di adolescenti [Optimal experience and female identity: a cross-cultural study on three adolescent groups]. In A. Delle Fave (Ed.), *La condivisione del benessere* (pp. 313–331). Milano: Franco Angeli.
Super, C. M., & Harkness, S. (1986). The developmental niche: A conceptualization at the interface of child and culture. *International Journal of Behavioral Development, 9*, 545–569.
Teichman, Y., & Lahav, Y. (1987). Expectant fathers: Emotional reactions, physical symptoms and coping styles. *British Journal of Medical Psychology, 60*, 225–232.
Thomas, J., & Daubman, K. (2001). The relationship between friendship quality and self-esteem in adolescent girls and boys. *Sex Roles, 45*, 53–65.
Thorpe, K. (2006). Twin children's language development. *Early Human Development, 82*, 387–395.
Thorpe, K., & Gardner, K. (2005). Twins and their friendships: Differences between monozygotic, dizygotic same-sex and dizygotic mixed-sex pairs. *Twin Research and Human Genetics, 9*, 155–164.
Tomlinson, P. (1987). Spousal differences in marital satisfaction during transition to parenthood. *Nursing Research, 36*, 239–243.
Tooby, J., & Cosmides, L. (1996). Friendship and the banker's paradox: Other pathways to the evolution of adaptations for altruism. *Proceedings of the British Academy, 88*, 119–143.
Towsends, J. M., Kline, J., & Wasserman, T. H. (1995). Low-investment copulation: Sex differences in motivations and emotional reactions. *Ethology and Sociobiology, 16*, 25–51.
Trethowan, W., & Conlon, M. F. (1965). The couvade syndrome. *Journal of British Psychiatry, 111*, 57–66.
Triandis, H. C. (1999). *Individualism and collectivism*. Boulder, CO: Westview.
Trivers, R. L. (1972). Parental investment and sexual selection. In B. Campbell (Ed.), *Sexual selection and the descent of man 1871–1971* (pp. 136–179). Chicago: Aldine.
UNICEF. (2005). *The State of the World's Children 2006*. New York: Unicef.
Valente Torre, L. (1998). Il paradosso dei fratelli gemelli [The paradox of twin siblings]. *Età Evolutiva, 56*, 77–84.
van Ijendoorn, M. H. (1992). Inter-generational transmission of parenting: A review of studies in nonclinical populations. *Developmental Review, 12*, 76–99.

van Wel, F., Linssen, H., & Abma, R. (2000). The parental bond and the well-being of adolescents and young adults. *Journal of Youth and Adolescence*, *29*, 307–318.

Von Bracken, H. (1934). Mutual intimacy in twins. *Character and Personality*, *2*, 293–309.

Vygotsky, L. (1978). *Mind in society*. Cambridge, MA: Harvard University Press.

Wang, S., & Tamis-Lemonda, C. S. (2003). Do child rearing practices in Taiwan and in the united states reflect cultural valued of collectivism and individualism? *Journal of Cross-Cultural Psychology*, *34*, 629–642.

Warren, M. P., & Shortle, B. (1990). Endocrine correlates of human parenting: A clinical perspective. In N. A. Krasnegor & R. S. Bridges (Eds.), *Mammalian parenting* (pp. 209–226). Oxford: Oxford University Press.

Weisz, C., & Wood, L. (2005). Social identity support and friendship outcomes: A longitudinal study predicting who will be friends and best friends 4 years later. *Journal of Social and Personal Relationships*, *22*, 416–432.

Wenk, D., Hardesty, C. L., Morgan, C. S., & Blair, S. L. (1994). The influence of parental involvement on the well-being of sons and daughters. *Journal of Marriage and the Family*, *56*, 229–234.

Whiting, B. B., & Edwards, C. (1988). *Children of different worlds: The formation of social behaviour*. Cambridge, MA: Harvard University Press.

Wigfield, A., Eccles, J. S., & Pintrich, P. R. (1996). Development between the ages of 11 and 25. In D. C. Berliner & R. C. Calfee (Eds.), *Handbook of educational psychology* (pp. 148–185). New York: Simon & Schuster Macmillan.

Wiggins, R. D., Higgs, P. F., Hyde, M., & Blane, D. B. (2004). Quality of life in the third age: Key predictors of the CASP-19 measure. *Ageing & Society*, *24*, 693–708.

Xiang, P., McBride, R., & Bruene, A. (2003). Relations of parents' beliefs to children's motivation in an elementary physical education running program. *Journal of Teaching in Physical Education*, *22*, 410–425.

Yogman, M. W. (1990). Male parental behavior in humans and nonhuman primates. In N. A. Krasnegor & R. S. Bridges (Eds.), *Mammalian Parenting* (pp. 461–481). Oxford: Oxford University Press.

Zani, B., Carelli, M. G., Benelli, B., & Cicognani, E. (1991). Communicative skills in childhood: The case of twins. *Discourse Processes*, *14*, 339–356.

Zani, B., & Kirchler, E. (1995). Pregiudizi ed emozioni nei rapporti interetnici [Prejudice and emotion in intergroup relationships]. *Giornale Italiano di Psicologia*, *22*, 65–85.

Zavattini, G. C., Tambelli, R., Volpi, B., Chiarolanza, C., & Macone, A. (2002). Rappresentazioni della famiglia e stili di attaccamento in adolescenti di famiglie unite e separate [Representations of family and attachment styles in adolescents with united and separated families]. *Psicologia Clinica dello Sviluppo*, *3*, 491–513.

Zazzo, R. (1960–2005). *Les jumeaux, le couple et la personne* [Twins, the couple, and the person] (5th ed.). Paris: Ed. PUF-Quadrige.

Zazzo, R. (1984). *Le paradoxe des jumeaux* [The twins' paradox]. Paris: Ed. Stock Laurence Pernoud.

Zhang, S., & Kline, S. L. (2009). Can I make my own decision? A cross-cultural study of perceived social network influence in mate selection. *Journal of Cross-Cultural Psychology*, *40*, 3–23.

Zick, C. D., & Bryant, W. K. (1996). A new look at parents' time spent in child care: Primary and secondary time use. *Social Science Research*, *25*, 1–21.

Chapter 11
Education, Learning, and Cultural Transmission

11.1 Education Across Cultures

Human beings are biologically equipped to learn from their environment in order to adapt to their living conditions in flexible and successful ways. Education represents a crucial unit in the set of challenges human beings and groups have to meet in life or in time (Chapters 2 and 3; Csikszentmihalyi & Massimini, 1985; Massimini & Delle Fave, 2000; Massimini, Inghilleri, & Delle Fave, 1996). The chief importance of learning in our species is related to its role as the primary means of cultural transmission. Throughout their lives, individuals build up a pool of information, which enables them to behave in accordance with the rules and values of the social systems they belong to. Since childhood, individuals receive behavioral instructions and information from other experienced members of the community, be they adults—parents, caregivers, teachers—or peers. Across cultures, education can be informal, in that it takes place in daily situations, such as the family setting or public contexts, in which the individual learns by imitation and by following social models (Bandura, 1986). Education can also be formal when it takes place in contexts, such as the school or ceremonies (e.g., initiation rites), that are culturally sanctioned and regulated. According to the type of culture, transmission can be primarily oral—for example, among illiterate societies—or predominantly written. In the former case, individuals mostly bequeath cultural information they have stored in their brains as intrasomatic culture; in the latter, they primarily pass on information over their cultural history that have been stored in books, as extrasomatic culture (see Chapter 2).

Education is not only crucial for the survival of individuals, it also plays a vital role for cultural systems. Though an independent paradigm, cultural selection requires the active engagement and resource investment of individuals in the transmission of memes (Csikszentmihalyi & Massimini, 1985; Massimini & Delle Fave, 2000). What distinguishes human groups from one another is the way in which the problem of education is solved (Massimini & Calegari, 1979; Massimini et al., 1996). A variety of educational systems and pedagogic strategies have been created in order to achieve this goal. By promoting the association of their memes with individuals' psychological selection, societies can successfully survive in the long term, and at the same time support individuals' development and well-being. For this

A. Delle Fave et al., *Psychological Selection and Optimal Experience Across Cultures*, Cross-Cultural Advancements in Positive Psychology 2,
DOI 10.1007/978-90-481-9876-4_11, © Springer Science+Business Media B.V. 2011

purpose, they have to provide their members with meaningful opportunities for action in relation to their cultural information (Delle Fave & Massimini, 2004; Delle Fave, 2006). This is extremely important in a world in which competition among cultures is fierce, and the globalized western model is predominant over indigenous or local cultural systems. It is ultimately the individual who contributes to the perpetration of culture, and an educational system allowing for the fruitful integration of memes from different cultures can sustain plurality, complexity, and differentiation in a new global society.

Given the importance of learning for both individuals and societies, flow researchers have devoted much attention to its investigation. In this chapter, we will sum up major findings related to the quality of experience reported during formal learning activities by individuals across cultures. We will identify the activities associated with optimal experience, the contextual and individual factors favoring flow in education, and we will outline the short- and long-term consequences of learning in relation to individuals' psychological selection.

11.2 The Quality of Experience of Learning Activities

The World Bank (2010) reporting data on enrollment in and attendance to schools as well as academic progression shows that huge discrepancies exist across countries, with a large share of individuals around the world being deprived of formal educational opportunities. For those individuals who have access to schools, a large number of studies on optimal experience have been performed across age, including children in primary, middle, and secondary school, as well as college students. Several countries have been investigated across the five continents: Argentina (Mesurado, 2008, 2009), Australia (Pearce, Ainley, & Howard, 2005), Canada (Sedig, 2007), Chad (Bassi, Coppa, & Delle Fave, 2008a), China (Moneta, 2004), Germany (Engeser & Rheinberg, 2008), Italy (Bassi & Delle Fave, 2004; Bassi, Steca, Delle Fave, & Caprara, 2007; Delle Fave & Bassi, 2000), Japan (Asakawa, 2004, 2010), Korea (Lee, 2005), Nepal (Cavallo, Lombardi, & Stokart, 2006; Delle Fave & Massimini, 2005), the Netherlands (Bakker, 2005; Delespaul, Reis, & deVries, 2004), Spain (Sanchez-Franco, 2010), Taiwan (Fu, Su, & Yu, 2009), Turkey (Inal & Cagiltay, 2007), Uganda (Careddu, 2001; Delle Fave, 2009), the United Kingdom (Clarke & Haworth, 1994), and the United States (Csikszentmihalyi & Larson, 1984; Csikszentmihalyi & Schneider, 2000; Shernoff & Csikszentmihalyi, 2009). Information was also gathered among Navajo youths living in Arizona and New Mexico (Delle Fave, 1999).

Research has shown that learning activities in terms of both academic tasks performed at school and studying at home, represent a large share of participants' daily time-budget, ranging between 40 and 78% according to ESM assessments (Hektner, Schmidt, & Csikszentmihalyi, 2007). Across all the investigated cultures, learning presents potentially challenging opportunities for self-expression and for building crucial skills and knowledge (Delle Fave & Massimini, 2005; Hektner et al., 2007; Shernoff & Csikszentmihalyi, 2009; Shernoff, Csikszentmihalyi, Schneider, &

Shernoff, 2003). In particular, students associate them with high cognitive investment, the perception of long-term goals and short-term stakes in the task at hand (see Table 5.2). However, they also describe low levels of happiness, intrinsic motivation, and short-term desirability. In addition, as shown in Chapter 5, when students report a match between high challenges and high skills (channel 2; Fig. 4.1), as in optimal experience, the quality of the learning experience improves in its cognitive, emotional, and motivational dimensions, even though short-term desirability and happiness still hit negative or average values (Table 5.2). The quality of experience while studying is also influenced by the social context: It improves when related activities are carried out in the presence of other people among Asian-American adolescents (Asakawa & Csikszentmihalyi, 2000), with the help or supervision of adults among Argentinian middle-school students (Mesurado, 2009), or while interacting with adults among US eighth graders (Shernoff & Vandell, 2007).

Important insights into learning and its associated experience can be drawn from the analysis of the distribution of self-reported studying activities in the eight channels of the EFM (Fig. 4.1). Distinguishing between homework and schoolwork tasks, such as lectures and taking notes, studies have shown that the former are more frequently associated with optimal experience, whereas the latter with apathy and disengagement. This is primarily true in western countries such as the United States, the Netherlands, and Italy (Bassi & Delle Fave, 2004; Delespaul et al., 2004; Hektner et al., 2007; Shernoff & Csikszentmihalyi, 2009). In Italy, for example, flow in schoolwork activities was reported in 13.2% of the ESM forms, and apathy in 17.8%; during study activities at home, flow accounted for 21.4% of the forms and apathy for 16.4% of them. By contrast, a study with Nepalese teenagers showed that both schoolwork and homework were predominantly associated with optimal experience, amounting to 24.5 and 22.4% of the forms, respectively (Lombardi, 2003), versus 6.7 and 13.4% for apathy. Similar differences between western and Asian cultures were observed by Asakawa and Csikszentmihalyi (1998a) who identified higher percentages of flow while studying among Asian-American adolescents than among Caucasian-American students.

Delving deeper into classroom activities of US adolescents, a study by Shernoff et al. (2003) showed that higher scores of flow were associated with individual and group work versus listening to lectures, watching videos, or taking exams. Additionally, comparing experiences in specific subject areas, it was shown that high school students generally felt more engaged in nonacademic subjects such as computer science, art, and vocational education than in academic subjects such as English, science, and mathematics. The use of computer and new technologies in school activities was also analyzed by Bassi and Delle Fave (2004) among Italian students. Findings showed that participants reported a higher frequency of optimal experience when they used the computer as a means for retrieving information or for preparing home assignments, compared to typical paper-and-pencil work or studying book chapters.

The analysis of learning activities with single-administration questionnaires allowed us to integrate information gathered through ESM. When asked to report the opportunities for optimal experiences they retrieved in their lives, students from western countries—e.g., Argentina, Italy, and the United States—predominantly described leisure activities, and quoted studying in lower percentages. This finding was confirmed among middle-school children (Mesurado, 2009) high-school adolescents (Csikszentmihalyi & Larson, 1984; Delle Fave & Bassi, 2003), and college students (Bassi et al., 2008a). For instance, Italian adolescents mentioned leisure—including activities such as sports, hobbies, and reading—51.1% of the times, and studying 30.4% of the times. Similar findings were obtained among Italian college students, who quoted leisure and studying in 57.5 and 17.5% of their answers, respectively. Among studying activities, participants distinguished between rote learning as a means to pass tests and exams, and studying as a means to gain knowledge and meet personal goals, the latter being associated with optimal experience. A 20-year-old Italian medical student reported: "Sometimes studying is stimulating: I can look at what I am studying with a critical and curious eye, so studying becomes a discovery, an experience. Other times, more often, studying is just mechanical; it implies reading, underlining, repeating, and above all it is aimed at getting a good grade at the exam".

In the analysis of non-western students, a different picture emerged, with learning activities representing the most frequently reported opportunity for optimal experience, and leisure having lower ranking (see Table 7.7). This was observed among Nepalese adolescents (Cavallo et al., 2006), Ugandan Karimojong pupils (Careddu, 2001; Delle Fave, Bassi, Cavallo, & Stokart, 2007), Navajo college students (Table 13.4; Delle Fave, 1999), and Chadian medical students (56.8% for studying and 8.1% for leisure; Bassi et al., 2008a). For all these participants, learning represented a privileged opportunity to gain knowledge, to prove one's skills, which could have a crucial impact on personal realization and community well-being. Here are some descriptions that were given by participants

> Studying teaches me to grow moral and it reforms you; and it will make you overcome ignorance and also to get a future after school (17-year-old Ugandan student)
>
> Studying means power of knowledge. It is as deep as the ocean. Once you dive into this ocean, you cannot come out. Those who reach the bottom will find those pearls which are so precious (18-year-old Nepalese high school student)
>
> To read is very interesting. I'll learn more words and about things I never heard before. It gives me the advantage while others don't get that kind of chance (18-year-old Navajo college student)
>
> Studying is a hard job that allows me to deeply acquire knowledge, and to start a profession which can serve mankind in a valid way (25-year-old Chadian medical student)

A deeper analysis of the data gathered among the Navajo and Nepalese participants allowed us to further distinguish between the different learning opportunities provided by more traditional school systems and fully westernized ones (Cavallo et al., 2006; Delle Fave, 1999; Lombardi, 2003; Massimini et al., 1996). Results showed that Navajo teenagers attending a western-style high school tended to reproduce typically western trends, with leisure representing the primary self-reported source of optimal experience. By contrast, older Navajo youths attending the Diné College (an institution providing both traditional knowledge and modern notions) primarily quoted learning activities as opportunities for flow. They referred to both Navajo traditional knowledge and western subjects, highlighting the adoption of a bicultural strategy developed by the Navajo people throughout the centuries (Delle Fave, 1999, Chapter 13). In particular Manuelito, one of the Navajo chiefs who signed the treaty with the United States at Fort Sumner in 1868, understood the importance of education as a crucial means to Navajos' cultural survival, and accordingly spurred his people to take on the challenge of a bicultural formal education system.

In the study conducted with Nepalese teenagers, participants were recruited from government-run, community-based, and private schools (Cavallo et al., 2006; Lombardi, 2003). Government-run schools are public, and grant free access for all students; community-based ones require an enrollment fee, but are run on no-profit principles by local community members; private schools are costly and exclusive institutions based on western educational principles. The community-based schools examined in this study belonged to a Buddhist minority group moved from Tibet to Nepal due to the conflict with China. Students attending the government-run and particularly the community-based schools quoted both western learning activities and traditional subjects, whereas teenagers from private schools mainly quoted western tasks.

11.2.1 Unraveling Cultural Differences

The findings illustrated thus far allow us to depict broad differences in the quality of experience and flow opportunities in learning between western and non-western cultures. Among western students, formal education is prominently characterized by apathy and boredom, and provides limited occasions for optimal experiences compared to leisure activities. This is a quite worrying finding, considering the importance of learning for cultural transmission and individuals' social adaptation. It is even more worrying if we consider the natural human tendency to learn and the thirst for knowledge in young children (Shernoff & Csikszentmihalyi, 2009). Once children enter the formal school system, they start to report lack of interest and disengagement toward learning, which can lead to poor concepts assimilation and eventually to school drop-out. On the one hand, disaffection with school can be interpreted as an aberrant consequence of the right to education for all. Western students take school access for granted, and do not perceive the challenges and opportunities they are provided with in such educational system (see also Chapter 15). On the other hand, the organization and the pedagogic strategies of the mainstream western educational model seem to fall short of students' needs for autonomy and self-regulation (Deci & Ryan, 2000; Vansteenkiste, Lens, & Deci, 2006). In particular, this is attested by the difference emerged between schoolwork activities—such as listening to lectures and taking notes—and homework tasks (Bassi & Delle Fave, 2004; Hektner et al., 2007; Shernoff et al., 2003). At school, learning activities are primarily directed by teachers, in terms of both lesson content and amount of time devoted to a given task. In this condition, participants mostly reported passively listening to lessons, perceiving the lack of meaningful challenges, and no room for skill investment. While at home, however, students are in control of learning activities, are free to decide how much time to devote to learning, and are thus more likely to experience flow and active engagement in the task at hand. The importance of autonomy in learning tasks is further attested by the experiential differences between passive school activities, such as listening to the teacher, and active participation in group and individual work: The former are commonly associated with apathy and boredom, the latter with optimal experience.

The findings obtained from non-western students highlighted different experiences at school as well as different concerns. Participants predominantly reported optimal experience during learning activities, both at school and at home. They recognized the importance of formal education to improve their living conditions and those of their community. In countries like Uganda and Chad education is a rare and costly opportunity for students. The participants interviewed in Uganda were girls attending high school at a Catholic mission (Careddu, 2001; Delle Fave, 2009). Differently from most girls in their region, who usually have unequal opportunities to school access compared to boys, these teenagers could improve their social condition; they could enjoy more independence and autonomy, while the majority of girls of their age do not attend school and are exchanged as brides in order to increase the cattle stock of the family. Participants from Chad were college students attending the medical school that was founded in N'Djamena in 2005 through the support of Italian and European institutions. Due to limited resources, only 25 students could be enrolled in the first medical program, in a country in which there are 345 physicians for 10 million people, i.e., 0.04 per 1,000 inhabitants (WHO 2006). These two African examples point to the fact that main concerns in some countries regard access to formal education. In addition, studies in other non-western countries such as Nepal and the Navajo nation highlighted the crucial instrumental role of education as a means to cultural integration through the adoption of a bicultural strategy (Delle Fave, 2006). The ability to draw opportunities for optimal experience both from one's traditional lore and from the dominant or globalized cultural system can favor individuals' adaptation to a plural environment, the development of tolerance among cultures, and the valorization of one's cultural identity.

11.3 Flow and Learning: The Influence of Individual and Contextual Factors

As shown in Chapter 5, several individual and contextual factors are associated with the retrieval of optimal experience in daily life. Some of them pertain to the learning environment (Bassi, Steca, & Delle Fave, 2010; Shernoff & Csikszentmihalyi, 2009).

11.3.1 Individual Characteristics

Among the individuals factors related to optimal experience and engagement in learning, studies have highlighted demographic variables. Among US adolescents, girls reported higher levels of flow in classrooms than boys (Shernoff, Kanuth, & Makris, 2000), even though this may reflect girls' tendency to report higher flow in all living contexts (Schmidt, Shernoff, & Csikszentmihalyi, 2007). Csikszentmihalyi et al. (1993) identified talents in specific subjects such as mathematics, science, music, art, or athletics, as important individual features. Comparing talented teenagers with their average peers, the researchers found that US talented students were significantly more engaged in classwork, but they did not spend any more time studying outside the school. They thus seemed to be able to study more efficiently both in and out of class. In addition, they felt happier and more cheerful in learning tasks, as well as more concentrated and engaged. Following up the talented sample 2 years later, the researchers also found that teens who showed standing commitment to their talent felt more positive affect, higher potency, and intrinsic motivation while performing in their talent area; they also perceived learning activities as highly important for their future goals, and reported optimal experience more often than those students who had not pursued their talents in the long term.

The perception of learning activities as opportunities for optimal experiences was also found to be related to students' academic self-efficacy beliefs, namely their self-beliefs in managing activities connected to learning processes and success at school (Bandura, 1997; Bandura, Barbaranelli, Caprara, & Pastorelli, 2001). In a study by Bassi et al. (2007), two groups of Italian secondary-school students were selected on the basis of their high and low perceived academic self-efficacy. High self-efficacy students were shown to devote significantly more time to learning, especially at home, than their counterparts. They also reported a more positive quality of experience during learning, primarily associating schoolwork (listening to lectures, taking notes), classwork (oral and written tests), and homework with optimal experience. On the contrary, low self-efficacy students did not perceive a great amount of opportunities for optimal experience in learning tasks. More specifically, they primarily associated schoolwork and homework with low challenging experiences, such as apathy and relaxation, and tests and exams with anxiety, reporting a perceived lack of skills in facing the task.

Beyond and above individual characteristics such as gender, talent, and levels in academic self-efficacy, investigations found that the most pervasive factor associated with optimal experience in learning was the perception of goals. Goals allow students to connect their daily engagement in educational tasks to their psychological selection and to the construction of a long-term life theme (Csikszentmihalyi & Beattie, 1979; Delle Fave & Massimini, 2005; Massimini & Delle Fave, 2000; Chapter 7) Across cultures, the pursuit of learning activities is sustained by clear goals about future career and life prospects. In some cases, these goals are focused on personal achievements, such as self-fulfillment, acquiring knowledge, finding a job. In other cases, goals have a broader scope, including family interests and the survival of the community. Research showed that students from western countries primarily associated self-related goals with learning activities, while participants from non-western countries reported both self- and community-related goals. For example, medical students from Chad predominantly quoted goals like helping those who suffer, and contributing to the development of their country, along with aims such as getting a degree, and becoming a good doctor (Bassi et al., 2008a). The most important goal perceived by Nepalese adolescents in learning tasks was the opening up of future job opportunities (Cavallo et al., 2006). Students from private schools additionally stressed the importance of personal growth, whereas participants from community-based schools mentioned social commitment. Ugandan girls primarily quoted work as a crucial future goal, which could improve personal conditions as well as the wealth of the extended family (Delle Fave et al., 2007). By contrast, US, Italian, and Japanese high-school students primarily reported self-related goals about future career (Asakawa & Csikszentmihalyi, 1998b; Hektner, 1996; Massimini et al., 1996). Similar results were obtained among Italian medical students who mainly connected study to work-related goals, such as becoming a good doctor and achieving professional self-actualization, together with life projects like doing what one likes most, and living serenely.

11.3.2 Cultural and Contextual Features

The studies illustrated in Section 11.2 detected broad cross-cultural differences in the quality of learning experience. Participants from countries like Japan, Nepal, and Chad retrieved more optimal experiences in learning activities than respondents from Italy and the United States. This dissimilarity can partly be related to the differential access to formal education or to personal factors such as the perception of long-term goals. Cultural factors can also influence the evaluation of learning as a means for personal achievement and social recognition. In a study by Shernoff and Schmidt (2008), for example, students from ethnic minorities—in particular African Americans—reported more flow in learning tasks than Caucasian students. Similar results were obtained by Asakawa and Csikszentmihalyi (1998a, 1998b) comparing Asian and Caucasian American adolescents.

As shown in a great number of studies, the family context plays a fundamental role in transmitting the cultural relevance of education and, simultaneously, in sustaining children's retrieval of optimal experience in learning (Bassi & Delle Fave, 2006). For example, studies examining parental practices concerning children's academic activities showed that Asian-American parents were more likely to decide whether their children should go to college, compared to Caucasian American parents (Asakawa & Csikszentmihalyi, 1998a; Asakawa, 2001). However, Asian-American parents seemed to allow their children more freedom in deciding what classes to take, and in doing homework, compared to their Caucasian counterparts. Among US adolescents, Rathunde (1997, 2001) highlighted that support and challenge were crucial family characteristics favoring children's resource investment in academic activities. Parents in a supportive family seemed to share some specific characteristics: They are warm and affectionate, they listen in open and non-judgmental ways, and they are helpful when their children are learning new skills or confronting obstacles. In a challenging family, parents are described as modeling self-directed behavior, setting rules and limits, and expecting the adolescent to take steps that will lead to individuation and goal achievement. The right balance between support and challenge helps adolescents demonstrate immediate involvement and an ability to focus their attention on goals. It further creates a growth-conducive environment, which is positively related to long-term engagement in learning activities (Hektner, 2001). Finally, a study by Steca et al. (2010) investigated parents' beliefs about their efficacy in carrying out their designed role behavior, and their children's psychosocial adaptation during adolescence. Findings showed that children of parents with high self-efficacy levels reported higher competence, freedom, and well-being in learning activities.

At the school level, various factors have been shown to impact on students' retrieval of optimal experiences: first and foremost, school types, pedagogies, and instructional practices (Nakamura & Csikszentmihalyi, 2009). Studies highlighted that the western traditional school system, that heavily rely on notion-centered educational strategies, can lead students to passive and compulsory learning. On the opposite, a learning environment that enables students to find meaningful relations between study contents and personal experience and goals can help them discover the rewarding features of knowledge, and the potential of learning tasks as opportunities for optimal experience. Such an environment is actively pursued in alternative institutions such as Montessori middle schools (see Shernoff & Csikszentmihalyi, 2009 for a review). It is also sustained by positive psychologists who believe that institutions should not only focus on building strengths to reduce negative outcomes such as academic failure, violence, or substance abuse, but they should implement programs that foster an equally broad range of positive outcomes (Clonan, Chafouleas, McDougal, & Riley-Tillman, 2004; Gillham, Reivich, & Shatté, 2002). Pedagogies focusing on cooperative learning provide more opportunities for optimal experience than passive pedagogies such as listening to lectures, in middle school (Mesurado, 2009), high school (Shernoff et al., 2003), as well as college (Beylefeld & Struwig, 2007). Another school feature that impacts on learning is the gamut of subjects being taught. As shown above, educational systems fostering biculturalism by integrating western knowledge and local traditional lore provide students with a varied choice of cultural instructions (Cavallo et al., 2006; Delle Fave, 1999). In particular, they allow students to develop their personal life themes by combining their traditional cultural identity and predominantly western models, thus favoring the understanding of and tolerance for cultural differences. Studies have further shown that the use of new technologies can also foster the retrieval of optimal experience in learning activities, in that they provide challenging opportunities for creatively applying one's skills (Delle Fave and Bassi 2004; Fu et al., 2009; Shernoff & Csikszentmihalyi, 2009). For example, an operational learnware for teaching geometry to Canadian middle-school children was shown to make mathematics a flow experience by gradually matching students' acquired skills with learning targets (i.e., challenges) (Sedig, 2007). Similar results were obtained among Australian college students with a software presenting learning exercises in physics (Pearce et al., 2005). In higher education, research has shown that a web-based learning environment can help universities reach increasing number of students, both in traditional distance education and continuing professional education. Findings among Spanish university students showed that the shift of focus away from traditional content-based learning to a more pro-active approach that embraces process-based learning promotes flow among participants (Sanchez-Franco, 2010).

As far as instructional strategies are concerned, teachers play a major role in promoting students' optimal experience at school through the support of learners' autonomy. A study among US elementary school pupils showed that participants retrieved more flow in math classrooms when teachers adopted a scaffolding role, provided feedback and clarification of concepts, supported autonomy, and encouraged children's learning for its own sake rather than being directive and evaluative (Schweinle, Meyer, & Turner, 2006). The importance of autonomy in fostering optimal experience in learning was also attested by a study on US adolescents (Hektner, 2001). Furthermore, analyzing Dutch music teachers and their students, Bakker (2005) showed that flow can cross over from teachers to their students on the basis of emotional contagion. Findings confirmed that the more flow experiences music teachers reported, the higher the frequency of comparable experiences that was observed among their students.

Teachers frequently report that students' engagement in academic activities supports their optimal experiences in teaching; in their turn, students indicate that their flow in learning is related to the teachers' enthusiasm (Hektner et al., 2007; Shernoff & Csikszentmihalyi, 2009). However, the simultaneous ESM assessment of students' and teachers' experience at school has shown an alarming discrepancy: While teachers mostly report flow while teaching, students mostly report apathy while listening to classes and taking notes. This was observed among Italian high school students (Bassi, Coppa, Sartori, & Delle Fave, 2008b) as well as US adolescents (DiBianca, 2000). Once again, this may be related to a difference in perceived autonomy. While teaching, teachers are fully responsible for their educational strategies and contents, but students are passive. This explanation can also apply to the different quality of experience students associate with various learning activities, as shown in Section 11.2 (Shernoff et al., 2003): Adolescents are more engaged in group and individual work than while listening to a lecture or watching TV or a video, since they play an active and creative role in the activities they are performing.

11.4 The Impact of Optimal Experience on Students' Well-Being and Development

Personal and cultural factors inextricably join in the construction of individuals' psychological selection (Massimini & Delle Fave, 2000). Studies have shown that the association of learning activities with optimal experience has both short- and long-term consequences (Hektner et al., 2007; Shernoff & Csikszentmihalyi, 2009). In the short-term, students derive enjoyment, gratification, and sense of mastery from learning tasks (Delle Fave & Bassi, 2000). They report high levels of positive affect and low levels of negative affect (Rogatko, 2009), as well as high levels of engagement and energy investment, which are reflected in high academic achievement and grades. These findings were confirmed by studies conducted among US high-school teens and German college students (Engeser & Rheinberg, 2008;

Shernoff & Schmidt, 2008). Findings among Korean undergraduate students also indicated that participants reporting optimal experience in learning activities tended not to procrastinate their academic work, but to take timely actions and to seize educational opportunities (Lee, 2005).

Benefits of flow in school activities extend beyond academic success and comprise other important life domains. For example, among British university students, Clarke and Haworth (1994) found that individuals reporting intense flow experiences at least twice during the tested week had higher scores of mental health than those reporting low-intensity flow. Among US college students, Steele and Fullagar (2009) showed that finding flow in attended courses impacted on psychological well-being. They also detected an indirect effect of flow on physical health, as measured in terms of pain, discomfort, medications, sleep, and fatigue. Engagement in academic activities thus seems to induce positive psychological states that increase physical resources and resilience, and enable students to cope more effectively with stress, and to function at an optimal level.

This interpretation also applies to the psychosocial sphere. Schmidt (2003) analyzed US adolescents who faced substantial adversity at home or at school, and who were thus at particular risk for increased misconduct. She found that time investment in challenging activities such as schoolwork (done both in and outside the school) and perceived success in daily challenges were associated with reduced misconduct both cross-sectionally and over time.

In the long term, research has highlighted the role of optimal experience in sustaining commitment to learn and in shaping individuals' psychological selection (Asakawa & Csikszentmihalyi, 1998b; Csikszentmihalyi et al., 1993; Delle Fave & Massimini, 2005). Flow was identified as a predictor of sustained motivation in specific subjects (Shernoff & Hoogstra, 2001) as well as of future intention to use web-based learning environments (Sanchez-Franco, 2010). For example, US students reported longitudinal coherence in the amount of time devoted to study over a 3-year period in secondary school (Hektner, 2001).

The association of flow with learning activities further contributes to predicting the level of academic career students are willing to pursue, and to shaping adolescents' long-term goals and future work interests (Csikszentmihalyi & Schneider, 2000; Hektner, 2001; Wong & Csikszentmihalyi, 1991). This is the case of US students who found flow in high-school math and science classes, and who were more likely to choose a science-related major in college (Shernoff & Hoogstra, 2001).

11.5 Learning Activities and Psychological Selection: A Comparison Between Italy and Nepal

In light of the findings presented above, in this section we will delve deeper into the role of learning in psychological selection of high school students by comparing data from Italy and Nepal. We have chosen these countries as representatives of western and non-western cultures, respectively, with the aim to identify similarities and differences among cultures in the investment in learning as a means of inculturation as well as of personal professional development. The Italian sample comprised 206 adolescents (62.6% girls) aged 15–19 ($M = 16.8$, $SD = 1.1$) coming from the metropolitan area of Rome; the Nepalese sample included 48 participants (60.4% girls) aged 13–17 ($M = 14.8$, $SD = 1.1$) from the capital city of Kathmandu and neighboring Lalitpur. Both groups were administered flow questionnaire and life theme questionnaire.

Some global findings were presented in Chapter 7, within an overview of flow in adolescence across cultures. Here we would like to point out more analytic results derived from the direct comparison of these two specific samples. As shown in Table 11.1, Italian adolescents primarily reported optimal experience in the category hobbies and sports, followed by studying, and to smaller extent by media (e.g., reading). By contrast, Nepalese participants predominantly quoted studying, followed by the other two leisure categories.

Among both Italians and Nepalese, the discrepancy between studying and leisure categories became even wider when participants were asked to select the activity in which optimal experience was more intense. However, this discrepancy had completely opposite directions in the two groups: Italians primarily quoted hobbies and sports, whereas Nepalese mainly reported studying. In all, 19.7% of Italians (28 participants) retrieved flow in studying, while 80.3% of them retrieved it other life domains (i.e., non-studying activities; 114 participants). Nepalese teens who reported studying amounted to 53% (18 participants) and those who reported non-studying activities equaled 47% (16 participants). Comparing scores between countries, we obtained a significant difference ($\chi^2 = 15.7, p<0.0001$), showing that more Nepalese teenagers reported studying as optimal activity, and more Italians reported other activities than their counterparts.

In order to explore the role of studying in participants' lives across countries, we next analyzed positive influences, present challenges, and future goals of participants reporting optimal experiences irrespective of whether they found it in studying activities or in other categories. In particular, we separated answers

Table 11.1 Percentage distribution of optimal activities among Italian and Nepalese students

	Optimal activities (%)		Selected optimal activities (%)	
Categories	Italy ($N = 142$)	Nepal ($N = 34$)	Italy ($N = 142$)	Nepal ($N = 34$)
Work	5	1.2	3.5	2.9
Study	30.4	43.2	19.7	53
Volunteering	–	1.2	–	2.9
Interactions	6.1	4.3	6.3	8.8
Hobbies and sports	37.5	15.6	52.1	17.7
Media	13.6	10.1	9.2	2.9
Family	5.7	8.6	8.5	–
Personal care	0.4	2.9	–	–
Introspection	1.4	5.8	0.7	2.9
Religious practice	–	1.2	–	–
Meditation	–	5.8	–	8.8
N answers	280	70	142	34

Table 11.2 Participants reporting productive activities (study or work) versus other activities across domains of psychological selection

	Italians		Nepalese	
	Study *N* (%)	Other *N* (%)	Study *N* (%)	Other *N* (%)
Positive influences	58 (40.8)	84 (59.2)	22 (64.7)	12 (35.3)
Current challenges	82 (57.7)	60 (42.3)	29 (85.3)	5 (14.7)
Future goals	124 (87.3)	18 (12.7)	30 (88.2)	4 (11.8)
N participants	142		34	

pertaining to productive activities (i.e., studying and work) from answers regarding other categories (such as family, leisure). This analysis allowed us to identify the relative weight or importance of productive activities in directing participants' developmental trend. Results are illustrated in Table 11.2.

Chi-square analyses showed significant differences between countries for positive influences ($\chi^2 = 6.3$, $p < 0.02$), and present challenges ($\chi^2 = 8.9$, $p < 0.003$), but not for future goals. These differences were due to the fact that a higher number of Nepalese students quoted productive activities among their positive influences and present challenges than their Italian counterparts. Vice versa, more Italians reported non-productive categories. Concerning goals, however, both groups predominantly described productive activities, as previously shown in Section 11.3.1 and in Chapter 7. These findings underline the importance individuals in these two countries assign to further studying and especially future profession as personal long-term goals. However, in the present, Nepalese adolescents recognize the effort as well as the resource investment entailed in studying, as a concrete and effective way to meet their future objectives. On the opposite, Italians are more focused on other present challenges regarding relations and leisure. They thus seem to overlook—or at best, to downplay the importance of—the relationship between seed time and harvest, postponing their commitment to their professional career to some indefinite future.

What can we say about those individuals who selected studying as their most intense optimal experience? Do they show congruence in reporting productive activities (study or work) across domains of psychological selection? In other words, are productive activities a *Leitmotiv* in the construction of their long-term life plan? Table 11.3 illustrates results.

Table 11.3 Participants' congruence in reporting productive activities (study or work) across time-related dimensions of psychological selection (past positive influences, present challenges, and future goals)

	Italians		Nepalese	
	Yes *N* (%)	No *N* (%)	Yes *N* (%)	No *N* (%)
Congruence	8 (28.6)	20 (71.4)	11 (61.1)	7 (38.9)
N participants	28		18	

Incongruence was more frequent for Italians, while congruence was more frequent for Nepalese, and this difference was significant ($\chi^2 = 4.8$, $p<0.03$). Italian adolescents reporting pervasive flow in studying activities derived enjoyment and engagement in learning, but primarily set a variety of positive influences, challenges, and goals pertaining to non-productive domains. By contrast, Nepalese teenagers who associated studying with the most intense optimal experiences identified most positive influences in the same domain, and pursued productive activities in the short and long term. These findings are in line with the ones illustrated in Table 11.2 about the whole samples, thus pointing to the presence of a pervasive cultural difference. Irrespective of whether participants associated studying with the most intense optimal experiences or not, Nepalese participants attributed a higher value to learning in the short and in the long term, whereas Italians primarily associated it with long-term objectives, but were daily involved in other activities and domains. Additionally, compared to Italians, a higher number of Nepalese teens identified opportunities for optimal experience in studying: In this case, greater short- and long-term commitment to productive activities was reported.

11.6 Concluding Remarks

Many crucial issues were brought forward in this chapter, and many fundamental questions were raised about the role of formal education for both individuals' psychosocial well-being and communities' thriving. In particular, findings highlighted how optimal experience in learning can promote short- and long-term constructive consequences in both these areas. They also underscored considerable differences across cultures, which deserve the attention of all those experts—psychologists, educators, pedagogists—as well as policy makers who believe that the formal school system should focus on building self-actualized and socially adapted individuals.

Findings from western countries repeatedly stressed students' growing disaffection for learning activities that mostly engender apathy and boredom. On the other hand, results from non-western populations pointed to the great investment in studying as a means to improve one's conditions, in the face of the limited resources available to provide education for all.

While the right and opportunity to instruction are a priority of the international community, this is not the only concern legislators should cope with. A broader concern regards the ability of the formal system to transmit education and enjoyment in learning, on the one hand, and the ability of students to seize the educational opportunities, on the other hand. This concern pertains to the entire social structure, and is related to the solutions that are found to promote optimal learning. As shown in this chapter, this entails fostering optimal experiences at school by providing challenging opportunities for action, autonomy, and creativity. It also implies successfully transmitting the value of formal learning in contexts such as the family and the local community, or through mass media such as television, which greatly provide young people with models and information.

To foster long-term commitment in educational activities, individuals should learn not only to look for short-term gratifications, but also to firmly connect present learning tasks with goals that can give meaning to their developmental path. Cultures can provide such a meaning-making system (see Chapter 7; Delle Fave, 2006; Massimini & Delle Fave, 2000; Triandis, 1995). In western societies, individualistic values prevail, with emphasis on personal achievement and success. In non-western societies, meaning is prominently linked to interpersonal and community well-being. Opening up to a broader framework of meanings encompassing individuals in the context of their society can provide higher and more valuable challenges in which children and youth could devote their effort and invest their resources. Meaningful opportunities for optimal experience can indeed be drawn from different cultural sources, as shown in the bicultural strategies of the Navajos (Delle Fave, 1999, 2009). Such strategies do not only favor the survival of traditional cultures that are threatened by modernization and globalization; they also show that it is possible, and enriching, to combine cultural information coming from different traditions for the construction of a plural society based on diversity and cooperation.

References

Asakawa, K. (2001). Family socialization practices and their effects on the internalization of educational values for Asian and white American adolescents. *Applied Developmental Science, 5*, 184–194.

Asakawa, K. (2004). Flow experience and autotelic personality in Japanese college students: how do they experience challenges in daily life? *Journal of Happiness Studies, 5*, 123–154.

Asakawa, K. (2010). Flow experience, culture, and well-being: how do autotelic Japanese college student feel, behave, and think in their daily lives? *Journal of Happiness Studies, 11*, 205–223.

Asakawa, K., & Csikszentmihalyi, M. (1998a). The quality of experience of Asian American adolescents in academic activities: an exploration of educational achievement. *Journal of Research on Adolescence, 8*, 241–262.

Asakawa, K., & Csikszentmihalyi, M. (1998b). The quality of experience of Asian American adolescents in activities related to future goals. *Journal of Youth and Adolescence, 27*, 141–163.

Asakawa, K., & Csikszentmihalyi, M. (2000). Feelings of connectedness and internalization of values in Asian American adolescents. *Journal of Youth and Adolescence, 29*, 121–145.

Bakker, A. B. (2005). Flow among music teachers and their students: the crossover of peak experiences. *Journal of Vocational Behavior, 66*, 26–44.

Bandura, A. (1986). Social foundations of thought and action. Englewood Cliffs, NJ: Prentice-Hall.

Bandura, A. (1997). *Self-efficacy: The exercise of control*. New York: Freeman.

Bandura, A., Barbaranelli, C., Caprara, G. V., & Pastorelli, C. (2001). Self-efficacy beliefs as shapers of children's aspirations and career trajectories. *Child Development, 72*, 187–206.

Bassi, M., Coppa, R., & Delle Fave, A. (2008a). Studiare medicina per condividere benessere: una ricerca transculturale in ciad e in italia [studying medicine to share well-being: A cross-cultural research in chad and italy]. *Psicologia della Salute, 1*, 93–107.

Bassi, M., Coppa, R., Sartori, R., & Delle Fave, A. (2008b). Condividere benessere per educare al benessere: l'esperienza quotidiana di insegnanti e studenti [sharing well-being to educate about well-being: daily experience of teachers and students]. In C. Guido e & G. Vernì (a cura di), *Educazione al benessere e nuova professionalità docente. Ricerca, profili, riflessioni* (pp. 19–66). Bari: Ufficio Scolastico Regionale Puglia.

Bassi, M., & Delle Fave, A. (2004). Adolescence and the changing context of optimal experience in time: Italy 1986–2000. *Journal of Happiness Studies, 5*, 155–179.

Bassi, M., & Delle Fave, A. (2006). The daily experience of Italian adolescents' in family interactions. Gender and developmental issues. In A. Delle Fave (Ed.), *Dimensions of well-being. Research and intervention* (pp. 172–190). Milano: Franco Angeli.

Bassi, M., Steca, P., & Delle Fave, A. (2010). Academic self-efficacy beliefs and optimal experience: merging perspectives in learning research. In R. Levesque (Ed.), *Encyclopedia of adolescence*. Dordrecht, NL: Springer.

Bassi, M., Steca, P., Delle Fave, A., & Caprara, G. V. (2007). Academic self-efficacy beliefs and quality of experience in learning. *Journal of Youth and Adolescence, 36*, 301–312.

Beylefeld, A. A., & Struwig, M. C. (2007). A gaming approach to learning medial microbiology: Students' experiences of flow. *Medical Teacher, 29*, 933–940.

Careddu, S. (2001). *Selezione e trasmissione femminile delle istruzioni culturali presso i Karimojong dell'Uganda* [Selection and female transmission of cultural instructions among Karimojong in Uganda]. Dissertation at IULM University, Milano, Italy.

Cavallo, M., Lombardi, M., & Stokart, Z. (2006). Complessità e sviluppo di opportunità: esperienza ottimale e selezione psicologica in un gruppo di adolescenti nepalesi [complexity and development of opportunities: optimal experience and psychological selection in a group of Nepalese adolescents]. *Passaggi, 11*, 77–100.

Clarke, S. G., & Haworth, J. T. (1994). 'Flow' experience in the daily lives of sixth-form college students. *British Journal of Psychology, 85*, 511–523.

Clonan, S. M., Chafouleas, S. M., McDougal, J., & Riley-Tillman, T. C. (2004). Positive psychology goes to school: are we there yet? *Psychology in Schools, 41*, 101–110.

Csikszentmihalyi, M., & Beattie, O. (1979). Life themes: A theoretical and empirical exploration of their origins and effects. *Journal of Humanistic Psychology, 19*, 677–693.

Csikszentmihalyi, M., & Larson, R. W. (1984). *Being adolescents: Conflict and growth in teenage years*. New York: Basic Books.

Csikszentmihalyi, M., & Massimini, F. (1985). On the psychological selection of bio-cultural information. *New Ideas in Psychology, 3*, 115–138.

Csikszentmihalyi, M., Rathunde, K., & Whalen, S. (1993). *Talented teenagers: The roots of success and failure*. New York: Cambridge University Press.

Csikszentmihalyi, M., & Schneider, B. (2000). *Becoming adult: How teenagers prepare for the world of work*. New York: Basic Books.

Deci, E. L., & Ryan, R. M. (2000). The "what" and "why" of goal pursuits: Human needs and the self-determination of behavior. *Psychological Inquiry, 11*, 227–268.

Delespaul, P. A. E. G., Reis, H. T., & deVries, M. W. (2004). Ecological and motivational determinants of activation: Studying compared to sports and watching TV. *Social Indicators Research, 67*, 129–143.

Delle Fave, A. (1999). Individual development and bicultural identity: The Navajo way. In A. Delle Fave & F. Meli (Eds.), *Modernization and cultural identity* (pp. 49–68). Milano: Edizioni dell'Arco.

Delle Fave, A. (2006). Selezione psicologica ed esperienza ottimale: applicazioni ed implicazioni transculturali [psychological selection and optimal experience: cross-cultural applications and implications]. *Passaggi, 11*, 35–54.

Delle Fave, A. (2009). Optimal experience and meaning: Which relationship? *Psychological Topics, 18*, 285–302.

Delle Fave, A., & Bassi, M. (2000). The quality of experience in adolescents' daily life: Developmental perspectives. *Genetic, Social, and General Psychology Monographs, 126*, 347–367.

Delle Fave, A., & Bassi, M. (2003). Italian adolescents and leisure: The role of engagement and optimal experience. In S. Verma & R. Larson (Eds.), *Examining adolescent leisure time across cultures: Developmental opportunities and risks. New directions in child and adolescent development* (pp. 79–93). San Francisco: Jossey-Bass.

Delle Fave, A., Bassi, M., Cavallo, M., & Stokart, Z. (2007). The cross-cultural investigation of optimal experience in learning: Implications for individual development and educational policies. Paper presented at *ESCAP XIII International Conference*. Florence, 26–29 August.

Delle Fave, A., & Massimini, F. (2004). The cross-cultural investigation of optimal experience. *Ricerche di Psicologia, 27*, 79–102.

Delle Fave, A., & Massimini, F. (2005). The investigation of optimal experience and apathy: Developmental and psychosocial implications. *European Psychologist, 10*, 264–274.

DiBianca, R. (2000). *Teaching adolescents: Relationships between features of instruction and student engagement in high school mathematics and science classrooms*. Doctoral dissertation, University of Chicago.

Engeser, S., & Rheinberg, F. (2008). Flow, performance and moderators of challenge-skill balance. *Motivation and Emotion, 32*, 158–172.

Fu, F. L., Su, R. C., & Yu, S. C. (2009). EGameFLOW: A scale to measure learners' enjoyment of e-learning games. *Computers & Education, 52*, 101–112.

Gillham, J. E., Reivich, K., & Shatté, A. (2002). Positive youth development, prevention, and positive psychology: Commentary on "Positive youth development in the United States". *Prevention & Treatment, 5, Article 18.*

Hektner, J. M. (1996). *Exploring optimal personality development: A longitudinal study of adolescents*. Doctoral dissertation, University of Chicago.

Hektner, J. M. (2001). Family, school, and community predictors of adolescent growth conducive experiences: Global and specific approaches. *Applied Developmental Science, 5*, 172–183.

Hektner, J. M., Schmidt, J., & Csikszentmihalyi, M. (2007). *Experience sampling method. Measuring the quality of everyday life*. Thousand Oaks: Sage.

Inal, Y., & Cagiltay, K. (2007). Flow experiences of children in an interactive social game environment. *British Journal of Educational Technology, 38*, 455–464.

Lee, E. (2005). The relationship of motivation and flow experience to academic procrastination in university students. *Journal of Genetic Psychology, 166*, 5–14.

Lombardi, M. (2003). *La qualità dell'esperienza di un gruppo di adolescenti nepalesi: applicazione transculturale di experience sampling method* [The quality of experience in a group of Nepalese adolescents: A cross-cultural application of ESM]. Doctoral Dissertation at Università degli Studi di Milano, Italy.

Massimini, F., & Calegari, C. (1979). *Il contesto normative sociale: teoria e metodo di analisi* [the social normative context: theory and method of analysis]. Milano: Franco Angeli.

Massimini, F., & Delle Fave, A. (2000). Individual development in a bio-cultural perspective. *American Psychologist, 55*, 24–33.

Massimini, F., Inghilleri, P., & Delle Fave, A. (Eds.). (1996). *La selezione psicologica umana - teoria e metodo d'analisi* [human psychological selection – theory and method of analysis]. Milano: Coop. Libraria IULM.

Mesurado, B. (2008). Factorial validity and reliability of optimal experience (flow) survey in children and teenagers. *Revista Iberoamericana de Diagnóstico y Evaluación Psicológica, 25*, 159–178.

Mesurado, B. (2009). Actividad estructurada vs. Actividad desestructurada, realizadas en solitario vs. En compañia de otros y la experiencia óptima [structured activities vs. Unstructured activities, performed alone vs. With others and optimal experience]. *Anales de psicología, 25*, 308–315.

Moneta, G. B. (2004). The flow model of intrinsic motivation in Chinese: Cultural and personal moderators. *Journal of Happiness Studies, 5*, 181–217.

Nakamura, J., & Csikszentmihalyi, M. (2009). Flow theory and research. In S. J. Lopez & C. R. Snyder (Eds.), *Handbook of positive psychology* (pp. 195–206). New York: Oxford University Press.

Pearce, J. M., Ainley, M., & Howard, S. (2005). The ebb and flow of online learning. *Computers in Human Behavior, 21*, 745–771.

Rathunde, K. (1997). Parent-adolescent interaction and optimal experience. *Journal of Youth and Adolescence, 26*, 669–689.

Rathunde, K. (2001). Family context and the development of undivided interest: A longitudinal study of family support and challenge and adolescents' quality of experience. *Applied Developmental Science, 5*, 158–171.

Rogatko, T. P. (2009). The influence of flow on positive affect in college students. *Journal of Happiness Studies, 10*, 133–148.

Sanchez-Franco, M. J. (2010). WebCT – the quasimoderating effect of perceived affective quality on an extending technology acceptance model. *Computers & Education, 54*, 37–46.

Schmidt, J. (2003). Correlates of reduced misconduct among adolescents facing adversity. *Journal of Youth and Adolescence, 32*, 439–452.

Schmidt, J., Shernoff, D., & Csikszentmihalyi, M. (2007). Individual and situational factors related to the experience of flow in adolescence: A multilevel approach. In A. D. Ong & M. van Dulmen (Eds.), *The handbook of methods in positive psychology* (pp. 542–558). Oxford: Oxford University Press.

Schweinle, A., Meyer, D. K., & Turner, J. C. (2006). Striking the right balance: Students' motivation and affect in elementary mathematics. *Journal of Educational Research, 99*, 271–293.

Sedig, K. (2007). Toward operationalization of 'flow' in mathematics learnware. *Computers in Human Behavior, 23*, 2064–2092.

Shernoff, D., & Csikszentmihalyi, M. (2009). Flow in schools. Cultivating engaged learners and optimal learning environments. In R. Gilman, E. Huebner, & M. Furlong (Eds.), *Handbook of positive psychology in schools* (pp. 131–145). New York: Taylor & Francis.

Shernoff, D., Csikszentmihalyi, M., Schneider, B., & Shernoff, E. (2003). Student engagement in high school classrooms from the perspective of flow theory. *School Psychology Quarterly, 18*, 158–176.

Shernoff, D., & Hoogstra, L. (2001). Continuing motivation beyond the high school classroom. *New Directions for Child and Adolescent Development, 93*, 73–87.

Shernoff, D., Kanuth, S., & Makris, E. (2000). The quality of classroom experiences. In M. Csikszentmihalyi & B. Schneider (Eds.), *Becoming adult: How teenagers prepare fro the world of work* (pp. 141–164). New York: Basic Books.

Shernoff, D., & Schmidt, J. (2008). Further evidence of an engagement-achievement paradox among U.S. high school students. *Journal of Youth and Adolescence, 37*, 564–580.

Shernoff, D., & Vandell, D. L. (2007). Engagement in after-school program activities: Quality of experience from the perspective of participants. *Journal of Youth and Adolescence, 36*, 891–903.

Steca, P., Bassi, M., Caprara, G. V., & Delle Fave, A. (2010). Parents' self-efficacy beliefs and their children's psychosocial adaptation during adolescence. *Journal of Youth and Adolescence*, published online 4 March 2010.

Steele, J. P., & Fullagar, C. J. (2009). Facilitators and outcome of student engagement in a college setting. *Journal of Psychology, 143*, 5–27.

Triandis, H. C. (1995). *Individualism and collectivism.* Boulder, CO: Westview.

Vansteenkiste, M., Lens, W., & Deci, E. (2006). Intrinsic versus extrinsic goal contents in self-determination theory: Another look at the quality of academic motivation. *Educational Psychologist, 41*, 9–31.

Wong, M. M., & Csikszentmihalyi, M. (1991). Motivation and academic achievement: The effects of personality traits and the quality of experience. *Journal of Personality, 59*, 539–574.

World Bank (2010). Education trends and comparisons. Resource documents. http://web.worldbank.org/WBSITE/EXTERNAL/TOPICS/EXTEDUCATION/EXTDATASTATISTICS/EXTEDSTATS/0,contentMDK:21605891~menuPK:3409559~pagePK:64168445~piPK:64168309~theSitePK:3232764,00.html. Accessed 23 April 2010.

World Health Organization (2006). Country health system fact sheet 2006. Chad. Resource document. http://www.who.int/countries/tcd/en/. Accessed 23 April 2010.

Chapter 12
Optimal Experience and Religious Practice

12.1 Religiousness and Spirituality: Looking for Definitions

Only very few studies have been published till now on the role of religious practice in promoting flow and in orienting psychological selection (Coppa & Delle Fave, 2007, 2009; Delle Fave & Bassi, 2004; Zaccagnini, Delle Fave, & Sanabria, 2010). Throughout the years our research group gathered information on this topic among participants following different religious traditions. This chapter is therefore an opportunity to provide new insight on this complex issue. In order to contextualize our findings, however, a brief though necessarily limited overview of the theoretical and empirical advancements on this topic is required.

Scholars interested in studying the dimensions of sacredness and transcendence have to face numerous challenges, both at the theoretical and methodological levels. First of all, ambiguity often arises in the use of two apparently overlapping terms: religiousness and spirituality. The definition of these two constructs is still controversial.

Spirituality was variously described as a subjective experience of sacredness and transcendence (Vaughan, 1991), the search for existential meaning (Doyle, 1992), a contact with the divine within the self (Fahlberg & Fahlberg, 1991), and as a broader conceptual system which also includes the feeling of connectedness and integration—with a transcendent power, with oneself, with nature, with one's community—and the process of meaning-making (Bellingham, Cohen, Jones, & Spaniol, 1989; King, Speck, & Thomas, 1995).

The term religiousness refers instead to the participation in a belief system, which comprises specific and institutionalized values, norms, and rituals aiming at the search for and connection with the divine (King, Speck, & Thoma, 2001; O'Collins & Farrugia, 1991). Religion represents a complex set of behavioral rules that can be actualized within the daily context, thus providing individuals with short- and long-term opportunities for action and goal setting (Emmons, 2005, 2006). It offers individuals an explanatory perspective of the environment and of their own life, thus supporting the process of meaning making (Park, 2005). It provides an answer to the human need for giving a sense and a meaning to daily events and circumstances, allowing individuals to transcend their own limited self toward a wider

A. Delle Fave et al., *Psychological Selection and Optimal Experience Across Cultures*, Cross-Cultural Advancements in Positive Psychology 2,
DOI 10.1007/978-90-481-9876-4_12, © Springer Science+Business Media B.V. 2011

vision of reality (Sperry & Shafranske, 2005). This process is influenced both by the cultural and religious context, and by personal predispositions, previous experiences and their appraisal, hierarchy of priorities and values that individuals ceaselessly build and shape throughout their lives.

Allport's seminal works distinguished between intrinsic and extrinsic religiosity (Allport & Ross, 1967) based on the essential and deep identification with a belief system, or on its instrumental use in situations of distress or as an opportunity for socialization. More recently Zinnbauer and Pargament (2005) highlighted that in western cultures the rise in popularity of the concept of spirituality, together with the decline of traditional religious practices and institutions, produced a theoretical tendency to juxtapose the two constructs in positive versus negative terms. Spirituality is currently perceived as dynamic, functional to the search for existential meanings, rooted in the subjective experience of transcendence and therefore more authentic and personalized; religion is described as a static and institutionalized system of prescriptions, dogmas, and formalisms that constrains the individual into well-defined pathways. However, empirical studies showed that the majority of people who define themselves religious also report being spiritual, even though an increasing number of respondents refer to be spiritual, but not religious (Shahabi et al., 2002).

Another challenge for researchers interested in religion and spirituality is that most studies on this topic have been conducted among western participants, thus focusing on the Judaic–Christian tradition with its specific implications for daily behavior and relationship with the divine. This is true even of the most recent extensive contributions in this domain (Paloutzian & Park, 2005; Sperry & Shafranske, 2005). A broader cross-cultural perspective is needed to understand the psychological and psychosocial roles of religiousness and spirituality (Tarakeshwar, Stanton, & Pargament, 2003).

The first systematic step toward this aim has been made within research on quality of life (QOL). Religion and spirituality were recently investigated as components of this multifaceted construct, defined by WHO as the individuals' perception of their position and role in their own life, culture, and value system, taking into account their personal expectations and goals (WHOQOL Group, 1994, 1995). The WHOQOL Group identified six domains as core components of the general concept of quality of life: physical health, psychological dimensions, independence, social relations, environment, as well as spirituality, religion, and personal beliefs (WHOQOL Group, 2006). The WHOQOL-100 scale was developed to evaluate perceived QOL in these six domains. Data gathered in 18 different countries showed that religion and spirituality play an independent role in influencing the perception of quality of life across cultures and traditions (WHOQOL SRPB Group, 2005).

12.1.1 Religion and Well-Being: Empirical Evidence

The importance of evaluating religiousness and spirituality among indicators of quality of life is confirmed by the abundant literature on the relationship between well-being and the cultivation of spirituality and religion. In particular, several studies emphasized the benefits of religiousness on both mental and physical health (Myers, 2000). In a broad review of the literature, Koenig and his colleagues (2001) showed that 79% of the studies conducted on this topic highlighted a significant and positive relationship between religiousness and well-being. The stability of this relationship was systematically confirmed by longitudinal studies.

In the domain of physical health, epidemiological analyses revealed a positive correlation between religious practice and low incidence of cardiovascular diseases, cancer, and mortality in general (Comstock & Partridge, 1972; Larson et al., 1989; McCullough et al., 1999). Various mechanisms can underlie this phenomenon (Mytko & Knight, 1999). First, most religious systems prescribe healthy lifestyles and food habits. Second, prayer and meditation foster psychophysical relaxation. Third, practicing religion promotes social support through more stable family ties and the participation to collective rituals and community activities. Finally, religiousness fosters the development of components of psychological well-being, such as the perception of meaning, optimism, hope, and a more active acceptance of negative events and chronic or fatal diseases (Bickel et al., 1998; Brady, Peterman, Fitchett, Mo, & Cella, 1999; Jenkins & Pargament, 1995; Park & Folkman, 1997; Spiegel & Fawzy, 2002).

This multifaceted role of religiousness in promoting well-being under stressful circumstances was repeatedly confirmed in both cross-sectional and longitudinal studies. Feher and Maly (1999) showed that women with breast cancer identified in faith and spirituality a major source of emotional support, social support, and meaning. Similar results were found by McClain and colleagues (2003) among patients in the terminal phase of a disease. Religiousness proved to be helpful also in dealing with bereavement. Walsh and colleagues (2002) followed, with a longitudinal assessment, people who had lost a family member. After 14 months, they found a positive correlation between faith and religiousness—on the one hand—and resolution of depressive symptoms related to bereavement—on the other hand.

However, few studies are currently available on the influence of religiousness on well-being in the context of ordinary daily life, and among participants who are not facing problematic situations. Even less information is available on the quality of experience people usually associate with religious practice. In the following pages we will offer some preliminary findings on these topics.

12.2 Religious Practice and Optimal Experience Across Cultures

In the next paragraphs we will investigate religious practice as it emerged through the administration of flow questionnaire and life theme questionnaire to participants coming from different cultures. We will first offer a general overview of this topic through findings derived from the cross-cultural sample described in detail in Chapter 7. We will then focus on findings obtained in specific cultures within this sample.

As concerns analyses, we will investigate the association of religious practice with flow, and its experiential features; the average quality of experience reported during ordinary religious practice (regardless of its association with flow); the meaning and role participants attributed to religion in their answers to the open-ended question "what does religious practice means for you?" Finally, we will investigate the impact of religion on participants' life influences, present challenges and future goals. However, for sake of synthesis not all these aspects will be discussed in detail for each group of participants: only results providing new or meaningful evidence will be selected for analysis and discussion.

12.2.1 Religious Practice and Flow: An Infrequent Association

The cross-cultural sample from which we will draw general results was described in detail in Chapter 7. It comprised women and men widely varying in their socio-economic and occupational status. The majority of participants reported optimal experience in their lives, but only 41 (5.6%) associated it with religious practice. An even lower number of participants (21, 2.9%) selected religious practice as opportunity for pervasive flow experiences.

Despite these very low percentages, significant cross-cultural differences were detected. We first compared the percentage of participants who did versus did not report religious practice as flow activity between western and non-western cultures (Table 12.1). A Chi-square test highlighted a significant difference ($\chi^2 = 15.3$, $p<0.0001$). The result was not surprising, since among the 41 participants who reported flow in religious practice, 29 (70.7%) belonged to non-western cultures. Similar results were obtained from the comparison of participants who did or did not select religious practice between the two groups ($\chi^2 = 8.1$, $p<0.01$). Also in this case, non-western participants accounted for 71.4% of those who associated religion with the most pervasive flow experience.

Results derived from the western sample are not surprising. As reported in the introductory section of this chapter, religious practice within the Christian tradition rapidly declined during the past three decades, leaving room to agnosticism or to other forms of spirituality (often related to Asian traditions, mainly to Buddhism). This is also true of Italy, homeland of the western participants in this sample. Recent statistics showed that, while 97.3% of the Italians report to be Catholic, only 45%

Table 12.1 Percentage of participants associating religious practice with flow across cultures

	Optimal activities		Selected optimal activities	
Cultures	Religion *N* (%)	Other *N* (%)	Religion *N* (%)	Other *N* (%)
Non-western	29 (9.7)	269 (90.3)	15 (5.0)	283 (95.0)
Western	12 (2.4)	426 (97.6)	6 (1.2)	492 (98.9)
Total *N* participants	736		736	

Note: *N* = Number of participants.

refer to attend church celebrations (http://www.nationmaster.com/country 2010). A similar trend is currently observed in most traditionally Catholic countries in Europe, with the exception of Ireland (in which church attendance hits 84%).

On the contrary, the non-western sample we examined comprises participants living in countries in which religious practice is still an integral part of the daily life. In India and Thailand people of any age and educational background regularly visit temples and often keep little altars in their own house for daily prayers. In Indonesia, Iran, and West Africa, where Islam is the predominant religion, the daily practice of prayer is widely spread across social classes.

12.2.2 Religion in Asian Cultures: Indonesia, India, and Thailand

We will now try to better disentangle the general information provided above, by looking closely to the results obtained from some specific groups comprised in the cross-cultural sample. We will start with findings gathered in three Asian countries greatly differing in their cultural and religious traditions: Indonesia, India, and Thailand.

The vast majority of the Indonesian population is presently Muslim. However, most of the world religions are represented in the country, some of them being concentrated in specific areas, such as Hinduism in Bali, Christianity in the islands of Flores and East Timor, animistic and tribal systems in Kalimantan. Although Indonesia is a secular state, throughout its history religion played an influential role at the political and economical levels (Williams, 1991). The 1945 Constitution acknowledged a natural tendency of the people to be deeply religious, and it endorsed the five philosophical principles (Pancasila) traditionally characterizing Indonesian society: the belief in one supreme God; a just and civil humanity; the unity of the country; democracy guided by wisdom; and social justice. The official assumption of people's natural tendency to religiousness leads to the obligation to report one's own religion in identity documents.

Within this peculiar context, we administered FQ and LT to 63 adult participants living in Java, comprised in the cross-cultural sample examined in Chapter 7. The vast majority of them (87.3%) were Muslims, the others being Christians and followers of Javanese cults. All participants except one reported flow in their lives. Religious practice accounted for 11 answers (10.9% of the total); seven participants selected it as opportunity for pervasive optimal experiences.

The psychological features of optimal experience were then compared through the Wilcoxon procedure between the 7 participants who selected religious practice, and the 55 participants who selected other domains. No significant group differences were detected. However, some differences were found in the average experience reported by the two groups during daily religious practice (evaluated through the same scaled items used for the assessment of flow). Table 12.2 illustrates these findings, distinguishing between participants who quoted religion as a flow activity (ROE) and participants who did not (RNOE). The ROE group reported

Table 12.2 The average quality of experience during religious practice across cultures

	Indonesia (ROE = 11, RNOE = 52)		India (ROE = 4, RNOE = 48)		Navajo (DC = 79, HS = 58)	
Variables	ROE *M* (*sd*)	RNOE *M* (*sd*)	ROE *M* (*sd*)	RNOE *M* (*sd*)	DC *M* (*sd*)	HS *M* (*sd*)
Involvement	7.4 (0.9)	6.0 (2.3)	7.5 (1.0)	2.6 (2.4)	2.7 (2.7)	1.9 (2.8)
Clear feedback	7.2 (1.0)	5.3 (2.5)	7.5 (1.0)	3.0 (2.4)	3.3 (2.6)	2.4 (2.5)
Intrinsic motivation	8.0 (0)	6.6 (2.4)	8.0 (0)	3.6 (3.1)	3.1 (2.8)	2.5 (2.6)
Excitement	7.8 (0.4)	6.6 (2.2)	8.0 (0)	5.2 (3.2)	4.8 (2.8)	4.3 (3.2)
Ease of concentration	7.6 (0.8)	6.1 (2.1)	6.5 (1.9)	4.6 (3.3)	4.3 (2.8)	3.4 (3.1)
Unselfconsciousness	–	–	7.0 (1.2)	5.2 (2.6)	4.2 (2.6)	3.4 (2.8)
Enjoyment	6.5 (1.5)	4.8 (2.3)	6.5 (1.9)	2.9 (2.6)	3.9 (2.5)	2.2 (2.7)
Concentration	7.5 (0.9)	6.2 (2.0)	7.0 (1.2)	3.9 (2.9)	4.6 (2.7)	3.6 (2.9)
Relaxation	6.9 (2.1)	6.9 (1.8)	6.0 (2.8)	6.3 (2.5)	3.3 (2.6)	2.5 (2.9)
Clear goals	6.9 (1.9)	5.2 (2.3)	7.5 (1.0)	4.4 (2.9)	2.7 (2.7)	2.2 (2.4)
Control of situation	6.9 (1.9)	5.6 (2.4)	7.5 (1.0)	3.6 (2.9)	3.6 (2.7)	2.3 (2.2)
Challenges	5.5 (2.4)	4.4 (2.5)	3.1 (3.6)	2.2 (2.4)	3.3 (2.8)	2.9 (2.5)
Skills	5.9 (1.7)	4.8 (1.9)	4.4 (3.8)	2.4 (2.4)	2.9 (2.7)	2.2 (2.6)

Note: ROE = Number of participants quoting religious practice as flow activity; RNOE = Number of participants not quoting religious practice as flow activity; DC = Diné College students; HS = High-school students.

significantly higher values of positive feedback from the activity ($Z = 2.4$, $p < 0.01$), intrinsic motivation ($Z = 2.2$, $p < 0.05$), ease of concentration ($Z = 2.6$, $p < 0.01$), enjoyment ($Z = 2.2$, $p < 0.05$), concentration ($Z = 2.1$, $p < 0.05$), and clear goals ($Z = 2.5$, $p < 0.05$). When experiencing flow during prayer, participants reported "to feel being in another world, to perceive a deep physical peace and concentration (35 year-old woman)."

As concerns the role attributed to religion in their lives, most participants referred to the importance of observing the five daily prayers prescribed by Islam. Some participants emphasized the thanksgiving role of prayer. A 40-year-old woman, teacher in a high school, answered, "I thank God every day for the joy He gives me through my family and through the satisfactions I get at school." Others stressed their expectations from God, like a 38-year-old woman who wrote, "I ask God to get peace into my heart and money." Eight participants reported religion as a positive life influence, and only one referred to it as a present challenge.

Similar results were found among Indian participants, though in a very different cultural and religious context. The sample (described in detail in Chapter 13) included 52 adults, 29 living in India and 23 migrated to Europe. Participants shared similar education level and socio-economic status: The majority got a University degree, and they worked as teachers, professionals, or managers. All but two had been raised within the Hindu tradition, and all reported to observe rituals and various form of religious practice in their life. Through FQ, they provided information on the role of religious practice as an opportunity for optimal experience, and on the associated quality of experience. Since migration did not exert any significant influence on participants' answer pattern concerning these issues, we will discuss results obtained from the analysis of the whole sample.

Out of the 243 answers provided by the participants when asked to list flow activities, only 6 referred to religious practice, with answers related to individual prayer and meditation. Moreover, only one participant, among the four who indicated religious practice as flow activity, selected it in relation to the most pervasive optimal experiences.

Participants were then asked to rate on 0–8 scales the quality of experience associated with habitual religious practice. As shown in Table 12.2, this allowed for a comparison between participants who reported flow during religious practice, and participants who did not. The four participants who associated religious practice with optimal experience (ROE in the Table) scored significantly higher than the other group (RNOE) for most variables: involvement (Wilcoxon, $Z = 2.9$, $p < 0.01$), clear feedback ($Z = 2.7$, $p < 0.01$), intrinsic motivation ($Z = 2.6$, $p < 0.05$), enjoyment ($Z = 2.4$, $p < 0.05$), concentration ($Z = 2.0$, $p < 0.05$), clear goals ($Z = 2.0$, $p < 0.05$), and control of the situation ($Z = 2.4$, $p < 0.05$).

The role of religion as a positive life influence was acknowledged by six participants. However, when asked about the meaning of religious practice for them, many participants stressed both its role as a source of psychological balance and its relation with personal and cultural identity. The following quotations exemplify the answers' typologies provided by the participants, "To me my religion is my culture. My thoughts, my expressions, my actions are formed and guided by my religion and its philosophy. It follows me as a shadow and is my learning post. To spend time in religious activities is a sort of self assessment and evaluation" (44-year-old man). "To me religious practice means prayers, reading religious books, visiting temples once in a week at least, listening to discourses by religious scholars once in a while, and participating in singing of Bhajans" (52-year-old woman); "It means doing pooja and meditation" (37-year-old man); "Through religious practice I get peace, self-confidence, inner strength, and derive energy" (43-year-old woman). In order to better understand these answers, we have to take into account the peculiarity of Hinduism, which is not based on strictly codified rituals or behavioral rules and rather emphasizes the importance of mind balance, and of the search for a personal pathway toward bliss and unity with the divine (Rao, Paranjpe, & Dalal, 2008).

Finally, we will briefly refer to information on flow and religious practice provided by 24 students and teachers at the University of Bangkok. All participants defined themselves as Buddhist, and 22 of them reported flow in their lives, associating it with various activities, for a total of 49 answers. Seven of these answers (14.3%) referred to prayer, meditation, and temple attendance. Six participants (22.7%) selected religious practice as occasion for pervasive optimal experiences. When asked to describe the psychological features of the experience associated with habitual religious practice on 0–8 scales, compared with participants who did not quote religion among flow activities, they reported higher values of involvement ($M = 5.3$ vs. $M = 2.8$, $Z = 2.9$, $p < 0.05$), clear feedback ($M = 4.8$ vs. $M = 2.6$, $Z=2.2$, $p < 0.05$), and skills ($M = 6.7$ vs. $M = 2.2$, $Z = 3.4$, $p < 0.01$). As for the meaning of religious practice, most participants highlighted the attainment of "inner peace and calmness, according to the aim of Dharma" (42-year-old woman). Others stressed the importance of serving the community, which is a peculiar feature of Buddhism, related to the opportunity for "making merit" in order to reach liberation from the rebirth cycle. A 28-year-old woman described this aspect of religion as follows: "Going to the temple, listening to the monk who speaks about the good way of life, making merit and doing charities."

12.2.3 Religious Ceremonies and Navajo Identity

In a post-industrial context, the survival of traditional beliefs and values strongly depends upon the awareness and active commitment of each individual in preserving them. This is especially true of low-institutionalized traditions, such as the religious systems of most Native American tribes living in the South West of the United States.

We gathered some information about this topic among Navajo adolescents and young people, through the administration of flow questionnaire (more details on these participants can be found in Chapters 7 and 13). Our sample included 58 adolescents attending Ganado high school, a public western-style institution, and 79 students and teachers of the Diné College, and therefore exposed to programs aimed at promoting the active participation in the preservation and transmission of Navajo traditions and values.

The essence of the Navajo religion is the relationship between the people and their land, which is considered sacred. The original Navajo myths and ceremonies belonged to the Athapaskan hunter tradition, centered on the sacredness of nature and of animals such as the buffalo, the main survival resource for the tribe.

According to Navajo belief system, each living being is provided with its own spirit, which gives it life and purpose. The universe is an orderly and harmonious system, in which everything is interrelated and interdependent. The purpose of Navajo existence is to maintain balance between the individual and the universe and to live in harmony with nature. In order to achieve this goal, the Navajos developed rituals connected to the Mother Earth (celebrated as Changing Woman), to sacred geographical sites, and to specific plants, particularly corn (Luckert, 1975; Reichard, 1950). Religious artifacts and customs comprise sand paintings, masks, offerings of turquoise, white and red shell, jet. The basic pattern of the Navajo rituals consists of 8 days of purification and offerings, and a ninth night of public celebration to partake the spirit blessing (Reichards 1950; Underhill, 1948). Ceremonies have often a healing purpose (Topper & Begaye, 1978). They are considered powerful means to bring dangerous powers under control and to restore balance in individuals suffering from physical or mental disorders. Rituals and ceremonies also represent very important opportunities for family and clan meetings, and for keeping the traditions and identity of the Diné people alive.

The data provided by Navajo participants who filled out the flow questionnaire offer some insight as concerns the association of optimal experience with religious practice, prominently consisting in ceremony attendance. Not surprisingly, this association was reported only by seven participants, all belonging to the Diné College group: As previously described, enrollment in this college promotes awareness of the individual's Navajo identity, and a strong sense of belonging to the Navajo culture and to its practices, which include ceremonies as a major component. Among these participants, one selected attending ceremonies in association with the most pervasive optimal experiences.

We assessed the quality of experience participants reported during ceremony attendance through the same 0–8-scaled items used to evaluate flow. As shown in Table 12.2, most items scored around 4 for Diné College participants, and around 2 for students, thus indicating that participation in ceremonies did not provide a particularly positive and complex experience. However, college participants reported significantly higher scores than Ganado adolescents in some of the variables. They perceived higher enjoyment ($Z = 3.2$, $p < 0.01$), control ($Z = 2.6$, $p < 0.01$), and relaxation ($Z = 2.1$, $p < 0.05$), as well as clearer feedback from the activity ($Z = 1.9$, $p < 0.06$).

The meaning these participants attributed to ceremonies was consistent with the bicultural approach promoted at the Diné College. A 22-year-old man reported, "In my point of view, our traditional ceremonies are very value to us. We don't go there just for fun. It's very sacred to us that we don't abuse it. I only attend for my belief, also give lots of respect for my culture as well for people." A 21-year-old woman described participation in Navajo Ceremonies as follows: "It makes me feel good and think clearly. I can learn more about it and I should not forget about it for the younger generations."

12.2.4 Migration from Africa and Religious Practice

Moving to a different cultural context in search for better life conditions implies sometimes radical changes in lifestyle and behavior that are discussed in Chapter 13. It can also require adjustments in religious practice, especially when the host country differs from homeland in belief system and related behavioral norms. To this purpose, we will discuss here findings on the religious experience of a group of 38 African participants immigrated in Italy (related findings are also reported in Chapter 13), who completed FQ and LT. Twelve of them came from Somalia, 13 from North Africa, and 13 from West Africa. They were prominently Muslim (92.1%), but their cultural background differed. Since decades Somalia is facing serious political and economical instability; Northern African countries are increasingly exposed to western influence and they are undergoing fast modernization; in many West African countries the traditional village lifestyle and ancient tribal cultures are still very lively.

None of the participants reported religious practice as an opportunity for optimal experience. Nevertheless, 75% of the Somalis and 80% of the West Africans referred commitment to regular prayer and attendance to rituals and ceremonies. On the contrary, only 30.8% of the Northern Africans reported to observe prayers and rituals, though not regularly, while another 53.8% referred having stopped practicing religion after childhood. Among the practicing participants, 28.6% described some change in their religious habits, primarily related to the difficulty to go to the Mosque; however, only two participants referred the interruption of religious practice as a consequence of migration.

When asked to describe the meaning they attributed to religion, participants highlighted the daily commitment to prayer required by Islam, as well as the role of religion in their lives. A Western African 25-year-old man reported, "Religion is very important for me. I pray five times a day. My only tie with Allah is prayer. If I do not pray this tie get broken. To pray is a duty, my soul forces me to pray." For a Somali 27-year-old woman to pray meant "to ask God for help. I pray five times a day. I do not feel forced to pray. I pray because this is my religion and I know I have to do it. I feel quiet when I pray. While I pray I feel the need for God." North Africans showed instead a generally low involvement in religious practice. A 29-year-old man traced his disengagement back during adolescence, "When I was a child I went to the Mosque with my father. When I grew up I started meeting girls, drinking alcohol, and thus I could not go to the Mosque anymore". Another 26-year-old man stressed the joys and sorrows of religious practice, "I do not practice religion. Religion makes you feel good, it gives you quietness. Our religion is beautiful, but it is difficult to follow it. When I practiced religion, I noticed that I was doing wrong things, and so I quitted."

Participants were also invited to describe through 0–8 scaled items the average quality of experience associated with religious practice before and after their migration in Italy. Results are reported in Table 12.3. No difference was detected within

Table 12.3 The average quality of experience reported by African immigrants during religious practice at home and in the host country

	Somalia		North Africa		West Africa	
Variables	Home ($N = 10$) *M* (*sd*)	Italy ($N = 11$) *M* (*sd*)	Home ($N = 6$) *M* (*sd*)	Italy ($N = 4$) *M* (*sd*)	Home ($N = 10$) *M* (*sd*)	Italy ($N = 11$) *M* (*sd*)
Involvement	4.5 (1.5)	4.8 (1.8)	4.7 (2.0)	3.8 (1.7)	6.8 (1.3)	6.7 (1.3)
Clear feedback	4.7 (1.2)	4.8 (1.2)	3.7 (1.5)	2.8 (1.0)	6.8 (1.5)	6.7 (1.4)
Intrinsic motivation	4.4 (1.5)	4.2 (1.4)	3.7 (2.7)	3.3 (2.8)	4.7 (3.7)	4.7 (3.5)
Excitement	5.7 (1.5)	5.5 (1.2)	5.5 (0.8)	5.0 (1.4)	6.8 (2.5)	6.8 (2.4)
Ease of concentration	4.9 (1.4)	4.6 (0.9)	5.3 (1.6)	5.3 (1.0)	5.9 (2.2)	5.9 (2.1)
Enjoyment	4.9 (2.3)	4.5 (2.0)	4.3 (1.0)	4.5 (1.3)	5.0 (2.0)	4.6 (1.8)
Concentration	4.9 (1.9)	4.5 (1.4)	5.3 (1.5)	4.8 (1.0)	6.0 (1.8)	6.0 (1.7)
Relaxation	6.0 (1.6)	5.9 (1.4)	5.8 (1.3)	5.3 (1.0)	7.3 (0.9)	7.2 (1.0)
Clear goals	5.0 (1.3)	4.8 (0.9)	5.3 (1.8)	5.0 (1.4)	6.8 (1.3)	6.6 (1.4)
Control of situation	4.3 (2.2)	3.9 (1.6)	5.0 (2.9)	4.5 (1.7)	6.2 (1.8)	6.1 (1.8)
Challenges	4.4 (2.1)	4.2 (1.7)	4.6 (1.2)	4.2 (1.4)	6.2 (1.8)	6.2 (1.2)
Skills	4.9 (1.7)	4.9 (1.7)	4.6 (1.3)	4.5 (1.8)	6.6 (0.9)	6.6 (0.9)

Note: N= Number of participants.

each group before and after migration; this result shows that the experiential features of religious practice were preserved, in spite of contextual changes. Significant differences in the religious experience across groups were detected instead through a nonparametric ANOVA. As concerns religious practice in the homeland, groups significantly differed in involvement ($F = 6.4$, $p < 0.01$), clear feedback ($F = 11.2$, $p < 0.001$), relaxation ($F = 3.4$, $p < 0.05$), and skills ($F = 4.0$, $p < 0.05$). After migration to Italy, significant differences emerged for involvement ($F = 6.9$, $p < 0.01$), clear feedback ($Z = 16.0$, $p < 0.001$), relaxation ($Z = 5.4$, $p < 0.05$), clear goals ($F = 7.1$, $p < 0.01$), control of the situation ($F = 4.6$, $p < 0.05$), challenges ($F = 5.2$, $p < 0.05$), and skills ($F = 4.8$, $p < 0.05$).

These group differences can be related to the different approach toward religion highlighted above. More specifically, if we look closer at the findings reported in Table 12.3, both at home and in the host country Western Africans associated religious practice with a substantially positive experience, characterized by high values of relaxation, involvement, excitement, clear feedback, and clear goals, whereas practicing participants in the other two groups reported similar and lower values for all the variables. These findings are consistent with the other information on religious practice provided by the three groups. All the practicing immigrants preserved their religious habits and the associated experience in the new context. Prayer thus emerged as an integral part of daily life, and its practice in the host country can be considered a powerful means to maintain and even reinforce one's own cultural identity in the face of the radical life changes produced by migration.

12.3 Religion and Faith as the Core of Psychological Selection

The results reported above suggest that in general religious practice represents only a marginal opportunity for optimal experience. However, what about people who have intentionally chosen to cultivate religion as a prominent activity of their daily life, and invest on it their energies and resources? How do they experience religious practice? What is its place in the process of psychological selection? To address this issue, we administered flow questionnaire and life theme questionnaire to 96 participants (54 women and 42 men) belonging to different Catholic religious orders and congregations, and to 70 lay people belonging to Catholic associations (Coppa & Delle Fave, 2007, 2009). Among consecrated people, the women's group comprised 27 nuns and 27 novices aged 18–59, belonging to different congregations and coming from different countries (Italy, Burundi, India). The men (aged 20–59, all Italian) comprised 8 seminarists, 10 diocesan priests, 14 Dominicans, and 10 Jesuits. The lay people (52 women and 18 men) were prominently young (65% below 30), unmarried (85,7%), and college students (55,7%).

As shown in Table 12.4, all participants except four consecrated people reported optimal experiences in their daily life. Both groups prominently associated optimal experience with religious practice, followed by hobby and sport. Religious practice mainly comprised prayer and contemplation (63% of the answers in this category), and to a lower extent preaching, teaching religion and catechism, visiting

Table 12.4 Percentage category distribution of optimal activities among members of religious orders and lay practicing Catholics

	Optimal activities		Selected optimal activities	
Categories	Religious ($N = 92$)	Lay ($N = 70$)	Religious ($N = 92$)	Lay ($N = 70$)
Work	9.8	9.5	2.2	2.9
Study	12.7	12.5	12.0	14.3
Volunteering	2.2	2.4	1.1	1.4
Social relations	14.2	7.1	5.4	7.1
Hobby, sport	15.8	19.9	10.9	10.0
Media	8.2	18.2	7.6	20.0
Family		2.0		1.4
Thoughts, introspection	1.6	7.8	1.1	10.0
Religious practice	35.4	20.6	59.8	32.9
N answers	316	296	92	70

Note: N= Number of participants.

families, formation meetings, youth education. Structured leisure mostly included playing music, painting, writing, and practicing sports. Although religious practice ranked first in both groups, a difference was detected in the related participant distribution. While 78 of the consecrated people (81.2%) reported religious practice as flow activity, 41 lay people (58.6%) did. This distribution difference was significant ($\chi^2 = 10.3$, $p<0.01$). A similar distribution pattern was detected as concerns the activities selected in relation to the most pervasive optimal experiences (Table 12.4). A conspicuous number of participants (59.8% among the members of religious orders and 32.9% of the lay people) indicated religious practice, while the others prominently referred to hobby and sports, studying, and the use of media. A significant difference was nevertheless detected in this percentage distribution between the two groups ($\chi^2 = 9.7$, $p<0.01$). However, the impact of religious practice as an opportunity for optimal experience among lay people clearly emerged in comparison with the cross-cultural findings previously described, where religion as an optimal activity reached only marginal percentages both in the western and non-western samples, and was reported by a very low number of participants.

Table 12.5 shows the features of optimal experience reported by the whole sample (religious and lay people) in the selected optimal activities, rated on 0–8 scales. Given the peculiarity of religious practice in its core dimension of individual prayer and contemplation, we decided to explore similarities and differences in the features of optimal experience as described by participants who selected religious practice ($N = 78$), and participants who selected other domains ($N = 84$). From a general point of view, optimal experience showed recurrent psychological features in association with both religious and non-religious activities: Participants reported high values of involvement and intrinsic motivation, excitement, relaxation, the perception of high challenges and moderately high skills, enjoyment, clear feedback, and goals. However, a Wilcoxon nonparametric comparison highlighted significant

Table 12.5 Optimal experience in religious practice and in other flow activities among members of religious orders and lay practicing Catholics

	Religious practice ($N = 78$)		Other OA ($N = 84$)			
Variables	*M*	*sd*	*M*	*sd*	*Z*	$p<$
Involvement	6.8	1.2	6.6	1.3	0.4	n.s.
Clear feedback	6.7	1.4	6.8	1.5	−1.3	n.s.
Intrinsic motivation	7.6	1.1	7.0	1.6	2.9	.05
Excitement	7.6	0.8	7.5	1.0	0.002	n.s.
Focus of attention	5.7	2.4	5.6	2.2	0.002	n.s.
Unselfconsciousness	4.0	2.8	5.0	2.8	−2.1	.05
Enjoyment	6.7	1.6	6.7	1.7	0.05	n.s.
Concentration	5.4	2.1	5.8	2.0	−1.6	n.s.
Relaxation	7.0	1.5	6.4	2.1	1.5	n.s.
Clear goals	6.4	1.9	6.8	2.0	−2.0	.05
Control of situation	5.5	2.1	6.0	2.0	−1.5	n.s.
Challenges	7.3	1.0	6.6	1.9	2.0	.05
Skills	5.5	2.0	5.9	1.9	−1.2	n.s.

Note: N= Number of participants.

differences for some variables. More specifically, religious practice as the preferential domain of optimal experience was associated with significantly higher values of intrinsic motivation, perceived challenges, and self-consciousness, as well as significant lower scores of clear goals.

How can we interpret these differences? As concerns intrinsic motivation, the significantly higher values associated with religious practice can be related to faith, which represents an inner and exquisitely self-determined source of commitment. Several participants emphasized their free adherence to a personal relationship with God, through prayer and through serving others. The intrinsic motivating power of faith emerged, however, more evidently among members or religious orders ($M = 7.8$, $sd = 0.5$) than among lay people ($M = 7.0$, $sd = 1.6$; Wilcoxon $Z = 2.7$, $p < 0.01$). Another peculiar result was the perception of challenges significantly higher than in other optimal activities, and exceeding the perceived skills. This result can again be referred to the specificity of religious practice, in which the believer faces transcendence, perceiving the limitations of human abilities and rational understanding. As quoted by the respondents, "Religion is not a matter of abilities," "there is awareness of one's own extreme limits," "I recognize to be a little nothing, however filled by His greatness." However, consecrated participants perceived significantly higher challenges in religious practice ($M = 7.2$, $sd = 1.2$) than lay people ($M = 6.7$, $sd = 1.2$; Wilcoxon $Z = 3.84$, $p < 0.0001$). Compared with other optimal activities, religious practice was also associated with a significantly lower perception of goals. This finding is consistent with the surrender to God's will and gifts: Praying means "staying in front of God. I do not care about how much I will be able to pray or meditate;" "it does not depend on me, it is something that comes from outside (from God?)." Finally, optimal experience in religious practice was characterized by levels of self-consciousness significantly higher than in other activities. This result is apparently inconsistent with the others, since the absence of self-monitoring is one of the core features of flow. However, due to its structural features, the practice of prayer requires sustained attention and self-awareness. In most religious traditions (see also Chapter 6) self-monitoring and watchfulness are substantial prerequisites for proper prayer and access to transcendence, while distraction is the major and most usual interference deviating the mind on worldly worries and desires as reported in the most recent compendium of the Cathechism of the Catholic Church (AA.VV. 2005). A certain amount of concentration effort and self-consciousness are therefore necessary to keep the attention focused on God.

All the lay participants and 94 religious people completed the life theme questionnaire. As reported in Table 12.6, both groups quoted religion as the prominent positive influence in their life, followed by family. In the domain of religion, the answers referred to the positive impact of the religious education received during childhood in the family and community environment, through the attendance of parish recreation centers, and through the behavioral models transmitted by consecrated people and spiritual masters. At a strictly personal level, having discovered faith, spiritual readings, religious conversion, and vocation were also quoted as positive influences.

As concerns negative life influences, the two prominent domains quoted by the participants were family and social relations, followed by personal experience and work/study. In the family domain, the answers mostly referred to death or severe disease of parents and close relatives, and to the separation from the family because of study or health reasons. Problems and conflicts within the family were also quoted, though to a lesser extent. A major peculiarity emerged in comparison with all the samples previously examined with the life theme questionnaire: a relevant percentage of participants (18% of the religious and 14.2% of the lay people) did not provide any answer to this question. In addition, 10.2% of the descriptions of negative influences was accompanied by comments such as "overcoming difficulties may become an enrichment" and "negative influences can be opportunities for growth."

As Table 12.6 shows, religion was prominent among the present challenges perceived by religious participants, followed by personal growth and social issues; lay people—as expected—were more focused on the productive life domains and on personal growth issues (this group was mainly composed by young people). For both groups, answers related to religion mostly referred to integration of faith within daily life, coherence between behavior and religious ideals, adequately witnessing one's own faith, developing one's own relationship with God, serving God through serving the neighbor, strengthening one's own vocation and faith. In the domain of personal growth, answers were largely consistent with the prominent role of faith in the life of the participants. They mostly referred to overcoming egoism and selfishness, mobilizing personal resources in facing daily challenges, developing awareness and coherence, putting ideals into daily practice and behavior.

As concerns future goals, religious practice and society issues (which comprised community service and helping others) grouped 84% of the consecrated people's

Table 12.6 Percentage category distribution of the prominent life influences, present challenges, and future goals among members of religious orders and lay practicing Catholics

	Positive influences		Negative influences		Challenges		Goals	
Categories	Religious ($N = 94$)	Lay ($N = 70$)	Religious ($N = 77$)	Lay ($N = 60$)	Religious ($N = 93$)	Lay ($N = 68$)	Religious ($N = 93$)	Lay ($N = 70$)
Work/study	9.6	18.2	13.1	14.6	7.8	33.3	3.5	30.8
Society issues	2.3	5.1	4.9	3.7	9.6	4.4	8.5	9.7
Social relations	14.2	13.4	25.1	18.9	7.0	3.5	4.2	3.2
Hobby, sport	1.6	2.8	2.2	1.8	–	–	–	1.6
Media	1.4	3.0	0.5	1.8	0.9	–	–	–
Wealth	–	0.3	–	–	–	0.9	–	0.5
Family	29.1	26.5	32.2	34.8	–	14.9	–	33.5
Health	0.2	0.5	2.7	4.3	2.6	0.9	–	0.5
Personal growth	2.1	3.0	12.0	15.2	17.4	21.9	8.4	8.7
Religious practice	39.6	27.3	7.1	4.9	54.8	20.2	75.4	11.4
N answers	437	396	183	164	115	114	142	185

Note: N= Number of participants

answers, while lay participants reported productive and family life as their prominent future achievements. However, religion and social issues represented almost 20% of the latter group's perceived goals, an absolutely unique finding in the cross-cultural investigation of flow and psychological selection. For both groups, within the religious domain future goals were largely consistent with present challenges: witnessing the love of God, doing God's will, living with completeness one's own religious vocation, becoming consecrated (for seminarists and novices), ceaselessly looking at God, aiming at perfection and holiness.

If we look at the percentage of participants quoting religion as a relevant dimension of their long-term psychological selection, the peculiarity of the consecrated group clearly emerges. Though in both groups religion ranked first among the positive life influences, it was quoted by 86.5% of the religious participants compared with the 72.9% of the lay people ($\chi^2 = 4.8$, $p < 0.05$). This difference increased for major present challenges, with 60.4% of the consecrated people quoting religion compared with 20% of the lay participants ($\chi^2 = 26.9$, $p < 0.0001$). Religion as a future goal recruited 83.3% of the consecrated participants, but only the 27.1% of the lay ones ($\chi^2 = 53.1$, $p < 0.0001$). These findings are not surprising: For the former group, following one's own religious vocation entailed a pervasive commitment to the pursuit of spiritual achievements. More specifically, the answers to FQ and LT highlighted that the psychological selection of religious participants unfolded around three major topics: the cultivation of a personal relationship with God; a ceaseless monitoring of one's own psychological resources, limitations, and developmental pathway; commitment and service to neighbor and community. Faith represented a unifying perspective to interpret life events and to build one's own identity. This was further confirmed by the finding—rather unique in flow research—that 37.5% of the consecrated people (compared with the 8.6% of the lay ones, $\chi^2 = 17.9$, $p < 0.0001$) showed a global congruence in the psychological selection trend, quoting religious practice as a selected flow activity, a positive life influence, a present challenge, as well as a future goal.

12.4 Believers and Followers, Disciples and Explorers

The results reported in the previous pages suggest that for the majority of people across cultures religion represents an aspect—even a major one—of individuals' cultural identity, but not a relevant opportunity for optimal experience in daily life. When asked about their religion, most participants did not hesitate to identify it, and—especially in non-western cultures—they reported to regularly perform individual prayer. However, the associated experience had prominently average features at the cognitive, emotional, and motivational levels. Only few participants perceived the deep engagement, enjoyment, and absorption that characterize optimal experience during religious practice.

Nevertheless, the supporting role of religion in facing stressful situations, its importance in shaping the person's behavior and interpretation of reality, and its relevance in providing individual and collective meanings and values are widely acknowledged (Emmons & McCullough, 2004; Geyer & Baumeister, 2005; McCullough, Pargament, & Thoresen, 2000). Our findings were consistent with this perspective, emerging from participants' descriptions of the meaning they attributed to religious practice.

These apparently contradictory findings require a broader interpretative framework. Considering the complex pathways through which individual development unfolds, good life is not necessarily related to good feelings. As reported by scholars from different disciplines (Bruni & Porta, 2006; Peterson, Park, & Sweeney, 2008; Sen, 1992), people often practice activities and pursue goals that they perceive as valuable, but that do not necessarily provide positive experiences in the short term (Delle Fave & Massimini, 2003, 2005). This tendency can be related to the overarching dimension of meaning making (Emmons, 2005, 2006), through which humans dynamically organize their experience moment by moment, ceaselessly integrating events and information into their own life history and developmental trajectory (Kunnen & Bosma, 2000; Singer, 2004). Meanings primarily stem from culture, allowing individuals to transcend their own limited self toward a wider vision of reality. In their turn, individuals actively transform collective-cultural meanings into a personal world outlook (Vaalsiner, 2007), which can be externalized through behaviors, goals, and strivings. Faith and religion, as meaning-providing systems, can deeply influence this process (Delle Fave, 2009; Koenig et al., 1997, 2001; Sperry and Shafranske 2005). Religion is part of the cultural network in which the person grows and develops its talents and potentials (Massimini & Delle Fave, 1991). It is not necessarily a challenge by itself, but it supports and orients psychological selection and the search for challenges.

However, some people do intentionally select religion as a domain in which putting their skills to the test and pursuing major goals. This is true of the consecrated people and practicing Catholics described in this chapter. This commitment creates a substantial difference between these individuals and the common believers, in that it implies a selective and long-term recruitment of attention and resources around one specific target, which deeply influences and globally orients psychological selection. As our results showed, this endeavor is highly complex. It requires awareness and self-monitoring, discipline, and self-control. However, it can give rise to authentic optimal experiences, which can be constantly pursued by virtue of their intimate relationship with the prominent values, goals, and meanings of the person.

John Martin Kuvarapu, an Indian Benedictine monk committed to the exploration Hinduism and Christianity in their shared aspects, distinguished among five different categories of people with respect to religious attitudes and practice: believers, followers, disciples, explorers, and discoverers (Kuvarapu, 2006). Believers are passively immersed in the belief system of their tradition; followers consciously adhere to and fight for it; disciples are open to deeper learning and religious experience; explorers engage in a personal search pathway, even overcoming the boundaries of institutionalized norms and rules; discoverers trace new pathways. Applying this categorization to our samples, we could define believers and followers as the participants who did not report optimal experience in religious practice, but who nevertheless perceived meaning in it. Participants who reported flow during prayer and religious activities can be classified as disciples, in that they personally and actively identify challenges and enjoyment in the daily practice of their religion. Finally, those consecrated people and lay practicing Catholics who were able to interconnect, within the complex meaning system of faith and religion, their opportunities for optimal experiences, present challenges, and future goals, can be labeled as explorers, in that –using the words of one of them—they found "a beautiful way worth betting your life on it."

References

AAVV. (2005). *The Catechism of the Catholic Church.* Rome: Libreria Editrice Vaticana.

Allport., G., & Ross, J. M. (1967). Personal religious orientation and prejudice. *Journal of Personality and Social Psychology, 5*, 432–443.

Bellingham, R., Cohen, B., Jones, T., & Spaniol, L. (1989). Connectedness: Some skills for spiritual health. *American Journal of Health Promotion, 4*, 18–31.

Bickel, C., Ciarrocchi, J., Sheers, N., Estdt, B., Powell, D., & Pargament, K. (1998). Perceived stress, religious coping styles, and depressive affect. *Journal of Psychology and Christianity, 17*, 33–42.

Brady, M. J., Peterman, A. H., Fitchett, G., Mo, M., & Cella, D. (1999). A case for including spirituality in quality of life measurement in oncology. *Psycho-Oncology, 8*, 417–428.

Bruni, L., & Porta, P. L. (Eds.). (2006). *Economics and happiness: Framing the analysis.* Oxford: Oxford University Press.

Comstock, G. W., & Partridge, K. B. (1972). Church attendance and health. *Journal of Chronic Disease, 25*, 665–672.

Coppa, R., & Delle Fave, A. (2007). Pratica religiosa ed esperienza ottimale: una prospettiva eudaimonica. [Religious practice and optimal experience: a eudaimonic perspective] In A. Delle Fave (Ed.), *La condivisione del benessere. Il contributo della psicologia positiva* (pp. 73–93). Milano: Franco Angeli.

Coppa, R., & Delle Fave, A. (2009). Esperienza ottimale nella pratica religiosa e processo di attaccamento nella relazione con Dio. [Optimal experience in religious practice and attachment relationship with God] In G. Rossi & M. Aletti (Eds.), *Psicologia della religione e teoria dell'attaccamento* [Psychology of religion and attachment theory] (pp. 95–106). Roma: Aracne Editrice.

Delle Fave, A. (2009). Optimal experience and meaning: Which relationship? *Psychological Topics, 18*, 285–302.

Delle Fave, A., & Bassi, M. (2004). Immigrati africani in italia: qualità dell'esperienza e pratica religiosa. In M. Aletti e & G. Rossi (Eds.), *Identità religiosa, pluralismo e fondamentalismi* (pp. 269–276). Torino: Centro Scientifico Editore.

Delle Fave, A., & Massimini, F. (2003). Optimal experience in work and leisure among teachers and physicians: Individual and bio-cultural implications. *Leisure Studies, 22*, 323–342.

Delle Fave, A., & Massimini, F. (2005). The investigation of optimal experience and apathy: Developmental and psychosocial implications. *European Psychologist, 10*, 264–274.

Doyle, D. (1992). Have we looked beyond the physical and psychosocial? *Journal of Pain and Symptoms Management, 7*, 302–311.

Emmons, R. A. (2005). Striving for the sacred: Personal goals, life meaning, and religion. *Journal of Social Issues, 61*, 731–745.

Emmons, R. A. (2006). *Spirituality.* In M. Csikszentmihalyi & I. Csikszentmihalyi (Eds.), *A life worth living. Contributions to positive psychology* (pp. 62–81). New York: Oxford University Press.

Emmons, R. A., & McCullough, M. E. (2004). *The psychology of gratitude.* New York: Oxford University Press.

Fahlberg, L. L., & Fahlberg, L. A. (1991). Exploring spirituality and consciousness with an expanded science: Beyond the ego with empiricism, phenomenology, and contemplation. *American Journal of Health Promotion, 5*, 273–281.
Feher, S., & Maly, R. C. (1999). Coping with breast cancer in later life: the role of religious faith. *Psycho-oncology, 8*, 408–416.
Geyer, A. L., & Baumeister, R. F. (2005). Religion, morality, and self-control. In R. F. Paloutzian & C. L. Park (Eds.), *Handbook of the psychology of religion and spirituality* (pp. 412–432). New York: the Guilford Press.
http://www.nationmaster.com/country/it-italy/rel-religion. (2010). Downloaded April 25, 2010
Jenkins, R., & Pargament, K. (1995). Religion and spirituality as resources for coping with cancer. *Journal of Psychosocial Oncology, 13*, 51–74.
King, M., Speck, P., & Thomas, A. (1995). The royal free interview for religious and spiritual beliefs: Development and standardization. *Psychological Medicine, 25*, 1125–1134.
King, M., Speck, P., & Thomas, A. (2001). The royal free interview for religious and spiritual beliefs: Development and validation of a self-report version. *Psychological Medicine, 31*, 1015–1023.
Koenig, H. G., Hays, J. C., George, L. K., Blazer, D. G., Larson, D. B., & Landerman, L. R. (1997). Modeling the cross-sectional relationship between religion, physical health, social support, and depressive symptoms. *American Journal of Geriatric Psychiatry, 5*, 131–143.
Koenig, H. G., McCullough, M., & Larson, D. B. (2001). *Handbook of religion and health*. New York: Oxford University Press.
Kunnen, E. S., & Bosma, H. A. (2000). Development of meaning making: A dynamic systems approach. *New Ideas in Psychology, 18*, 57–82.
Kuvarapu, J. M. (2006). *The hindu Christ. Jesus message through eastern eyes*. Alresford, Hants: O-Books.
Larson, D. B., Koenig, H. G., Kaplan, B. H., Greenberg, R. S., Logue, E., & Taylor, H. A. (1989). The impact of religion on men's blood pressure. *Journal of Religion and Health, 28*, 265–278.
Luckert, K. W. (1975). *The Navajo hunter tradition*. Tucson, AZ: The University of Arizona Press.
Massimini, F., & Delle Fave, A. (1991). Religion and cultural evolution. *Zygon, 1*, 27–47.
McClain, C. S., Rosenfeld, B., & Breitbart, W. (2003). Effect of spiritual well-being on end-of-life despair in terminally-ill cancer patients. *The Lancet, 361*, 1603–1607.
McCullough, M. E., Larson, D. B., Hoyt, W. T., Koenig, H. G., & Thoreson, C. E. (1999). *Religious involvement and mortality: a meta-analysis review*. Communication to the *107th Convention of the American Psychological Association*, Boston, MA.
McCullough, M. E., Pargament, K. I., & Thoresen, C. E. (2000). *Forgiveness: Theory, research, and practice*. New York: Guilford Press.
Myers, D. G. (2000). The funds, friends and faith of happy people. *American Psychologist, 55*, 56–67.
Mytko, J. J., & Knight, S. J. (1999). Body, mind and spirit: Towards the integration of religiosity and spirituality in cancer quality of life research. *Psycho-Oncology, 8*, 439–450.
O'Collins, G., & Farrugia, E. G. (1991). *A concise dictionary of theology*. New York: Paulist Press.
Paloutzian, R. F. & Park, C. L. (Eds.). (2005). *Handbook of the psychology of religion and spirituality*. New York: The Guilford Press.
Park, C. (2005). Religion as a meaning-making framework in coping with life stress. *Journal of Social Issues, 61*, 707–729.
Park, C., & Folkman, S. (1997). The role of meaning in the context of stress and coping. *Review of General Psychology, 1*, 115–144.
Peterson, C., Park, N., & Sweeney, P. J. (2008). Group well-being: morale from a positive psychology perspective. *Applied Psychology, 57*, 19–36.
Rao, K. R., Paranjpe, A. C., & Dalal, A. K. (Eds.). (2008). *Handbook of Indian psychology*. New Delhi: Cambridge University Press India.
Reichard, G. (1950). *Navaho religion. A study of symbolism*. New York: Bollingen.

Sen, A. (1992). *Inequality reexamined*. Oxford: Oxford University Press.

Shahabi, L., Powell, L. H., Musick, M. A., Pargament, K. I., Thoresen, C. E., Williams, D., et al. (2002). Correlates of self-perceptions of spirituality in American adults. *Annals of Behavioral Medicine, 24*, 59–68.

Singer, J. A. (2004). Narrative identity and meaning making across the adult life span: An introduction. *Journal of Personality, 72*, 438–459.

Sperry, K. & Shafranske, E. P. (Eds.). (2005). *Spiritually oriented psychotherapy*. Washington, DC: American Psychological Association.

Spiegel, D., & Fawzy, I. F. (2002). Psychosocial interventions and prognosis in cancer. In H. G. Koenig & H. J. Cohen (Eds.), The *link between religion and health. Psychoneuroimmunology and the faith factor* (pp. 84–100). New York: Oxford Univ. Press.

Tarakeshwar, N., Stanton, J., & Pargament, K. J. (2003). Religion. An overlooked dimension in cross-cultural psychology. *Journal of Cross-Cultural Psychology, 34*, 377–394.

Topper, M. D., & Begaye, C. (1978). "Not Navajo life": Clinical anthropology, "mental illness" and psychotherapy among the Navajo. In Steinberg, J. L. (Ed.), *Cultural factors in the rehabilitation process* (pp. 83–120). Los Angeles: California State University.

Underhill, R. M. (1948). Ceremonial patterns in the greater Southwest. *American Ethnological society Monographs, XIII*.

Vaalsiner, J. (2007). Personal culture and conduct of value. *Journal of Social, Evolutionary, and Cultural Psychology, 1*, 59–65.

Vaughan, F. (1991). Spiritual issues in psychotherapy. *Journal of Transpersonal Psychology, 23*, 105–119.

Walsh, K., King, M., Jones, L., Tookman, A., & Blizard, R. (2002). Spiritual beliefs May affect outcome of bereavement: Prospective study. *British Medical Journal, 324*, 1551–1555.

WHOQOL Group. (1994). Development of the WHOQOL: Rationale and current status. *International Journal of Mental Health, 23*, 24–56.

WHOQOL Group. (1995). The world health organisation quality of life assessment (WHOQOL): Position paper from the world health organisation. *Social Science and Medicine, 41*, 1403–1409.

WHOQOL Group. (2006). A cross-cultural study of spirituality, religion, and personal beliefs as components of quality of life. *Social Science and Medicine, 62*, 1486–1497.

WHOQOL SRPB Group. (2005). A cross-cultural study of spirituality, religion, and personal beliefs as components of quality of life. *Social Science and Medicine, 62*, 1486–1497.

Williams, W. (1991). *Javanese lives: Men and women in modern Indonesian society*. New Brunswick, NJ: Rutgers University Press.

Zaccagnini, J. L., Delle Fave, A., & Sanabria, E. (2010). Religious practice and optimal experience in a Spanish Catholic sample. Presentation at the *5th European Conference on Positive Psychology*, Copenhagen, June 23–26.

Zinnbauer, B. J., & Pargament, K. I. (2005). Religiousness and spirituality. In R. F. Paloutzian & C. L. Park (Eds.), *Handbook of the psychology of religion and spirituality* (pp. 21–42). New York: the Guilford Press.

Chapter 13
Acculturation and Optimal Experience

13.1 Acculturation

The acculturation process was originally described as the modifications individuals and groups undergo at the psychological and social levels when a continuous contact between two cultures is established (Redfield, Linton, & Herskovits, 1936). However, as chronicles and social studies have systematically highlighted, acculturation only seldom occurs as a bi-directional process (Berry & Sam, 1997; LaFromboise, Coleman, & Gerton, 1993). More often, cultural modification concerns the changes a cultural group has to introduce in collective as well as individual behavior, in order to coexist and interact with the norms and habits of a dominant social system. It usually applies to ethnic minorities, immigrants, indigenous peoples exposed to colonization, and refugees, which can be globally considered as acculturating groups (Berry, 1997).

According to Tajfel (1978), one's social identity is "that part of an individual's self-concept which derives from his knowledge of his membership in a social group (or groups), together with the value and emotional significance attached to that membership" (p. 63). In multicultural contexts groups usually distinguish themselves and are distinguished by others on the basis of ethnicity. This can create conflicts and discrimination, but can also become a richness for the host culture, provided that immigrants and minorities are allowed to follow an adaptive acculturation pathway (Berry, 2001).

Acculturation mostly concerns minorities within a dominant social context. Moreover, the involuntary character of the process has been stressed: minorities are mostly forced to adapt to the cultural system they live in, in order to cope with the dominant environment and to become active parts in it.

Acculturation implies two forms of change: socio-cultural adjustment (Searle & Ward, 1990; Ward, 2001; Ward & Kennedy, 1994) and psychological adaptation (Berry, 1997). Socio-cultural adjustment is conceptualized as the degree of immigrants' acquisition of new skills and behaviors; it implies a learning process and the opportunity to interact with host citizens. Several studies highlighted some key predictors of socio-cultural adjustment of immigrants, namely the length of residence in the new culture, the relationships with host nationals, the immigrant status

A. Delle Fave et al., *Psychological Selection and Optimal Experience Across Cultures*, Cross-Cultural Advancements in Positive Psychology 2,
DOI 10.1007/978-90-481-9876-4_13,

(having residence permit versus being "illegal"), and the education level (Ataca and Berry 2002; Ward & Kennedy, 1993; Zlobina, Basabe, Paez, & Furnham, 2006). Psychological adaptation refers to emotional well-being and satisfaction; however, it is mostly investigated in the perspective of stress and coping, In particular, research has highlighted the mental and psychosomatic disorders, such as the acculturative stress syndrome, affecting people living in close contact with a foreign dominant environment (Berry, Kim, Minde, & Mok, 1987; Finch & Vega, 2003; Kazarian & Evans, 2001) or in cultures undergoing rapid modernization changes (Al-Issa, 1995).

Four strategies of acculturation have been recognized (Berry, 1997): assimilation, separation, marginalization, integration. Here we will refer to them in terms of psychological acculturation, that is, the changes arising in the acculturating individual's patterns of interaction with the new environment.

Assimilation occurs when, within the acculturating group, individuals lose their ties with the original cultural background, and acquire values, habits, and behaviors from the dominant culture. In the *separation* pattern, people belonging to the acculturating minority maintain strong relationships within their group. They keep their own traditions, behaviors, values. They create a separate sub-culture, which is minimally influenced by the dominant group. The contacts between the two social systems are subsequently very restricted. The Amish of Pennsylvania represent a typical example of this kind of strategy. *Marginalization* occurs when individuals originating from the acculturating group are not accepted as members of the dominant culture. They are not given opportunities to join the majority as concerns education, employment, civil rights; they are segregated (Berry & Sam, 1997) by the dominant group, regardless of their wish to integrate and/or to assimilate. Finally, in the *integration* pattern, acculturating individuals manage to acquire values and behaviors characterizing the dominant culture where they live, at the same time preserving their own traditions and habits. This strategy, by and large the most adaptive one, allows individuals to become full-fledged members of the acculturating society, without losing their original cultural identity.

This last kind of interaction with a dominant culture has also been labeled as biculturalism (Delle Fave & Massimini, 1991). Also, LaFromboise and colleagues (1993) employ the term "biculturalism," but they include it within a model of second culture acquisition which they define alternation. It is different from integration in that it does not necessarily imply that two given cultures are continuously interacting as components of a single social structure. A bicultural individual knows and understands two different cultures, and he/she is able to show dual modes of social behavior that can be alternately used depending upon which culture the individual is interacting with (LaFromboise & Rowe, 1983). This does neither automatically imply that a bicultural individual daily comes into contact with the dominant culture, nor that the two cultures share a common geographical area.

The ability to preserve original traditions and, at the same time, to introduce new information is the best strategy to maintain flexibility and increase complexity both in individuals and in cultural systems (Delle Fave & Massimini, 1999). It allows an individual or a culture to successfully cope with environmental changes, thanks to the introduction of new memes and their integration with the already existing ones. However, coping with the demands of a dominant culture is a complex challenge. In different parts of the world we can see the various results of the acculturation process at the psychological as well as at the social levels. There are cases of complete assimilation, be it forced or voluntarily: this is, for example, what often happens among some of the American-Indian populations. Especially the youngest generations find it easier to cut the ties with their original cultural pool, in the effort to be accepted in the European-American teenager groups.

Bicultural competence is a laborious task: it requires the creation of effective interpersonal relationships with both cultures without losing personal identity. It implies knowledge of the dominant values, positive attitude to both cultural patterns, communication through the use of the dominant language, adequate role repertoire, sense of being grounded in both cultures (LaFromboise et al., 1993). Nevertheless, a growing number of studies have highlighted its adaptive role in promoting well-being and in enhancing individual cognitive complexity (Benet-Martinez, Lee, & Leu, 2006; Matsunaga, Hecte, Elek, & Ndiaye, 2010; Tadmor & Tetlock, 2006; Tadmor, Tetlock, & Peng, 2009).

However, till now few studies have focused on the perceived level of well-being and goal pursuit among immigrants, and on their implications for psychological adaptation and socio-cultural adjustment. Among the factors which promote adequate integration, the most relevant ones at the psychological level seem to be a strong personal identity and the availability of one's own ethnic group to search for assistance in case of need (Jasinskaja-Lathi et al., 2006; Noh & Kaspar, 2003; Phinney, Horenczyk, Liebkind, & Vedder, 2001).

13.2 Optimal Experience and Migration

In this section, we will provide evidence of the occurrence of optimal experience among immigrants. To this purpose, we will refer to studies mainly conducted among first-generation immigrants settled in Italy from different countries.

In a comparative study conducted with flow questionnaire and life theme questionnaire, we gathered information among immigrants from Africa, India, South America, and Eastern Europe. We investigated the opportunities for optimal experience they retrieved in the new cultural context, the experience they associated with daily domains, their present challenges, and future goals (Delle Fave & Bassi, 2009).

The great majority of Indian and Eastern European, who were living in Italy since a longer period, reported optimal experience in their daily life, mostly associating it with work, leisure, and interactions. Their major present challenges referred to the achievement of professional advancements, family development, and personal growth. A lower percentage of South American and African participants reported flow (63 and 42%, respectively). South Americans prominently associated optimal experience with work and interactions, Africans with leisure activities. The prominent challenges of both groups of participants were related to basic survival needs, such as finding a stable job and a decent housing.

Findings confirmed the theoretical expectations concerning the role of socio-cultural components of adaptation in supporting the retrieval of optimal experiences and the identification of current challenges. In particular, we took into account participants' length of stay in Italy, their immigrant status, the cultural distance between the homeland and the hosting country, their job opportunities, and the availability of a social and family network providing support.

Overall, Indians and Eastern Europeans reported optimal experience in a higher percentage, and associated it with a wider range of activity categories. In fact, these two groups could rely on more resources in their process of socio-cultural adjustment. Indians were highly educated professionals, had achieved good job positions, and lived together with their families. Eastern Europeans had a job, though not always corresponding to their expectations, but at the same time they enjoyed little cultural distance from the host country, they spoke Italian fluently, some of them lived with their families, or could visit them relatively often.

Africans and South Americans, on the contrary, shared shorter length of residence in Italy and lower educational level. Their immigrant irregular status negatively affected their chances to get a stable and adequately paid occupation, and their access to social and health services. They prominently lived alone, far from their beloved ones.

In spite of these differences related to their levels of socio-cultural adjustment, participants in the four groups did not show substantial differences in long-term expectations, unanimously reporting the pursuit of personal, professional, and relational goals. In particular, they quoted satisfaction and fulfillment in job, children's well-being and success in life, inner harmony and self-actualization. These findings suggest that, regardless of the difficulties they had to cope with in the new environment, participants perceived self-concordance and self-determination in their goal orientation (Gong & Chang, 2007; Sheldon et al., 2004), and they pursued eudaimonic well-being.

A more in depth analysis of the experience of migration will be offered in the following sections, through the closer examination of two groups of immigrants.

13.2.1 Living in India and Living Abroad

The impact of migration on daily life and experience can be investigated from a comparative perspective, collecting information among people living in their homeland and among their fellow citizens living abroad. We adopted this strategy to investigate optimal experiences and life theme in a sample of Indians, 16 men and 36 women, 23 of them (2 men and 21 women) living in Europe and 29 (14 men and 15 women) living in India (Swarup & Delle Fave, 1999). Although participants were raised in different parts of India, they shared similar levels of education and socio-economic status: most of them got a University degree, and they worked as teachers, professionals, or managers. This provided a reasonable basis for drawing comparisons between the two groups.

In order to better interpret the results obtained in this study, we have to preliminarily take into account some characteristics of the recent migration flows from India to Southern Europe, and more specifically to Italy, where 80% of the migrated participants lived. During the second half of the previous century, two subsequent migratory waves could be distinguished. The first group of Indians left their homeland during the 1960s, within the "brain drain" phenomenon that attracted to western countries young and highly educated professionals who aspired to expand their professional knowledge and find better job opportunities. In the same period, an increasing amount of college students earned scholarships abroad. Almost all of them spoke English fluently, were hardworking, belonged to socially and economically well-settled families, and had been raised according to the traditional Indian values. Some were already married, some got married soon after. The social and political conditions in Europe and Italy allowed them to achieve a good level of integration in the new environment. A second wave of migration from India took place during the 1980s and 1990s, mainly comprising people with lower education and SES levels, who looked for better life conditions. Since most of them could only speak their regional language, after migration they prominently adopted a separation pattern of acculturation, both in the interaction with Europeans and with previously migrated Indians. However, with time, in the multicultural urban environment they were able to develop healthy identities and positive inter-group attitudes, by virtue of the strong affiliation and social support they could find in the local Indian communities.

The participants in this study belonged to the first migration shift. Thanks to their educational and professional background, they could pursue and achieve integration in the host culture. Participants showed interest and motivation in learning the new language, and in building work and personal relationships with members of the hosting countries. They attained good levels of social participation and acquired customs and activities from the dominant culture, at the same time maintaining a strong original identity, by virtue of their solid socialization background within the Indian culture.

The participants were administered flow questionnaire and life theme questionnaire. We will analyze findings adopting a comparative perspective with the aim of detecting similarities and differences between the two groups.

As concerns optimal experience, all participants reported its occurrence in their lives, and associated it with various activities. As Table 13.1 shows, leisure ranked first among optimal activities. Over half of the answers in this domain (64%) referred to the use of media, that primarily comprised reading and listening to music. Migrated participants clearly highlighted the cultivation of a bicultural competence, quoting listening to Indian music and watching films in their native language, together with reading newspaper and books in Italian, and following Italian TV programs. Within the remaining 36% of the answers, immigrants mainly reported typically western sports and individual hobbies, while participants living in India primarily referred to activities that were more social in nature, such as playing cards and other collective games, playing music, dancing, and singing.

Table 13.1 Percentage distribution of optimal activities among participants living in India and migrated to Europe

	Optimal activities		Selected optimal activities	
Categories	India	Europe	India	Europe
Productive activities	38.7	35.6	41.4	47.8
Leisure	48.6	50.0	44.8	39.1
Interactions	8.1	11.3	3.5	8.7
Introspection	4.6	3.1	10.3	4.3
N answers	111	132	29	23

Work that ranked second among the optimal activity categories, primarily referred to intellectual tasks such as planning, developing new projects, solving problems, and teaching. Migrated women, who represented the majority of the participants in this group, reported household tasks more often than their counterparts living in India. This finding can be related to the different household management in the two countries. In India, women belonging to upper classes—as those here examined—can rely upon several people helping in the chores and doing most part of them. For migrated women, therefore, domestic tasks were a rather new activity, and it represented a potential opportunity to develop new competences and skills. For women in both groups, however, cooking ranked first activity among optimal activities in the domestic sphere. Migrated participants had to learn Italian recipes beside the Indian ones: due to the substantial differences in food habits between the two cultures, this task was a relevant component of the integration process, together with language acquisition and the development of social relations and friendships with the local people. As concerns Indian participants, cooking is a very important aspect of girls' education before marriage, and much attention is paid to it. Other activities recorded by women in both groups were stitching, knitting, and embroidery. This finding confirms the tendency of migrated women to preserve and cultivate activities learned at home outside of their native context.

The percentage of optimal activities associated with interactions and with introspection was similar in the two groups, and it also reflected the findings of the general cross-cultural sample examined in Chapter 7. As a specific remark, six participants reported religious practice in this domain, and all of them lived in India. A more detailed discussion of the role of religion in this sample is provided in Chapter 12.

As concerns selected optimal activities, work prevailed in both groups compared with the other categories. A reversed pattern was observed for interactions and introspection: migrated participants prominently selected the former, while people living in India selected the latter in greater percentage. However, due to the limited sample size, no group differences could be detected in the participants' distribution across domains.

Table 13.2 shows the quality of experience participants in the two groups associated with selected optimal activities. Participants in both groups reported high

Table 13.2 The quality of experience during selected optimal activities and family life in Europe and in India

	Optimal activities		Family	
Variables	India *M* (*sd*)	Europe *M* (*sd*)	India *M* (*sd*)	Europe *M* (*sd*)
Involvement	7.5 (1.3)	6.2 (1.9)	5.2 (2.6)	6.6 (1.6)
Clear feedback	6.8 (1.8)	6.7 (1.5)	4.8 (2.4)	6.4 (1.8)
Intrinsic motivation	6.5 (2.2)	6.1 (2.4)	5.4 (2.1)	7.3 (1.3)
Excitement	7.9 (0.4)	7.4 (1.1)	7.0 (1.3)	7.7 (0.7)
Ease of concentration	7.1 (1.2)	6.9 (2.3)	5.8 (2.4)	6.8 (1.7)
Unselfconsciousness	6.6 (2.6)	6.3 (2.4)	5.5 (2.1)	4.6 (2.9)
Enjoyment	7.4 (1.3)	6.8 (2.1)	6.0 (1.8)	7.0 (1.3)
Concentration	6.5 (1.6)	6.5 (1.6)	5.7 (1.8)	6.2 (1.5)
Relaxation	7.1 (1.7)	5.7 (3.2)	4.9 (2.9)	5.5 (2.6)
Clear goals	7.3 (1.2)	7.0 (2.0)	6.3 (1.9)	7.1 (1.2)
Control of situation	6.7 (1.7)	7.0 (1.2)	5.7 (2.1)	6.4 (1.8)
Challenges	4.7 (2.8)	5.5 (2.5)	4.3 (2.5)	5.1 (2.7)
Skills	6.8 (1.1)	6.1 (2.0)	5.8 (1.9)	5.9 (1.6)

Note: Number of participants in India = 29; Number of participants in Europe = 23.

levels of clear goals, control of the situation, enjoyment, focus of attention, unselfconsciousness, excitement, and wish to do the activity. Only involvement scored significantly higher among participants living in India ($Z = 2.81$, $p < 0.01$), consistently with the findings obtained in Chapter 7.

An intriguing finding concerns the relatively low values participants in both groups attributed to perceived challenges. Other works conducted with flow questionnaire and ESM in different cultures highlighted that the strictly literal translation of the term was well-suited for situations characterized by competition, external evaluation, and high social expectations, such as sport contests, work, and study. However, it did not fit situations such as reading, painting, contemplating a landscape, talking to a friend (Delle Fave & Massimini, 2004; Chapter 4). The Indian participants in this study, who filled out the original English version of the flow questionnaire, repeatedly remarked this difficulty. This can partly explain their peculiar answer pattern. Further investigations are needed to better disentangle this topic, which is apparently related to the more or less marked cultural emphasis on the dimension of competition/achievement versus personal growth/self-expression.

As concerns the quality of experience associated with daily contexts, we will focus on the family domain, in which interesting differences were detected between the two groups. As shown in Table 13.2, both groups associated with family a globally positive experience, in many respects similar to flow. A paired *t* test comparison allowed for detecting discrepancies between the two conditions. Participants living in India associated family daily life with significant lower values of involvement ($t = 3.58, p < 0.01$), clear ideas ($t = 3.27, p < 0.01$), wish to do the activity ($t = 2.36$, $p < 0.05$), excitement ($t = 3.03, p < 0.01$), enjoyment ($t = 2.58, p < 0.05$), relaxation

($t = 3.29$, $p < 0.01$), clear goals ($t = 2.93$, $p < 0.01$), and skills ($t = 2.51$, $p < 0.05$). On the contrary, participants living in Europe reported an almost overlapping quality of experience in flow activities and in family life, except for two variables: the wish to do the activity, scoring significantly higher with family ($t = 2.2$, $p < 0.05$), and unselfconsciousness, scoring higher during optimal activities ($t = 2.7$, $p < 0.05$). A nonparametric comparison of the family experience in the two groups highlighted significantly higher values of intrinsic motivation ($Z = 3.4$, $p < 0.001$), excitement ($Z = 2.2$, $p < 0.05$), and clear ideas ($Z = 2.4$, $p < 0.05$) among migrated participants.

This is an apparently paradoxical result, given the extreme importance of family ties and roles in Indian society. However, a more complex picture emerges if we take into account the impact of cultural change on immigrants' daily life and relations. In India the family is organized as an extended network of relatives, usually living together or in very close contact: the traditional joint family system still persists in spite of modernization pressures (Juthani, 1992). It implies a higher frequency of daily interaction with various family members, and a lower probability for parents to spend time with their children alone. Migration to western countries brought about a substantial change for participants in this study, who were forced to adjust to the dominant pattern of nuclear family. Immigrants, and especially mothers, had to learn to take care of family needs single handedly. At the same time, however, they were more free to plan, to take decisions, and to set goals without the sometimes unwelcome control and advice of other family members. The Indian and European characterization of family clearly emerged from the descriptions provided by the participants to the question "What do you mean with being with family?" As an exemplary quotation, a woman migrated to Italy answered, "It means sitting, talking about day's activities, and deriving satisfaction from it"(female, Italy). A woman living in India reported instead, "To me family is like a 'stream', with whom I move to fulfill my commitments in life. Being with family means sharing the moments-both tender and tense- with other members."

As concerns findings from the life theme questionnaire, we only highlight that family was identified as the prominent positive influence, present challenge, and future goal in both groups, followed by work. Using the congruence approach described in Chapter 7 (Table 7.7), work was recurrent at congruence level 1 among 28% of the participants living in India and among 13% of those migrated to Europe, at congruence level 2 among 10.3 and 8.7% of the participants in the two groups, respectively, and at congruence level 3 among 17.2 and 8.7% of them. Family recurred at congruence level 1 among 31% of the participants living in India and among 39% of the migrated ones, and at congruence level 2 among 27.6 and 30.4% of the participants in each group, respectively. Only two migrated participants quoted family at congruence level 3. In general, these findings are consistent with the cross-cultural analysis described in Chapter 7. In particular, both groups of Indian participants examined here showed a similar pattern of congruence in relation to family, thus confirming the pervasive role of intimate relationships in orienting psychological selection, in spite of their low frequency as opportunities for optimal experience.

All together, findings highlighted a substantial similarity in optimal experiences and psychological selection between the two groups. In particular, immigrant Indians managed to find meaningful and gratifying opportunities for action in their daily life abroad, seemly developing a bicultural identity.

13.2.2 The Daily Life of East European Women in Italy

The percentage of women migrating around the world steadily increased from 46.6% during the 1960s to 48.8% in 2004; in some countries they represent 70% of the immigrants. The prominent reasons for women to migrate are poor socio-economic conditions in the homeland, family reunification, and the search for higher opportunities for autonomy, emancipation, and financial independence. However, women migration is also related to prostitution and illegal work exploitation. In Italy, female presence among immigrants increased from 42% in 1991 to 50% in 2005 (Caritas 2005). These women prominently come from South America and Eastern Europe, and find most work opportunities as home helpers and household staff, taking care of elders and children. In particular, women from Eastern Europe are often highly educated, but they accept domestic jobs in order to provide financial support to their parents, husband, and children still living in the homeland, with the risks for psychosocial maladjustment that this forced decision implies (Aycan & Berry, 1996).

Migration under these circumstances often causes family disruption and divorces, which force migrated women to search for other caregivers for their children at home. Their maternal role becomes also problematic, due to their economical presence but affective absence.

In a recent study, we explored the experience fluctuation in daily life among women migrated to Italy from three Eastern European countries (Fianco & Delle Fave, 2006). As per our knowledge, this was the first study conducted with ESM among migrants. Participants were 11 women aged 28–56, 5 of them coming from Moldova, 4 from Ukraine, and 2 from Romania. All lived in Italy since 3 years at least, and the majority of them worked as home help or family caregiver. As for their educational level, eight women had got a University degree, two had a high school diploma, and one was a professional nurse.

Six participants had arrived in Italy alone, leaving their husband and children in the homeland; all of them divorced after migration, and at the time of the study they economically supported their children and parents. Two participants were able to obtain family reunification, and three participants, who were single before migration, built a couple relationship in the host country.

The immigrant women completed the ESM weekly session providing a total of 263 valid self-reports (25 each on average). Due to their tight daily schedule, filling out forms at signal reception was often problematic; therefore, their active collaboration in this project was highly appreciable.

Their daily activities mostly comprised work (35.4% of the forms), followed by maintenance (14.1%, including eating, resting, personal care), and house chores

Table 13.3 East European immigrant women: percentage distribution of the self-reports in the EFM channels throughout the sampling week, and during work

Channels	Overall	Work
1. Activation	24.0	24.6
2. Optimal experience	14.8	20.4
3. Control	4.5	6.5
4. Relaxation	14.0	10.8
5. Boredom	14.5	9.6
6. Apathy	15.6	17.3
7. Worry	5.8	3.1
8. Anxiety	6.8	7.6
N self-reports	263	93

(12.5%). Participants' free time prominently comprised watching TV (9.2%) and reading (4.9%). Interactions with employers and friends accounted for 13.7 of the self-reports.

As concerns locations, participants prominently reported being at work and at home (51.9 and 36.4% of the forms, respectively). However, in 30% of the self-reports they expressed the wish to be somewhere else, mostly at home (41.8%) and in their homeland (21.5%). Their social context proved to be very limited: participants reported to be alone in 37.7% of the forms, and with people they took care of in 26.8%. In 31% of the forms they wished to be with someone else, mostly the partner (34.2%), children (20.3%), and family (17%).

Participants' daily quality of experience was investigated through the experience fluctuation model (see Chapters 4 and 5 for a detailed description). Table 13.3 shows the percentage distribution of the self-reports across the EFM channels in the whole dataset, and during work. In general, conditions characterized by perceived high challenges (Channels 1, 2 and 8) and conditions characterized by perceived low challenges (Channels 4, 5, and 6) were balanced throughout the week. While working, participants perceived high challenges in over half of the self-reports. Optimal experience and its closest condition, arousal (Channel 1) accounted together for 45% of the forms. The perception of below average challenges, on the contrary, was prominently associated with maintenance, home chores, and TV watching (Fianco & Delle Fave, 2006).

We subsequently analyzed the percentage distribution of self-reports in the three conditions of high, average, and low challenges in each participants' answers. As detected in other ESM studies and discussed in Chapter 5, the perception of high challenges is usually associated with a globally positive experience, while low challenges are prominently connected to negative states. Figure 15.3 illustrates the findings obtained from the immigrant women. This kind of analysis, together with the evaluation of the activity domains most recurrent in the three conditions for each participant, allowed us to distinguish among four different distribution patterns.

Pattern 1. Participants A, B, and J prominently reported high challenges in their daily life, and mostly referred them to work. These three women had a University degree, and worked as household staff. Two of them left their family in the homeland, while the third one lived in Italy with husband and children.

Pattern 2. Participants C, D, and I showed a more uniform answer pattern across low and high challenge conditions. They prominently associated the perception of high challenges with leisure and interactions, and to a lesser extent to house chores. Each of them worked as house help and baby sitter for several families, being thus forced to devote a high amount of time to transportation every day, and saving little room for rest and privacy. Participants C and I left their families in east Europe, while D lived with an Italian partner.

Pattern 3. Participants E and F also showed an overall homogeneous distribution of answers between high-challenge and low-challenge conditions. However, they mostly associated the former with work. Both were college graduates; one was social worker, lived with the family and planned to definitely settle in Italy. The other one, a biologist, was employed in a pharmaceutical company and had left a child in the homeland.

Pattern 4. Participants G, H, and K prominently perceived low challenges in their lives. H had worked as a high school teacher in Moldova, and in Italy she found a job as elders' caregiver. Her children lived in the homeland. K was a young journalist, she had moved to Italy in search for better job opportunities, and she worked as domestic aid. Both H and K were dissatisfied with their present occupation, which was very different from what they had expected to do according to their educational and professional background. Finally, G practiced her profession as nurse, and lived with her husband and children. She prominently associated low challenges with house chores, while the self-reports related to work were homogeneously distributed across the channels.

Which suggestions can we derive from these findings? At a first glance, we could assume that among immigrant women in this study the perception of high challenges—and thus of positive experiences—was related to an adequate match between work opportunities and educational background. This assumption was verified among participants showing answer pattern 3 and 4 (the latter from a reversed perspective). It was also consistent with the situation of participants showing answer pattern 2, who indeed perceived high challenges in daily life, but in leisure activities. What about participants showing answer pattern 1, who prominently reported high challenges during work in spite of its discrepancy with their educational level? We propose to take into account the meaning and long-term goals these women attached to work (Emmons, 2005) as a means to support their families and to guarantee their children a better future. As suggested in Chapters 1 and 3, people can commit themselves to the cultivation of activities or to the pursuit of goals that they perceive as valuable, even though they undermine or limit in various ways their quality of life in the short term (Sen, 1992). This eudaimonic interpretation of the findings is also consistent with the bulk of evidence gathered on flow and psychological selection among people living under difficult circumstances (see Chapter 15, Sections 2.5.4 and 2.6).

13.3 Navajos: The Bicultural People

The history and present life conditions of American-Indian populations are very often taken as examples of the struggle for survival of preindustrial societies, facing the challenges of modernization and acculturation within the dominant western world. The assimilation trend promoted by the Euro-American domination and the numeric and technological weakness of most tribes have caused a great amount of social and psychological difficulties as concerns individual development, culture preservation, and chances of integration into the modern world.

American-Indians are often considered as a homogeneous group of tribes, regardless of the differences in language, traditions, and social organization. On the contrary, they show a great variety of customs and biocultural adaptation strategies, as regards their settlement in the United States and Canada and their interaction with the Anglo-American modernized context (Trimble & Medicine, 1993). This section will specifically focus on the Navajo people, one of the most numerous and integrated Native tribes in the United States. The whole history of the Navajos, as well as their present interaction pattern with the western culture, represent a peculiar example of bicultural strategy which allowed them to survive and to adapt to modernization changes, without losing their original identity.

The Navajos are presently settled in a wide territory mostly located in Arizona, and for smaller portions in New Mexico, Colorado, and Utah. They descend from an ancient Sino-Mongolian population, the Nadene (Downs, 1972; Kluckhohn & Leighton, 1974), migrated to America through Bering lands during the seventh millennium BC (Collins, 1991). With time, the Nadene split into distinct groups according to different language affiliations; one of them was the Athapaskan, comprising the Navajos and the Apaches, which separated from the other groups around the fifth century AD, and moved to the southwest.

The presence of the Navajos in New Mexico has been presumably established around 1300 AD (Luckert, 1975). Since their early settlement, the Diné (the people, as the Navajos define themselves in their native language) showed a distinctive style of interaction with the local cultures. They originally were a nomadic hunter-gatherer society, equipped with basic artifacts such as baskets, bows, and arrows. In the southwest they met the Pueblos, a group of sedentary populations also originating from Asia, organized in villages and practicing agriculture and handicraft. The Navajos rapidly absorbed these skills, and started to extensively raise corn, beans, and squash, to weave and to produce pottery.

The introduction of these activities produced some changes in the religious practices and rituals. The original Navajo myths and ceremonies belonged to the Athapaskan hunter tradition, and were centered on the worship of sacred animals such as the buffalo, the main survival resource for the tribe. After the contact with Pueblos, the Navajos developed rituals connected to Mother Earth, sacred sites and plants, particularly corn (Luckert, 1975; Reichard, 1950). They borrowed Pueblo religious artifacts and customs: sand paintings, ceremonial masks, prayer-sticks, offerings of turquoise, jet, white and red shell. They also adopted the Pueblo pattern of rituals, consisting in 8 days of purification and offerings, and a ninth night of public celebration to partake the spirit blessing, attaching to them their own meanings (Topper & Begaye, 1978; Underhill, 1948). They lived in hogans, consisting in a conical frame of logs covered with earth, which subsequently became hexagonal or octagonal. The Navajo territory is still disseminated with thousands of these buildings, which are often used as ceremonial places, while the main dwelling is usually a brick house or a trailer (Underhill, 1967).

Their strategy of borrowing information from neighbors and of integrating it in their culture led them to overcome the Pueblos in the skill of agriculture. In fact, "Navajo" was a later name given to the tribe by the Tewa Indians, meaning "great cultivated fields." They also brought to extreme refinement the art of sand painting, which is still today one of the most renowned expressions of Navajo religious and cultural beliefs.

During the seventeenth century, Spanish farmers invaded the southwestern territories and subjugated most Pueblo groups, while the Navajos, settled in remote canyons, and thanks to their warrior and nomadic tradition, were able to escape direct dominance: Spaniards never succeeded in controlling the whole tribe and its land (Trafzer, 1978a). Form Spanish settlers, the Navajos acquired the skill of animal husbandry (mainly goats, sheep, and horses), perfectly suited to their semi-nomadic lifestyle centered on the extended family as the basic social unit. At the same time, they continued to practice extensive agriculture, raids, and hunting expeditions. The integration of herding and horse riding techniques in their cultural system provided the Navajos with higher mobility and more powerful war strategies. These changes contributed to the significant growth in complexity of the Navajo culture and to the strength and power of the tribe. The increasing wealth of the Navajos was connected with their combined ability as herders and raiders. Livestock and silver works were often stolen or traded with Spanish and later with Mexicans: livestock was subsequently used to enlarge flocks, and silver works to exchange goods with other peoples.

In 1846, the US army invaded the southwestern territories with the purpose to settle boundaries with Mexico; the subsequent war eventually led to the inclusion of New Mexico in the United States (Trafzer, 1978b). Later on, campaigns were started against the tribes settled in this area. Navajos were valid warriors, but Kit Carson's soldiers attacked their survival resources. Fields were burned out, orchards were destroyed, animals were slaughtered. The Navajos took shelter in the most remote canyons of their land, but starvation ultimately defeated them, and they had to surrender.

In 1863, a so-called humanitarian plan was started, and the Navajos were taken to Fort Sumner, in New Mexico: they were expected to adopt a sedentary way of life, to become peaceful farmers and to be converted to Christianity (Downs, 1972). During this period of seclusion, interspersed with famines and epidemics, the Navajos were confronted with the necessity to find a compromise with the US government. Manuelito, one of the most famous chiefs of the tribe, played a crucial role in persuading the people to accept the conditions posed by the Americans in exchange for freedom. Above all, he understood that, due to the numeric and technological inferiority of the Navajos, fighting Americans with weapons would not lead to success. Instead, the fight had to be promoted through education, encouraging children to study and to become acquainted with the white men's culture. Economists, politicians, lawyers were needed to engage in legal and political disputes to defend Navajo identity and rights. This is an additional example of the bicultural strategy adopted by the tribe throughout its history. The words Chief Manuelito addressed to his grandchild Chee Dodge in 1893, few days before dying, have become legendary (Fuchs & Havighurst, 1972, p. 39)

> My grandchild, the whites have many things which we Navajo need. But we cannot get them. It is as though the whites were in a grassy canyon an there they have wagons, plows, and plenty of food. We Navajos are up on the dry mesa. We can hear them talking but we cannot get them. My grandchild, education is the ladder. Tell our people to take it.

In 1868 a treaty was signed, and the Diné settled in a small area, working as farmers and herders, and sending their children to schools. They acquired from Mexicans the skills of silversmithing and of forging iron. Thanks to the exchanges with American traders, they also developed commercial skills: they sold blankets, rugs, cattle, and silver ornaments; they bought steel tools and unfortunately alcohols.

The transition to modernization was a difficult process. The reservation was too small for the needs of a growing population. Drought, epidemics, and frost recurrently damaged harvests and cattle. A federal agent, after his visit to the Navajos, wrote, "... The country is almost entirely rock. An Illinois or Iowa or Kansas farmer would laugh to scorn the assertion that you could raise anything there ..." (Reports of Commissioners of Indian Affairs 1883, 129). The rigid discipline, the foreign language and the stranger notions taught in the schools did not appeal to the Navajo children, who had been raised in the open air and educated to different values. In 1886 school was made compulsory for Navajo children, but still many parents were not persuaded to send their sons and daughters away, under strangers' control and norms.

The Navajo territory was gradually enlarged until 1934. Diné people were offered new opportunities for work and employment in factories and commercial enterprises. In 1923, the first Tribal Council was proclaimed, and the land officially became property of the tribe. Since 1923 the political and administrative structure of the Navajo Nation was developed. Tribal offices were located in traditionally eight-sided buildings; the inner walls of the tribal council chamber were frescoed by Navajo artists with images summarizing the history of the tribe. In 1924, the Navajos were given voting rights as US citizens. A tribal code of laws, which endorses Navajo customs and traditions, was adopted in 1937; today, legal disputes and minor crimes and offenses taking place on the Navajo territory are tried on the basis of this code by the tribal court. Window Rock (Tsenghah-odzani), a sacred Navajo site for centuries, became the capital of the new territory.

After the formalization of the tribal code, the growing claims for independence of the Navajo nation led to self-government. The underground resources of the area allowed the tribe to get oil's and minerals' royalties from federal industries. The use of the land for traders and missions was permitted under payment of a rent. The income provided by these practices allowed the tribe to improve farming and herding techniques, and to start new enterprises, such as coal mines, timber mills, handicraft centers, motels, coffee shops and other tourists' facilities (Locke, 1976).

During the twentieth century, the Navajos have gradually improved their material, economic, and political conditions. The process of modernization did not destroy the traditional system of values and the basic structure of the society, as often happens with assimilation. Formal education, and the acquisition of skills in the fields of management, technology, and commerce are slowly contributing to the emancipation of the people; at the same time, the awareness of "Navajoness" is kept alive among young people by means of the traditional family organization, religious ceremonies, and a growing production in literature, arts, and handicrafts.

Since 1975, the Indian Self-Determination and Educational Assistance Act has enabled American-Indian communities to enact self-determination through community-based schooling. Several studies have shown the chief role of these institutions to promote individual and collective self-determination (Manuelito, 2005). In this domain the Diné College (first named Navajo Community College, NCC) is the most prominent actualization of the tribe's bicultural strategy. Established in 1968, it is a public institution, which offers certificates and credits to attend 4-years colleges. The architectural structure of the buildings and the educational programs are designed to meet the challenges of biculturalism and integration. The former is based on the circle and the octagone, the two traditional and sacred shapes Navajo dwellings and ceremonial buildings are based on. The latter is centered on the implementation of Navajo self-identity: vocational and technical training, courses in mathematics, natural science, business, humanities, and social sciences are combined with the study of the Navajo language, mythology, philosophy, and with applied research programs specifically dealing with the needs and problems of the American-Indian cultures. One of the chief missions of the college is to provide post-secondary education for Navajos as individuals and as a nation, in order to increase their productive participation in the larger society and their capacity to control their own destiny. This is a bicultural goal par excellence, and it reveals the effort to give the students self-awareness both as members of the tribe, and as citizens of a modern western nation.

During the last decades, the Navajo population steadily increased to 255,000 people (2001 tribal enrolment data). The numbers of hospitals, schools, and tribal government offices have increased. Many wage jobs are available in the Navajo Nation, mostly comprising are clerical and service occupations filled by women. Men have been able to find jobs in strip mining, forestry, and large-scale agriculture, even though these jobs have been declining. Many Navajos commute daily to towns outside the reservation, to work in fast food restaurants, grocery stores, gas stations, and motels (Lamphere, 2007).

During several visits to the Navajos, we tried to detect the bicultural traits embedded in subjective experience and personal growth patterns. To this purpose, we collected data through the flow questionnaire in two groups of participants: 58 students at Ganado High School (34 girls and 24 boys aged 14–19), and 79 students

Table 13.4 Percentage distribution of optimal activities among Navajo participants

Optimal activities	High school	Diné College
Work	8.3	11.5
Studying/reading	25.0	30.9
Interactions	11,1	7.9
Leisure	43.1	27.3
Media	5.6	5.0
Introspection	6.9	10.8
Religious practice	–	6.6
N answers	72	139

Note: N high school participants = 37; N Diné College participants = 69.

and teachers at the Diné College (51 women and 28 men aged 19–44). Ganado High School is a western-style institution: most of the teachers are European-Americans, the teaching language is English, the curricula and recreation activities are typical of any US high school. But the students are Native Americans, and when they come back home they often live in a traditional joint family environment. Among the participants in our study, 63% spoke both Navajo and English, while 34% spoke only English: modernization had a strong influence on the transmission of cultural information through the generations, undermining the original knowledge and habits. Among participants at Diné College the percentage of native language speakers hit 87.3%. Today, an increasing number of Navajo students learn their native language at college for the first time. Thus, formal education seems to successfully counterbalance the impoverishment of the culture provoked by assimilation. This very fact points out the key role of Diné College in fostering the preservation and development of the Navajo culture.

Among high-school students, 37 (63.8%) reported optimal experiences in their lives, while the percentage increased to 82.2% at Diné College. This difference can be partially explained with the age of the participants (see Chapter 7). The distribution of optimal activities also differed between the two groups, as shown in Table 13.4.

Leisure was the prominent opportunity for optimal experience among adolescents, followed by studying and reading, but with a much lower percentage of answers. Diné College participants reported a more homogeneous distribution of the answers in the different categories: studying and reading—the Navajo bicultural activities par excellence—prevailed, closely followed by leisure; working and thinking came next.

Differences between the two groups also emerged in the specific activities quoted within each domain. Among adolescents, leisure mostly included western sports, such as football, basketball, jogging, and volleyball, while Diné College participants quoted both traditional practices, such as hunting, fishing, and wandering in the countryside, and modern sports and hobbies.

Additional group differences were detected in the domains of work and religion. Not surprisingly, college members had more opportunities and necessity to work.

Navajos still marry very young: several students at Diné College were married and had children, the campus offers dormitories for families. Interestingly enough, however, the work activities more often associated with optimal experience by these participants were traditional ones: silversmithing, weaving, and cooking. Only four answers related to modern tasks, such as typewriting, welding, and repairing cars. As for religious practices—participating in Navajo ceremonies and praying—they were uniquely quoted by Diné College participants (as specifically discussed in Chapter 12).

The category "introspection" was associated with optimal experience by both groups. Among the Navajos, there is a deep respect for the individual. Although group and family ties are the essential woof of society, the integrity, and freedom of the single person are very important values (Chisholm, 1995; Kluckhohn & Leighton, 1974). In addition, the nomadic pastoralist tradition and the dispersion of the home sites throughout wide spaces and prairies encourage the habit of solitude and the attitude toward lonely reflections and meditation (this aspect was discussed in detail in Chapter 10). Children's raising practices are characterized by a close physical contact with the mother, but by limited verbal interaction. This custom is spread in most southern and eastern Asian cultures; it is not surprising that it is retained by a society originally settled in Asia. The attitude toward silence, quietness, and meditation can moreover be partially traced back to a biological trait shared with Sino-Mongolian populations, as research studies on Navajo newborns have highlighted (Freedman, 1979).

Table 13.5 proposes a description of these findings based on the traditional, bicultural, or modernized features of the optimal activities. Traditional activities comprise work, leisure, and religious practices strictly belonging to the Navajo culture: herding sheep, weaving rugs, attending healing ceremonies, meditating in solitude, hunting, wandering in the prairie. Bicultural activities include studying and reading, which Navajos decided to use as "the ladder" to face the challenge of integration. Modernized activities consist of originally Western jobs, sports, and hobbies, such as repairing cars, playing basketball or football, watching TV, going to the movies, and listening to rock music. As the table shows, high-school students reported a slight prevalence of modernized activities, but the percentage differences between the three activity categories were substantially irrelevant. Diné College members reported bicultural optimal activities with a comparatively higher percentage than modernized activities. These results confirm that the bicultural strategy is deeply rooted in Navajo individual behavior. This peculiar cultural feature allowed

Table 13.5 Percentage distribution of the optimal activities reported by Navajo participants according to cultural typologies

Optimal activities	High school	Diné College
Traditional	26.4	29.5
Modernized	29.2	23.7
Bicultural	27.8	33.8
Interactions	8.3	3.6
Other	8.3	9.4
N answers	72	139

the Navajos to resist the persistent and potentially disruptive impact of westernization. Participants interviewed in this study had been exposed to modernization and western values since their childhood, due to the contents and teaching style of most primary and secondary schools within the Navajo nation (Ismail & Cazden, 2005). Experiencing the gap between their Navajo traditions and the culture acquired at school, Navajo children precociously learn to find a compromise between the two sets of information, cultivating the sense of belonging to their own tradition, and at the same time developing the skills and behaviors which will allow them to successfully integrate into the American life (Dole & Csordas, 2003; Jones & Galliher, 2007).

In these pages, we deliberately overlooked the social and psychological problems Navajos have to face in their daily life, as US citizens, tribe members, and human beings. A large amount of essays have dealt with health care problems such as alcoholism (Kunitz, 1996, 2008; Kunitz & Levy, 1994; May et al., 2002) and with the psychological difficulties faced by Native adolescents and adults living in a modernized and multiethnic setting (Garrett & Myers, 1996; Rieckmann et al., 2004; Topper & Curtis, 1987; Zimmerman, Ramirez-Valles, Washienko, Walter, & Dyer, 1996). On the contrary, our aim was to point out the strengths of Navajo culture, emphasizing the evolutionary advantages of the Navajo bicultural strategy at the social level, and the fundamental role of daily psychological selection in supporting this bicultural trend.

13.4 Concluding Remarks

The findings obtained from these studies suggest that, independent of predictors of socio-cultural adjustment and of acculturation patterns, the opportunities for retrieval of optimal experience available to immigrants and members of ethnic minorities can shed light on their overall quality of life, and on the acculturation strategies they are adopting.

Moreover, findings suggest the need for taking into account the individual long-term expectations in acculturation research. The data gathered among East European women highlighted that in spite of similarities in daily life, job, and social roles, and also in spite of similarities in experience fluctuation, the long-term dimensions of goals, life projects, and meaning have to be taken into account in order to understand the role of flow—and of the other daily experiences—within the process of psychological selection.

Acculturation should not to be considered only in negative terms: it can provide individuals with new opportunities for learning and growth, as the studies on biculturalism and our own findings have highlighted. However, the effort an individual has to perform in the acculturation process is too often not rewarded. In several cases integration remains a remote goal, or—even worse—an unrealistic ideal.

The main problem for immigrants and minority members is represented by social stereotypes and prejudices, not necessarily developed out of previous historical contacts, which may heavily obstacle their integration. As pointed out by Brislin and

Horvarth (1997), "the willingness to empathize and to comprehend is not universal" (p. 330), and members of the dominant groups are often not aware of the migrants' efforts and of the complexity of the integration pathway.

More systematic studies on cultural differences are welcome in the affluent countries of Europe and North America. It is also important to develop intervention programs concerned with multiculturalism, at the occupational and educational levels, to facilitate job participation of immigrants and minority members, and school integration of their children. This is a necessary tribute to the improvement and enrichment citizens from abroad are bringing to western knowledge and experience of the reality.

References

Al-Issa I. (Ed.). (1995). *Handbook of culture and mental illness: An international perspective*. Madison, CT: International Universities Press.

Ataca, B., & Berry, J. W. (2002). Psychological, sociocultural and marital adaptation of Turkish immigrant couples in Canada. *International Journal of Psychology, 37*, 13–26.

Aycan, Z., & Berry, J. W. (1996). Impact of employment-related experiences on immigrants' adaptation to Canada. *Canadian Journal of Behavioral Science, 28*, 240–251.

Benet-Martinez, V., Lee, F., & Leu, J. (2006). Biculturalism and cognitive complexity. Expertise in cultural representations. *Journal of Cross-Cultural Psychology, 37*, 386–407.

Berry, J. W. (1997). Immigration, acculturation, and adaptation. *Applied Psychology: An International Review, 46*, 5–34.

Berry, J. W. (2001). A psychology of immigration. *Journal of Social Issues, 57*, 615–631.

Berry, J. W., Kim, U., Minde, T., & Mok, D. (1987). Comparative studies of acculturative stress. *International Migration Review, 21*, 491–511.

Berry, J. W., & Sam, D. L. (1997). Acculturation and adaptation. In J. W. Berry, M. H. Segall, & C. Kagitçibasi (Eds.), *Handbook of cross-cultural psychology: Vol. 3. Social Behavior and Applications* (pp. 1–49). Needam Heights, MA: Allyn & Bacon.

Brislin, R., & Horvarth, A. -M. (1997). Cross-cultural training and multicultural education. In J. W. Berry, M. H. Segall, & C. Kagitçibasi (Eds.), *Handbook of cross-cultural psychology: Vol. 3. Social behavior and applications* (pp. 327–369). Boston: Allyn & Bacon.

Caritas/Migrantes. (2005). *XV dossier statistico sull'immigrazione*. Roma: Centro Studi e Ricerche IDOS.

Chisholm, J. S. (1995). Learning 'respect for everything': Navajo images of development. In L. J. Crockett & A. C. Crouter (Eds.), *Pathways through adolescence*. Mahwah, NJ: Lawrence Erlbaum Associates, Inc.

Collins, R. (Ed.). (1991). *The native Americans: The indigenous people of North America*. London: Salamander Books.

Delle Fave, A., & Bassi, M. (2009). Sharing optimal experiences and promoting good community life in a multicultural society. *Journal of Positive Psychology, 4*, 280–289.

Delle Fave, A., & Massimini, F. (1991). Modernization and the quality of daily experience in a southern Italy village. In N. Bleichrodt & P. J. D. Drenth (Eds.), *Contemporary issues in cross-cultural psychology* (pp. 110–119). Amsterdam: Swets & Zeitlinger B.V.

Delle Fave, A., & Massimini, F. (1999). Inter-cultural relations: A challenge for psychology. In A. Delle Fave & F. Meli (Eds.), *Modernization and cultural identity* (pp. 11–22). Milano: Edizioni Dell'Arco.

Delle Fave, A., & Massimini, F. (2004). The cross-cultural investigation of optimal experience. *Ricerche di Psicologia, 27*, 79–102.

Dole, C., & Csordas, T. J. (2003). Trials of Navajo youth: identity, healing, and the struggle for maturity. *Ethos, 31*, 357–384.

Downs, J. F. (1972). *The Navajo*. New York: Holt, Rinehart and Winston, Inc.
Emmons, R. A. (2005). Striving for the sacred: personal goals, life meaning, and religion. *Journal of Social Issues, 61*, 731–745.
Fianco, A., & Delle Fave, A. (2006). Donne migranti e qualità dell'esperienza soggettiva: uno studio con experience sampling method. *Passaggi. Rivista Italiana di Scienze Transculturali, 11*, 101–122.
Finch, B. K., & Vega, A. W. (2003). Acculturation stress, social support, and self-rated health among Latinos in California. *Journal of Immigrant Health, 5*, 109–117.
Freedman, D. G. (1979). *Human sociobiology*. New York: Academic Press.
Fuchs, E., & Havighurst, R. J. (1972). *To live on this earth. American Indian education*. Garden City, NY: Doubleday and Company, Inc.
Garrett, M. T., & Myers, J. E. (1996). The rule of opposites: A paradigm for counseling Native Americans. *Journal of Multicultural Counseling and Development, 24*, 89–104.
Gong, Y., & Chang, S. (2007). The relationships of cross-cultural adjustment with dispositional learning orientation and goal setting. *Journal of Cross-cultural Psychology, 38*, 19–25.
Ismail, S. M., & Cazden, C. B. (2005). Struggles for indigenous education and self-determination: Culture, context, and collaboration. *Anthropology & Education Quarterly, 36*, 88–92.
Jasinskaja-Lathi, I., Liebkind, K, Jaakkola, M., & Reuter, A. (2006). Perceived discrimination, social support networks, and psychological well-being among three immigrant groups. Journal of Cross-Cultural Psychology, 37, 293–311.
Jones, M. D., & Galliher, R. V. (2007). Ethnic identity and psychosocial functioning in Navajo adolescents. *Journal of Research on Adolescence, 17*, 683–696.
Juthani, N. V. (1992). Immigrant mental health: Conflicts & concerns on Indian immigrants in the U.S. *Psychology & Developing Societies, 4*, 133–148.
Kazarian, S. S., & Evans, D. R. (2001). *Handbook of cultural health psychology*. San Diego, CA: Academic Press.
Kluckhohn, C., & Leighton, D. (1974). *The Navaho*. Cambridge, MA: Harvard University Press.
Kunitz, S. J. (1996). The history and politics of US health care policy for American Indians and Alaskan natives. *American Journal of Public Health, 86*, 1464–1473.
Kunitz, S. J. (2008). Risk factors for polydrug use in a Native American population. *Substance Use & Misuse, 43*, 331–339.
Kunitz, S. J., & Levy, J. E. (1994). *Drinking careers: A twenty-five year follow-up of three Navajo populations*. New Haven, CT: Yale University Press.
LaFromboise, T., Coleman, H. L. K., & Gerton, J. (1993). Psychological impact of biculturalism: Evidence and theory. *Psychological Bulletin, 114*, 395–412.
LaFromboise, T., & Rowe, W. (1983). Skill training for bicultural competence. Rationale and application. *Journal of Counseling Psychology, 30*, 589–595.
Lamphere, L. (2007). Migration, assimilation and the cultural construction of identity: Navajo perspectives. *Ethnic and Racial Studies, 30*, 1132–1151.
Locke, R. F. (1976). *The book of the Navajo*. Los Angeles: Mankind Publishing Company.
Luckert, K. W. (1975). *The Navajo hunter tradition*. Tucson, AZ: The University of Arizona Press.
Manuelito, K. (2005). The role of education in American Indian self-determination: Lessons from the Ramah Navajo community school. *Anthropology & Education Quarterly., 36*, 73–87.
Matsunaga, M., Hecte, M. L., Elek, E., & Ndiaye, K. (2010). Ethnic identity development ad acculturation: A longitudinal analysis of Mexican-heritage youth in the southwest United States. *Journal of Cross-Cultural Psychology, 41*, 410–427.
May, P. A., Van Winkle, N. W., Williams, M. B., McFeeley, P. J., DeBruyn, L. M., & Serna, P. (2002). Alcohol and suicide death among American Indians of new Mexico: 1980–1998. *Suicide and Life-Threatening Behavior, 32*, 240–255.
Noh, S., & Kaspar, V. (2003). Perceived discrimination and depression: Moderating effect of coping, acculturation and ethnic support. *American Journal of Public Health, 93*, 232–238.
Phinney, J. S., Horenczyk, G., Liebkind, K., & Vedder, P. (2001). Ethnic identity, immigration, and well-being: An interactional perspective. *Journal of Social Issues, 57*, 493–510.

Redfield, R., Linton, R., & Herskovits, M. J. (1936). Memorandum on the study of acculturation. *American Anthropologist, 38*, 149–152.

Reichard, G. (1950). *Navaho religion. A study of symbolism*. New York: Bollingen.

Rieckmann, T. R., Wadsworth, M. E., & Deyhle, D. (2004). Cultural identity, explanatory style, and depression in Navajo adolescents. *Cultural Diversity and Ethnic Minority Psychology, 10*, 365–382.

Searle, W., & Ward, C. (1990). The prediction of psychological and sociocultural adjustment during cross-cultural transitions. *International Journal of Intercultural Relations, 14*, 449–464.

Sen, A. (1992). *Inequality reexamined*. Oxford: Oxford University Press.

Sheldon, K. M., Elliot, A. J., Ryan, R. M., Chirkov, V., Kim, Y., Wu, C., et al. (2004). Self-concordance and subjective well-being in four cultures. *Journal of Cross-cultural Psychology, 35*, 209–223.

Swarup, W., & Delle Fave, A. (1999). From India to Europe: migration and the quality of experience. In A. Delle Fave & F. Meli (Eds.), *Modernization and cultural identity* (pp. 103–120). Milano: Edizioni Dell'Arco.

Tadmor, C. T., & Tetlock, P. E. (2006). Biculturalism. A model of the effects of second-culture exposure on acculturation and integrative complexity. *Journal of Cross-Cultural Psychology, 37*, 173–190.

Tadmor, C. T., Tetlock, P. E., & Peng, K. (2009). Acculturation strategies and integrative complexity. The cognitive implications of biculturalism. *Journal of Cross-Cultural Psychology, 40*, 105–139.

Tajfel, H. (1978). *Differentiation between social groups*. London: Academic Press.

Topper, M. D., & Begaye, C. (1978). "Not Navajo life": clinical anthropology, "mental illness" and psychotherapy among the Navajo. In J. L. Steinberg (Ed.), *Cultural factors in the rehabilitation process* (pp. 83–120). Los Angeles: California State University.

Topper, M. D., & Curtis, J. (1987). Extended family therapy: A clinical approach to the treatment of synergistic dual anomic depression among Navajo agency town adolescents. *Journal of Community Psychology, 15*, 334–348.

Trafzer, C. E. (1978a). *Navajos and Spaniards*. Tsaile, AZ: Navajo Community College Press.

Trafzer, C. E. (1978b). *The Navajos and the first Anglos*. Tsaile, AZ: Navajo Community College Press.

Trimble, J. E., & Medicine, B. (1993). Diversification of American Indians. In U. Kim & J. W. Berry (Eds.), *Indigenous psychologies* (pp. 133–151). Newbury Park, CA: Sage.

Underhill, R. M. (1948). Ceremonial patterns in the greater Southwest. *American Ethnological Society Monographs, XIII*.

Underhill, R. M. (1967). *The Navajos* (Rev. Ed.). Norman: University of Oklahoma Press.

Ward, C. (2001). The A, B, Cs of acculturation. In D. Matsumoto (Ed.), *The handbook of culture and psychology* (pp. 411–445). Oxford: Oxford Univ. Press

Ward, C., & Kennedy, A. (1993). Where's the "culture" in cross-cultural transitions? Comparative studies on sojourner adjustment. *Journal of Cross-cultural Psychology, 24*, 221–249.

Ward, C., & Kennedy, A. (1994). Acculturation strategies, psychological adjustment, and sociocultural competence during cross-cultural transitions. *International Journal of Intercultural Relations, 18*, 329–343.

Zimmerman, M. A., Ramirez-Valles, J., Washienko, K. M., Walter, B., & Dyer, S. (1996). The development of a measure of enculturation for Native American youth. *American Journal of Community Psychology, 24*, 295–310.

Zlobina, A., Basabe, N., Paez, D., & Furnham, A. (2006). Sociocultural adjustment of immigrants: Universal and group predictors. *International Journal of Intercultural Relations, 30*, 195–211.

Chapter 14
Flow and Health: A Bio-psycho-social Perspective

14.1 Introduction

More than any other topic we have dealt with in this book, health is *par excellence* related to the biological survival of the human species. Disease, treatment, and prevention have been prominent objects of investigation and resource investments in all cultures (Delle Fave & Massimini, 2001, 2005). Disease, in both its physical and mental components, represents a privileged topic of psychology, which—throughout its history—has primarily focused on identifying pathologies and strategies and procedures to cope with them. This chapter proposes a cultural revolution in the approach to health, stemming from the positive psychology movement. To this purpose, we will focus on the constructive side of disease, outlining the individual and environmental resources that can promote well-being and life fulfillment in spite of biological limitations. Optimal experience can play a prominent role in this process (Delle Fave & Massimini, 2005; Delle Fave, 2006).

14.2 The Three Dimensions of Health

Definitions of health vary according to cultures and historical grounds (Delle Fave & Bassi, 2007; Jones, 2004). We can identify different conceptualizations whether we ask the layman or the expert, a person from Europe or from Asia, a sociologist or an economist. Moreover, these definitions undergo constant changes over time (Levin & Browner, 2005).

Western medicine, which has become the predominant approach throughout the world, has been based for decades on a strictly problem-centered *biomedical model.* Physicians pay attention to the specific symptoms reported by their patients, and try to trace these symptoms back to a well-defined pathology, involving a specific body organ or apparatus. Patients are therefore treated for a specific illness, irrespective of how their environment, social context, and subjective experience influence the onset and the outcomes of disease. Based on the superiority of science over bodies of lay knowledge, the biomedical model emphasizes objective measurement of disease through, for example, the assessment of physiological parameters

A. Delle Fave et al., *Psychological Selection and Optimal Experience Across Cultures*, Cross-Cultural Advancements in Positive Psychology 2,
DOI 10.1007/978-90-481-9876-4_14, © Springer Science+Business Media B.V. 2011

(Arnold, Ranchor, Koëter, De Jongste, & Sanderman, 2005). From this deterministic perspective, health is synonymous with objective health, considered as a physical condition, which can be measured objectively.

This model has provided important advancements in understanding and treating disease, as well as in planning social and international policies aimed at granting adequate standards of health and assistance to all (Hernández-Quevedo, Jones, López-Nicolás, & Rice, 2006). However, limitations were first pointed out by Engel (1977, 1982), who formalized the *bio-psycho-social model* in which a systems approach to illness and health was applied. In particular, Engel's model emphasizes the active role of the individual both in the etiopathogenesis and in the treatment process. It focuses on the patient as a person, that is a complex living system, an individual with a subjective interpretation of health, disease, quality of life, and well-being, and also a carrier of a specific cultural background and a member of a particular society.

The multidimensional nature of health was promptly acknowledged by most international health agencies and institutions. However, it had already been highlighted by WHO in 1946 that health is a state of complete physical, mental, and social well-being, and not merely the absence of disease or infirmity. More recently, an analogous definition was provided for mental health, described as a state of well-being in which the individual realizes his or her own abilities, can cope with the normal stresses of life, can work productively and fruitfully, and is able to make a contribution to her community (WHO 2004).

14.3 A Positive Perspective on Health and Disease

The international endorsement of the bio-psycho-social model led to a thorough revision of the existing classifications of diseases and disabilities, which brought forth the new International Classification of Functioning (ICF; WHO 2001). ICF includes a marked shift in terminology, from pathology and constraints (impairments, disabilities, handicaps) to health and resources (functioning), from the consequences of disease to the components of health. Far from being a pure linguistic convention, a relevant conceptual change underlies this shift, namely the need to evaluate any health condition from a constructive, subjective, and substantially positive perspective. ICF aims at investigating what people with different health conditions can do in their daily life and in their social context, emphasizing the active role of the person in interacting with the environment, in terms of physical resources, daily activity performance, and social participation.

It is worth noticing that this shift from objective measurement to subjective evaluation, from absence of disease to presence of well-being, from the negative to the positive, from cure to prevention and health promotion is at the core of positive psychology, as illustrated in Chapter 1 (Seligman & Csikszentmihalyi, 2000). Researchers in positive psychology and, before them, pioneer scholars in the study of well-being have focused on two issues (Delle Fave & Bassi, 2007). First of all, health and disease are not opposite ends of a continuum; rather, they represent at least partially independent dimensions, which, in principle, can be simultaneously present and can exert mutual influences. For example, studies have shown that in expressing a judgment about their conditions, individuals take into consideration qualitatively different factors. Sick people usually mention somatic symptoms such as pain or fatigue, whereas healthy individuals commonly refer to their overall level of functioning in daily activities (Kaplan & Baron-Epel, 2003). Among patients with a chronic disease, the physical disorder by itself is not directly related to perceived health: Such judgment is rather connected to a number of variables, including the level of functioning and perceived control (Arnold et al., 2005). The distinction between health and disease at the physical level has also been proposed at the mental level (see Section 14.4.1). According to Keyes (2002, 2007), mental health and mental illness lie on separate continua, and identifying mental health with absence of psychiatric disorder is not correct. For example, each year 90% of the adult population in the United States does not report episodes of major depression, but we cannot consequently conclude that these individuals are mentally healthy. Based on these findings, the absence of disorder can be a necessary but not sufficient criterion for mental health evaluation.

The second issue in well-being research regards the attempt to operationalize health and disease as complex bio-psycho-social constructs, and not as separate life domains, in order to promote individuals' thriving in their living context. To this purpose, a wide range of quality of life indicators were identified (WHOQOL Group, 2006), including physical health, psychological well-being, independence, social relations, environmental factors, spirituality, religion, and personal beliefs. Other models were fully described in Chapter 1: They range from the strictly hedonic approach of subjective well-being (Diener, 2009) to broad eudaimonic theories of personal growth. In particular, the latter have provided interesting results in the health sector, as positive emotions are often not compatible with physical illness and suffering. Quality of life should be considered as a relative and subjective concept, involving perceived opportunities for action and skill development in the daily environment, social relations, and the setting and pursuit of goals, which are not necessarily dependent on physical functioning or on material affluence (Fitzpatrick, 2000). Individuals develop a personal evaluation of what a good quality of life means, according to criteria such as values, beliefs, goal hierarchy, personality, and idiosyncratic styles of interaction with the environment (Delle Fave Massimini 2004a). Objective indicators, and in particular physical health conditions, only partially influence this evaluation.

Several studies supported this approach. For example, Albrecht and Devliger (1999) found that 54.3% of people with serious disablement rated their quality of life as excellent or good. Sodergren and Hyland (2000) interviewed people currently sick or recovering from disease about the positive consequences of their illness. Participants reported answers such as improved interpersonal relationships, positive personality changes, life reappraisal and restructuring. These results are related to processes such as benefit finding (Tennen & Affleck, 2002) and post-traumatic growth (Tedeschi & Calhoun, 1995). In their turn, positive consequences influence physical health in the long term (King & Miner, 2000). Affleck, Tennen, Croog, and

Levine (1987) found that 8 years after experiencing a heart attack, participants who had reported benefits had better cardiac functionality and were less likely to have suffered another attack. Analogously, the perception of positive changes contributes to mobilizing the immune system defense (LeShan, 1994).

Positive psychology is greatly contributing to the identification of the personal and social resources underlying adjustment to illness conditions, benefit finding, and post-traumatic growth. One of the first researchers interested in the psychological factors involved in the adaptation to disease was Antonovsky (1987), who developed the concept of *salutogenesis* (as opposed to pathogenesis). From his perspective, individuals differ in their reaction to negative events and conditions, based on the strategies they use to cope with stress. Some people report a good quality of life in adverse situations, such as disease. This positive adaptation is related to the *sense of coherence* (SOC), a general orientation of the individual toward reality, according to which people who believe that any life event or situation can ultimately be comprehensible, manageable, and meaningful—at least to a certain extent—are able to find and bring order and organization in apparently ambiguous and disruptive situations. Particularly relevant in SOC is the attribution of meaning to life events (Baumeister & Vohs, 2002; see Section 1.2.1.2), and the ability to transform one's narrative identity in the wake of traumatic events, in order to gain new insights about the self (Bauer, McAdams, & Pals, 2008).

Interesting results also stem from *Self-Determination Theory* (SDT; Deci & Ryan, 2000; Ryan, Patrick, Deci, & Williams, 2008; Chapter 1). The fulfillment of the needs for autonomy, competence, and relatedness fosters well-being in adverse health conditions, and facilitates the adoption of preventive behaviors in healthy individuals (Sheldon, Williams, & Joiner, 2003). In particular, the support of patients' autonomy proved to promote their better adherence to medical treatments (Williams, Rodin, Ryan, Grolnick, & Deci, 1998). Autonomy-supportive physicians encourage their patients to take part in the therapeutic process, involve them in the active sharing of responsibility in the selection of treatment, and foster their capacity of self-monitoring and awareness (Williams & Deci, 1998). The benefits of this approach were highlighted in studies with obese patients and heavy smokers: Increased levels of self-determination and autonomy were correlated with weight and smoking reduction, respectively, and with the long-term maintenance of related healthy habits (Williams & Deci, 2001; Williams, Grow, Freedman, Ryan, & Deci, 1996).

Other constructs that were fruitfully applied in the health sector comprise optimism, resilience, hope, and self-efficacy. *Optimism* can be described as a generally positive orientation toward life, characterized by positive expectations for the future (Peterson, 2000). It can be indirectly related to a genetic component (Schulman, Keith, & Seligman, 1993); however, it can also be learned, thus representing an important basis for intervention in well-being promotion. Schwarzer (1994, 1998) distinguished between defensive optimism and functional optimism. The former includes the unrealistic overestimation of the person's control of an adverse condition, for example, an uncontrollable disease, with a consequent biased risk perception. In contrast, functional optimism involves the belief in the person's ability to cope with the demands of the situation, and it is therefore an adaptive component of health behavior. Several studies confirmed the positive impact of optimism in promoting health and well-being in conditions of disease. Optimism proved to play a protective role against the development of post-partum depression (Carver & Gaines, 1987), and was associated with lower levels of distress after the diagnosis of breast cancer (Carver et al., 1993). Optimism also fostered faster recovery and better quality of life in patients undergoing coronary bypass surgery (Scheier et al., 1989). It proved to be useful also in facing temporary and controllable disease conditions. Research work highlighted that optimists were more active and engaged in solving a problem than pessimists. Similarly, in situations of chronic or degenerative disease, characterized by low controllability and impossibility to solve the problem, optimists were more effective in finding positive ways to cope with the situation, through active acceptance of the related changes and constraints, and through the re-definition of goals and life meanings (Greer, Morris, Pettingale, & Haybittle, 1990; Scheier & Carver, 2001; Shepperd, Maroto, & Pbert, 1996). Individuals with an optimistic attributional style reported higher levels of physical and mental health (Peterson & Park, 1998), a healthier lifestyle (Peterson, Seligman, & Vaillant, 1988) and a lower exposure to risky behaviors (Peterson, Seligman, Yurko, Martin, & Friedman, 1998).

Hope was defined as the ability to identify goals, to detect adequate and realistic ways to achieve them, and to mobilize the motivational resources needed to accomplish this task (Snyder, 1994, 1998; Snyder, Rand, & Sigmon, 2002). Several studies have investigated the impact of hope on well-being. Individuals high in hope showed better and faster adaptation to stress conditions; moreover, in situations of change that required a revision and a modification of previous goals and plans, they showed higher flexibility in identifying alternative goals (Michael, 2000). These characteristics of hope turn out to be especially relevant in the domain of health. Individuals high in hope follow a healthier lifestyle and are more concerned with prevention behaviors. In case of disease, high levels of hope showed to be positively correlated with a better adaptation and a more effective coping style in facing the consequences of medullary lesions (Elliott, Kurylo, & Rivera, 2002), fibromyalgia (Affleck & Tennen, 1996), and blindness (Jackson, Taylor, Palmatier, Elliott, & Elliott, 1998). From the emotional point of view, sick people who report high levels of hope tend to invest their attention and resources on attainable goals, rather than on the disease itself, and on the negative feelings that can arise in this condition (Snyder & Pulvers, 2001). Similarly, other studies showed that hope was positively correlated with positive affect, and negatively correlated with negative emotions (Snyder et al., 1996).

Resilience has been described as a state of optimal functioning and successful adaptation in spite of adverse environmental conditions (Masten & Reed, 2002). Little research has so far been conducted on the role of resilience in coping with adverse health conditions. However, available studies suggest the importance of supporting resilience in patients and their families. For example, an investigation was conducted among people with amyotrophic lateral sclerosis (ALS) and their family caregivers (Rabkin, Wagner, & Del Bene, 2000). No significant correlations were detected between perceived level of functioning and the severity of the disease outcomes. On the contrary, a positive correlation was found between the levels of adaptation and functioning of the patients and those of their family members. This finding confirms the pivotal role of satisfying family relationships as a resource in the process of adaptation to adverse health conditions. Moreover, one of the basic aspects of resilience is its dynamic structure. Resilience is not a personality trait; people can be trained to become resilient in the face of difficult situations. This is an important prerequisite to develop intervention programs addressed to patients and their families, especially when the patient is a child, and the impact of parents' behavior and attitude toward disease is of primary importance. The family system illness, an intervention model based on the promotion of patients' and caregivers' resilience in coping with disease, was developed and fruitfully applied (Rolland, 2005; Rolland and Walsh 2005; Walsh 2003).

Individuals usually decide whether to engage in a specific behavior or to avoid it, on the basis of two main evaluations: their perception of control of the situation, and their perceived level of competence in pursuing and attaining desired achievements. *Self-efficacy* can be defined as the level of competence an individual perceives in facing a specific situation (Bandura, 1997, 2004); therefore it is strictly related to the perceived locus of control. In particular, high levels of self-efficacy are associated with the perception of an internal locus of control. This can be useful in coping with adverse health conditions, since people high in self-efficacy face negative life events in an active way, perceiving themselves as directly responsible for their outcomes. Moreover, in situations characterized by low controllability—such as permanent disabilities or the terminal stage of a disease—self-efficacious individuals are also advantaged, in that their perception of an adequate level of competence allows them to develop effective coping strategies, a good management of emotions and the capacity to set and attain realistic goals (Hurley & Shea, 1992; Merluzzi & Sanchez, 1997; Schwarzer & Fuchs, 1996). Self-efficacy can be enhanced and implemented through the gradual building of competences and perceived mastery (Moore, 2002), and through the observation of exemplary models. In the domain of health, and especially in chronic diseases, this is particularly important to promote patients' well-being and positive adjustment in the long term (Kuijer & deRidder, 2003).

Finally, religiosity and spirituality have been linked to the promotion of health, and to the positive interpretation and acceptance of disease, as outlined in Chapter 12.

14.4 Retrieving Optimal Experience in Extraordinary Circumstances

Can people with chronic health conditions experience flow? Can they build their autonomous life theme over time? To what extent do disease and trauma affect individuals' psychological selection? Does mental health influence the opportunities for and the contents of optimal experiences? What social and cultural resources can patients have access to? These are some of the questions we tackle in the following sections.

14.4.1 Living with Chronic Disease

One of the crucial findings repeatedly obtained in our field research is that people with chronic health conditions, such as motor or sensory disabilities, can retrieve opportunities for optimal experience in their lives, like any other individual in good health, and can build their own life themes, based on personal goals, meaningful challenges, and available skills (Delle Fave & Massimini, 2004a; Delle Fave, 2010). In spite of the widespread prejudice according to which physical disability is synonymous with lack of satisfaction and well-being (Weinberg, 1988), objective physical impairments do not prevent individuals from living a full life. As reported by Saravanan et al. (2001), people with disabilities perceive themselves as ordinary persons coping with extraordinary circumstances.

In particular, this is the case of individuals who have developed disabilities in early age, and have ever since coped with their physical conditions on a daily basis. In a pilot study in collaboration with AIAS (Italian Association for Assistance to People with Spastic Diseases), we administered a shortened version of flow questionnaire (FQ) and life theme questionnaire (LT) to a group of ten adolescents diagnosed with infant cerebral palsy (ICP) (see Chapter 4 for questionnaire description). These teenagers had attended rehabilitation sessions at the AIAS center ever since childhood, in order to improve or at least maintain their motor functioning. To this purpose, the great majority of them also underwent a series of invasive surgical interventions during adolescence, primarily aiming at elongating tendons, rotating bones and muscles, thus favoring walking.

For exemplification purposes, in Boxes 14.1 and 14.2 we report the answers of two participants to some relevant questions included in FQ and LT.

The analysis of the participants' answers highlighted some common themes, as well as perceived resources and barriers. Teenagers identified optimal experiences in their lives and related them not only to typical adolescents' activities such as studying, reading, meeting friends, but also to activities they had discovered because of their health conditions, such as horse riding, which is part of the therapy program. Disability posed them difficult challenges to be faced with courage and persistence, and they were proud to quote integration and school success as personal accomplishments. Their prominent future goals—finding a job and having a family—were shared by most participants examined with the two questionnaires across cultures, and represented essential elements of a meaningful life (Chapter 7; Delle Fave, 2009; Delle Fave, Brdar, Freire, Vella-Brodrick, & Wissing, 2010).

Participants further reported the crucial role of family and friends in facing the challenges and problems connected with disability. Disability did not negatively affect important relations with beloved ones, even though parents may become overprotective toward their sick children. At the same time, ignorance and prejudice at

Box 14.1

Participant	Boy, 18 years old
Diagnosis	Spastic paraparesis (initially quadriparesis)
Education	Secondary school degree (social worker)
Optimal activities	Reading Studying
Positive influences	My parents My grandparents
Negative influences	My grandfather's death
Accomplishments	Having had a normal life Having succeeded in integrating
Current challenges	To overcome architectural barriers To use public means of transport
Future goals	To have a family To find a job
Disability	
Has disability influenced your life till now?	I have problems in moving
Do you think it will influence your future? How?	Yes. My condition lasts for the whole life, but it can be attenuated
Does it influence your family relations? How?	No
Does it influence the relations with your friends? How?	Yes, again in moving . . . and I am lazy. . .

Box 14.2

Participant	Girl, 17 years old
Diagnosis	Spastic paraparesis
Education	Attending secondary school (tourist operator)
Optimal activities	Riding
Positive influences	The last operation; it changed my life My grandmother Beloved ones
Negative influences	Friends at the elementary school who made fun of me
Accomplishments	The love of those people I care for Having shown teachers that I can make it even with my physical problems
Current challenges	To be able to walk like anybody else so that I can take a revenge on those who laughed at me

Future goals	To travel To have a family To have many dogs
Disability	
Has disability influenced your life till now?	Yes
Do you think it will influence your future? How?	No, because the worst is over
Does it influence your family relations? How?	Positively: they give me a lot of attentions Negatively: my brothers envy me because they do not receive the same amount of attentions
Does it influence the relations with your friends? How?	No

the social level as well as environmental barriers were identified as obstacles in the process of becoming autonomous, restricting participants' opportunities to explore the wider world outside the family circle. Particularly interesting are the answers provided to the direct questions on the influence of disability on their present and future lives. These adolescents were aware of their disability as a lifelong condition, they did not spend their time in wishful thinking; they rather showed optimism and hope in what they could realistically do to improve their physical conditions.

Some of the themes we identified among young people with ICP were also recurrent in the answers provided by adults who had been affected by motor and perceptual disabilities since birth or at an early age (Bassi & Delle Fave, 2007; Delle Fave & Maletto, 1992; Delle Fave & Massimini, 2004a); Delle Fave, 2010). We collected data among individuals with motor impairments such as paraplegia and quadriplegia, and among blind persons. Data analysis showed that 94.7% of blind people and 92% of people with motor disabilities retrieved optimal experiences in their lives.

While physical conditions per se did not hamper the retrieval of optimal experience in participants' lives, they certainly influenced the kinds of activities individuals could engage in. Blind people primarily reported media-related activities (35.4%) and work tasks (25.3%). The first category comprised reading in Braille, listening to music, "watching" TV; the second one included activities such as typing, knitting, making sweeps and stuffing chairs. Both categories played a relevant role in participants' lives. Media were described as important instruments to get into contact with the outer world, to retrieve information and to keep oneself updated. As for work, the preference for manual activities attested to participants' investment in the sense of touch and to the cultivation of manual dexterity since childhood. People with motor disabilities primarily clustered their answers in the domains of work (29.2%), leisure (27.7%), and to a smaller extent family relations (9.2%). This group placed a characteristic emphasis on relations. Not only were they quoted within the family domain, they also emerged in answers related to work domain (such as talking/helping customers), and in free time (playing chess with a friend; social past time activities).

The participants' descriptions of life theme issues, such as current challenges, personal accomplishments, and future goals, were consistent with findings obtained among adult participants across cultures (Chapter 7), with emphasis placed on family, work, and personal growth. In these categories, however, we also identified semantic areas pertaining to participants' physical conditions. Daily life was perceived as a constant challenge due to environmental barriers, or difficulties in performing simple daily tasks such as cooking and cleaning. For both groups of participants the major accomplishment regarded having obtained a certain degree of autonomy. In addition, blind people reported having found a job they liked, and in which to invest their personal skills. While blind participants were affected by a stable health condition which could hardly worsen, people with motor impairments were constantly confronted with insidious health problems such as pressure ulcers, poor bladder functioning, and limb pain which were reflected in their concern for future autonomy and independent functioning, as well as on preserving health through physical exercise and a healthy lifestyle.

To delve more deeply in the daily lives of people with motor disabilities, we administered ESM to a group of 35 participants aged 22–70, primarily diagnosed with paraplegia (69%) and quadriplegia (17%) (Bassi, Preziosa, & Pozzoli, 2007). The analysis of their daily time-budget highlighted the chief role of maintenance activities (23.3% of the self-reports), the small percentage of time devoted to work (12.5%; only 68.6% of participants had a job), the relatively low frequency of social interactions (11.7%), and the relatively high frequency of watching TV (13.5%). Analyzing daily locations and companionships, we further observed that the participants mostly spent time at home (64.5% of the self-reports) and alone (48.1%). Motor disability as well as environmental and social barriers clearly affected participants' ability to move, limiting the occasions for meeting friends or making new ones. By contrast, the participants attributed utmost importance to relations, which represented the most frequent optimal activity in their daily life (18.4%), in spite of its overall low frequency. Similar results were also obtained among people with achondroplasia (Sessa et al., 2006), the most common form of dwarfism. This condition is associated with the onset of moderate to severe physical impairments during adulthood, including a higher incidence of chronic back problems, allergies, arthritis/rheumatism, hearing impairment, and spine deformity (Mahomed, Spellmann, & Goldberg, 1998). A group of 18 participants aged 23–48 was administered ESM for 1 week. Compared with people with para and quadriplegia and tetraplegia, these participants spent more time interacting with other people (19.8% of the self-reports), but devoted very little time to socializing with friends (6%), which was, however, reported as a prominent optimal activity. Findings with ESM were consistent with results stemming from the administration of FQ and LT to the same group of people: Relations with friends (22.6%) and with family (13.1%) accounted for the most frequently reported optimal activity (35.7%), followed by work (32.1%).

14.4.2 Positive Growth After Trauma

The unexpected onset of adverse health conditions has been the object of our investigations in order to assess individuals' ability to pursue their psychological selection in the face of changed physical and psychological conditions. As shown in Section 14.3, disease can represent a threat to people's well-being, disrupt their lives, and cause adjustment problems. However, it can also represent an occasion for restructuring life priorities and meanings, providing important challenges in which to invest personal resources. Indeed, the ability to adjust is not strictly dependent on objective physical conditions. Two persons with the same degree of physical health can have different levels of functioning (Delle Fave & Massimini, 2004), based on variables such as individual psychological features, family and social support, material and economic resources, educational background, cultural representations, and social policies (Ingstad, 1999; Simeonsson, Lollar, Hollowell, & Adams, 2000; Űstün et al., 2001). In particular, there are situations in which full functioning in terms of performance, productivity, and efficiency cannot be completely restored, as not all situations can be changed or controlled. In these cases, *being* takes precedence over *doing*, through the mobilization or development of resources such as relatedness, love, gratitude, search for meaning, spirituality, wisdom, and equanimity (Delle Fave and Fava, in press).

Considering the importance of flow in the promotion of psychological well-being and physical and mental health (Delle Fave & Bassi, 2007; Massimini & Delle Fave, 2000; Steele & Fullagar, 2009), we investigated the potential for positive growth in two groups of individuals: persons who had acquired physical disability in adulthood and patients who were diagnosed breast cancer.

In our study on motor and perceptual impairments (Bassi & Delle Fave, 2007; Delle Fave & Maletto, 1992; Delle Fave & Massimini, 2004a); Delle Fave, 2010), besides interviewing individuals with congenital health conditions, we administered FQ and LT to a group of individuals having acquired disabilities in the wake of accidents or diseases: 25 people with spinal cord injuries and 12 blind persons. For these individuals, the so-called process of *transformation of optimal experience* was identified. Physical impairments can make activities previously associated with flow unavailable to the individual, who is thus forced to modify optimal activities on the basis of the new physical conditions, or to look for new areas of commitment and skill development. Most participants in our study successfully managed to identify new opportunities for optimal experience after the onset of disability, sometimes in areas very different from their previous interests, proving behavioral flexibility and resilience in adapting to the environment, and being able to pursue developmental goals despite biological constraints. Among people with spinal cord injuries, for example, a higher percentage of participants found flow after than before the disabling event (88% vs. 80%). Before disability onset, leisure was the most frequent optimal domain (37.8%), with activities such as soccer, swimming, skiing, and dancing; after the onset, this category was reduced by half (19.1%), and it primarily included hobbies like painting and playing guitar. Additionally, higher percentages of optimal activities in the domain of work (22.1%), reading (17.6%), family (13.2%), and social relations (14.7%) were reported. A shift in optimal activities was also identified among blind individuals: Leisure accounted for 35.5% of the answers before onset, and to 16.1% after onset. Similarly to participants with congenital blindness, individuals with acquired perceptual impairment primarily associated the use of media with optimal experience (29%). In particular, for them reading in Braille was extremely challenging as it implied a skill they had never cultivated before. These participants also reported a low percentage of work activities (12.9%), since some of them became unemployed after the disabling event; the activities they now reported were primarily intellectual. These findings challenge the assumptions of adaptation theory (see Chapter 1; Brickman & Campbell, 1971), which states that within few weeks after a trauma individuals tend to psychologically adapt to the new condition and that their average mood gets back to the levels reported before trauma. Research findings highlighted that after the onset of a chronic disease, individuals can attain even higher levels of well-being and actively search for new interests, meanings, and life goals (Delle Fave & Massimini, 2003). Optimal experience plays a crucial role in this process, supporting resource investment, skill development, and personal growth.

Interesting results were also obtained by analyzing participants' life themes. Personal accomplishments like serenity, self-acceptance, strong will power, and higher awareness in facing life events were most frequently reported by both people with spinal cord injury (48%) and blindness (31.8%). Among current challenges and future goals participants quoted personal growth, referring to autonomy and satisfaction with oneself, thus showing that adjusting to disability is a process requiring constant effort and renegotiation of one's priorities in the life context. Moreover, compared to individuals who developed disability at an early age, individuals with acquired impairments more frequently reported health among current challenges and future goals. This was particularly true of individuals with spinal lesions who, as shown before, constantly have to preserve good health conditions through physical exercise and preventive lifestyles, in order not to lose their conquered autonomy. Finally, the urge to integrate into a "normal life" was made explicit through participants' description of their future goals, mostly referring to getting married and having children. For exemplification purposes, Box 14.3 summarizes the personal accomplishments, current challenges, and future goals reported by two participants.

Positive growth after traumatic events was also investigated in a group of 46 women, aged 39–76, who were diagnosed breast cancer, and consequently underwent quadrantectomy (78.3%) or mastectomy (21.7%) (Nosenzo et al., 2008). An ad hoc questionnaire, also including the first section of FQ, was prepared for this study, in order to explore optimal experiences and activities, available resources in facing disease, and positive and negative consequences of illness. The majority of participants (65%) identified optimal experiences in their lives, primarily in free time activities (42%), work (40%), religious practice (9%), social relations (6%), and volunteering (3%). Most of them (90.5%) reported having successfully coped with cancer, primarily mobilizing personal resources such as courage, optimism and positive evaluation of the situation, and serenity (67% of the answers). They also quoted social support (21%) from family members, physicians, and volunteers, and faith (12%) to much lesser extents. Only four participants stated that they negatively tackled the situation, but did not provide any further clarifications.

Patients' positive and negative consequences of disease are reported in Table 14.1.

Box 14.3

Participant	Woman, 30 years old
Diagnosis	Acquired visual impairment
Education	Music school
Current challenges	"Keeping my autonomy and independence"
Future goals	"I try to engage in life integrating my goals (getting a degree, becoming a music teacher, having a child) into a broader view of my life"
Accomplishments	"The greatest accomplishment is having found peace and joy in this condition. You can do many things even if you can't see, you can play, you can find a job . . . you can have a life like other women"
Participant	Woman, 34 years old
Diagnosis	Acquired motor impairment
Education	High school degree
Current challenges	"my major challenges are autonomy and building a family"
Future goals	"the same as challenges"
Accomplishments	"Being quadriplegic and not having lost the ability to smile, nor friends, nor love, nor the will to live"

Table 14.1 Positive and negative consequences of disease reported by women having undergone breast cancer surgery

Positive consequences	%
Personality improvement	58
Rediscovering small things	27
Attention to health	15
N answers	37
N patients	25
Negative consequences	%
Awareness of change	37
Fear of relapse	31
Non-acceptance	19
Relational problems	13
N answers	36
N patients	33

Over half of the participants (54.3%) identified at least one positive consequence in their pathological condition. Positive changes primarily regarded personality, including existential courage and strength, and acceptance of the course of the disease. Participants next quoted rediscovering and valuing small things in daily life, and paying more attention onto health and active prevention. Negative consequences were identified by 71.7% of the participants, which also means that 28% of the respondents did not report any. Psychological problems prevailed, including awareness of physical changes, fear of relapse, and non-acceptance of the disease. To a smaller extent, relational problems were also reported. In general, negative consequences did not pertain to external symptoms or changes, rather they referred to a different perception of one's self and body.

These findings suggest that the psychological sphere plays a crucial role in adjusting to the onset of a disease. Besides supporting patients' trust in the healing power of medical therapies—embedded in the biomedical model—treatments should also rely on patients' inner resources to foster positive recovery.

14.4.3 Body Image and Eating Disorders

As shown at the beginning of this chapter, health is a universal value at the core of international legislations. Nevertheless, discrepancies exist across countries in terms of access to basic services, such as water supply or vaccination campaigns. Also, eating habits—a crucial factor favoring good physical health—present wide national and regional variations, ranging from food shortage and people's undernourishment to food surplus and excessive emphasis on body shape. In western countries, in particular, unhealthy eating habits and obsession for physical shape have led to the rapid spread of eating disorders. In a study with 394 women, aged 18–64, Greenleaf (2005) investigated disordered eating in relation to the self-objectification process, according to which women are socialized to view their own bodies as objects. The author replicated previous findings, showing that body shame mediated the relationship between self-objectification and disordered eating (Tiggemann and Slater, 2001). She also highlighted the relationship between self-objectification and optimal experience, which was used as an indicator of well-being. In particular, flow in physical exercise, as measured with the flow trait scale (see Chapter 4), was negatively correlated with self-objectification, body shame, and disordered eating. Among older women flow was positively correlated with physical activity. Younger women—who were assumed to have more body concerns than older women—reported lower scores at the flow subscale "loss of self-consciousness."

Our research group investigated the quality of experience of obese people during hospital treatment with the aim to understand the mechanisms involved in weight loss and maintenance (Preziosa, Riva, & Delle Fave, 2008). A group of 28 patients, aged 18–70, was longitudinally monitored with two ESM sessions during their stay in a hospital specialized in the treatment of obesity and, 3 months later, in their home environment. During hospitalization, participants reported high investment in physical exercise, and commitment to modify eating habits, and to monitor their health status. Once back home, however, individuals were primarily engaged in family and work matters, showing reduced attention to their health. In hospital and at home, maintenance (comprising eating and personal care) was the most frequently daily thought, accounting for 25.4% of the self-reports during hospitalization and 15.9% during follow-up. Answers primarily referred to eating, health, physical exercises, and weight problems. Social relations and personal care activities were the primary opportunities for optimal experience during hospitalization (23% and 21.7% of the self-reports, respectively), showing that patients could find meaningful challenges in the treatment process and the interaction with other patients and hospital staff. However, returning to their home environment, the percentage of optimal experiences during personal care dropped (13.8%), while interactions were more frequently reported (26.6%), followed by work (14.9%). The analysis of participants' optimal experiences through FQ administered during hospitalization further stressed their high investment in work and household tasks (42.8%) compared to leisure (30.3%), which included physical activities such as gymnastics, aerobics, and swimming in 35.3% of the answers, and hobbies such as gardening, painting, and reading in 64.7% of them. Answers to LT showed that patients' current challenge was primarily losing weight (57.4%); however, in the long-term perspective of future goals, family prevailed (37.5%), followed by work and health (being in good shape) in equal percentages (21.4%).

Overall, results of this study highlighted the potentials of associating optimal experience to hospital treatment and personal care as a means to motivate individuals in losing weight. However, they also point to the importance of taking into account contextual factors in people's everyday lives in order to sustain perseverance in pursuing weight loss and to favor maintenance of physical shape in the long term.

14.4.4 Mental Health

In the domain of psychopathology, only scattered studies are available on daily quality of experience and flow. The major contribution to these topics comes from Marten deVries and his collaborators, who investigated the fluctuations of experience and pathological symptoms in daily life and in relation to activities and social contexts among people suffering from various mental disorders. Merrick (1992) detected that clinically depressed participants reported sadness, loneliness, and boredom more frequently and in higher intensity than non-depressed people. They also spent more time at home, alone, and watching TV, and less time in productive and relational activities. Similarly, psychotic patients more often reported delusional thoughts while being alone with nothing to do (Delespaul & deVries, 1992a; Myin-Germeys, Nicolson, & Delespaul, 2001). These participants reported optimal mental states in presence of one to three other persons. On the contrary, highly anxious patients—but not agoraphobic ones—reported better quality of experience while alone, and higher thought disorganization in social contexts (deVries, Delespaul, & Dijkman-Caes, 1992; Dijkman-Caes & deVries, 1992).

A longitudinal study with ESM investigated the impact of pharmacological treatment on the quality of experience among depressed participants (Barge-Schaapveld, Nicolson, van der Hoop, & deVries, 1995). Treatment was associated with an increased frequency of ESM forms reporting positive mood and a decrease of forms referring to negative affect. In addition, participants progressively spent more time in structured activities and less time in passive entertainments.

Similar findings were obtained through the longitudinal ESM assessment of the quality of experience reported by a woman with panic disorder and agoraphobia undergoing psychotherapy (Delle Fave & Massimini, 1992). The repeated administration of ESM was integral part of the psychotherapy program, characterized by a cognitive behavioral approach combined with the promotion of optimal experiences, goal setting, and meaning development. The ESM assessment extended over one and a half year, during which the woman completed nine ESM sessions. A comparison of the findings obtained in the first and in the ninth session highlighted a significant increase in the occurrence of optimal experience from 15 to 51% of the ESM forms, and a decrease in apathy from 61 to 35% of the forms. In the course of the psychotherapy treatment, the client progressively devoted more time to complex and structured activities, such as volunteering, reading, and socializing, and reduced the time spent watching TV. Consistently with the above-reported findings on agoraphobia, at the beginning of the treatment she felt highly uncomfortable alone, and thus avoided this condition, reporting it in 19% of the ESM forms. By the end of the treatment, however, her need for social support—especially in public places and while walking in the streets—decreased, and she reported to be alone in 43.9% of the self-reports.

A more recent study (Lanfranchi et al., submitted) investigated optimal experience in a group of 54 schizophrenic participants, all of them undergoing pharmacological treatment and stabilized in the chronic phase of the disease. Most participants (67%) lived with their family, and were followed as outpatients by public mental health services, while a minority lived in a residential community.

Patients were involved in a psychiatric rehabilitation program based on mountain therapy: they regularly practiced trekking and mountain walks, accompanied by psychiatrists and expert alpine guides. They were administered flow questionnaire and a shorter version of the life theme questionnaire. All the participants except two identified flow in their lives, and prominently associated with it structured leisure activities (64%), followed by work and socialization with friends in much lower percentages (11 and 8%, respectively). Their ratings of the experiential features of flow were consistent with the theoretical expectations and the empirical evidence. Within the leisure category, 68% of the activities referred to mountain therapy. Participants were also asked to describe the most relevant features of mountain activities. In 40% of their answers they referred to the social and physical environment, highlighting the importance of sharing with others the challenges related to mountaineering and the associated positive experiences.

These findings showed that individuals identify complex and gratifying experiences of engagement and skill development even in suboptimal mental health conditions. They also provided evidence of the role of highly structured and challenging activities in promoting well-being and effective rehabilitation (Glick, Kamm, & Morse, 2009; Rohricht et al., 2009).

All together, these studies highlight the importance of analyzing the quality of experience patients associate with daily contexts and rehabilitation activities. This information can help health professionals cope with the treatment challenges together with the patient, through a co-construction of intervention based on the identification of daily domains and social contexts associated with optimal experiences, and orienting the process of identity building and meaning construction around these sources of well-being. Moreover, this approach sets off the original and active contribution of the individuals to the promotion of their own well-being and development.

14.4.5 Contextual Influences and Cultural Differences

According to the systems approach of the bio-psycho-social model (Section 14.1), the biological and psychological components interact with relevant social factors in influencing health. Socio-cultural influences are pervasive in all health-related aspects: they contribute to shape individuals' illness and health beliefs (Furnham, Akande, & Baguma, 1999; Leventhal, Diefenbach, & Leventhal, 1992), to determine the availability of health services (Engel, 1977), to offer chronically ill people support and opportunities for integration into the socio-economic system (Delle Fave & Massimini, 2004a, 2005), and to shape treatment practices and doctor–patient communication (Delle Fave & Bassi, 2007). Paradoxically, these same socio-cultural factors can cause or promote the onset of illness under certain circumstances (Berry & Sam, 1997).

Each community has developed traditions and beliefs concerning the body and its functions, the causes and the treatment of diseases, and the impact of physical and mental impairments on the person's functioning potential (Dasen, Berry, & Sartorius, 1988). In spite of the predominance of the biomedical model in western medicine, various human communities around the world rely on the person-centered approach. Most traditional non-western medicines, such as Ayurveda in India, the Unani medicine of the Islamic tradition, and the Chinese practice of acupuncture and phytotherapy, consider any physical or mental disease from a holistic perspective, as an imbalance of the whole individual's functioning, taking into account psychological dimensions and the quality of relationships between the person and her natural and social environment (Beardsley & Pedersen, 1997). In other words, traditional medicine throughout the world is substantially grounded in the bio-psycho-social model (Delle Fave & Massimini, 2001; Delle Fave, 2005).

Studies have shown that in non-western developing countries, despite limitations in health services, logistic facilities, and material resources, people with disabilities or chronic illnesses are often more integrated in society than in industrialized countries. Social cohesion and lower levels of individualism enhance the chances for at least some people to actively participate in the daily life of their community (Brown et al., 1998; Tanaka-Matsumi & Draguns, 1997).

Our cross-cultural studies supported these findings. We administered FQ and LT to 20 young people, with congenital or early occurring disabilities, living in the area of Bhaktapur, in the Kathmandu Valley in Nepal (ages 14–29) (Delle Fave & Massimini, 2004a; Delle Fave, 2010; Delle Fave, Lombardi, & Massimini, 2003). Participants had motor impairments either due to hereditary diseases such as osteogenesis imperfecta and Duchenne's muscular dystrophy, or acquired at birth and during infancy as a consequence of poliomyelitis, intra-partum asphyxia or premature birth. These young people benefited from a CBR project first launched in 1986 by a group of Jaycees volunteers. CBR (community-based rehabilitation) programs are intervention schemes, often supported by local and international non-governmental organizations, designed to provide medical treatment and psychosocial support to ill and disabled people. Main features of CBR are decentralization and involvement of families and local communities in the rehabilitation process (Atkinson, Rolim Medeiros, Lima Oliveira, & Dias de Almeida, 2000): Therapists and nurses pass on their competences to the families and the communities so that rehabilitation can take place at home.

All the young participants recognized optimal experience and associated it with a variety of daily activities. Work was quoted as a flow opportunity in 46.4% of the answers; it included both traditional activities such as woodcarving, knitting, and tailoring, and modern jobs, such as using the computer and printing. The use of media ranked second (21.4%), mostly referring to watching films. Studying followed (17.9%), quoted by the participants who attended school. To a smaller extent, also leisure activities (7.1%), personal care (3.6%), and thinking (3.6%) were reported. These results emphasize the successful integration of the participants in their social context, and their exposure to enjoyable and challenges opportunities for action in daily life. In particular, the association of optimal experience with work had several implications for social integration. It allowed participants not only to gradually improve personal skills and performance in the activity, but also to play an active role in the productive life of the community, and to contribute to the family income.

Disabled persons will only be disadvantaged in a social, cultural, or attitudinal environment in which their condition brings about disadvantageous consequences (Bickenbach, Chatterji, Badley, & Űstün, 1999). The problems connected to solitude and to limited social relations that were reported by Italian people with disabilities in our studies were not mentioned by the Nepalese young participants. Besides environmental and intrapersonal factors, interpersonal resources moderated the effects of chronic illness, with family and community offering opportunities for action and self-expression which have a tremendous impact on participants' physical and psychological development (Saraswathi, 1992; Tripathi & Agarwal, 2000; Ünalan et al., 2001). The social capital represents a powerful resource in handling disease and promoting well-being (Helliwell & Putnam, 2005).

However, in line with the bio-psycho-social model, the cultural features of a community not always favor people's psychophysical well-being; they can also hamper it. Scholars and practitioners in the health domain have detected the so-called *acculturative stress syndrome* (Berry & Sam, 1997) among people living in urban areas and immigrants to western countries who are exposed to fast cultural changes that can trigger maladjustment and disease. In daily life these people often have to face harsh contrasts between traditional habits and modernization demands (see Chapter 13). Cultural change can prevent individuals from retrieving optimal experience in traditional activities, and the lack of complex and meaningful activities in which to invest personal resources can have dangerous physical and psychological consequences (Bassi & Delle Fave, 1999; Delle Fave & Bassi, 2009; Delle Fave, 1999; Massimini, Inghilleri, & Delle Fave, 1996). Bicultural integration strategies have been shown to favor psychological well-being (Delle Fave & Massimini, 2004b; Chapter 13). However, a great number of studies have underlined how difficult it is for traditional values to coexist with modernization pressures. Indeed, the acculturative stress syndrome was identified in a wide range of populations. It can manifest itself in the form of alcoholism, as happens for instance among American Indians and Australian Aborigines (Brady, 1995), or in the form of epidemic psychological disorders (EPD) characterized by violent behavior and psychophysical symptoms such as cephalea, inappetence, hallucinations, as observed in Malawi and other countries (McLahan et al., 1995; Tseng & Hsu, 1980).

Finally, health-related cultural norms also regulate daily interactions between doctors and patients. As shown in Chapter 8, these relations can contribute to physicians' well-being when they are associated with optimal experience (Delle Fave & Massimini, 2003; Delle Fave, 2006). Physicians' work satisfaction and constant skills cultivation, in their turn, can impact on patients' satisfaction with the quality of treatment (Leiter, Harvie, & Frizzell, 1998), treatment adherence (Stewart, 1996), and adjustment to illness (Mager & Andrykowski, 2002).

In the study on women with breast cancer previously illustrated, participants were also invited to evaluate doctors' communication styles, assessed as the perceived amount of information provided in the various stages of treatment (Nosenzo et al., 2008). They filled in the need for closure scale (Kruglanski, 1989), assessing patients' decisional style in critical situations with 42 Likert-type items ranging from 1 "strongly disagree" to 6 "strongly agree." Need for closure (NFC) refers to the person's need to close or interrupt the decisional process, avoiding to explore other possible alternatives. Subscale components are as follows: preference for order and structure, intolerance to ambiguity, decisiveness, predictability, close-mindedness. Research showed that some individuals need to gather a great amount of information before taking a decision (low NFC), while others prefer to decide on the basis of few essential information (high NFC).

As shown in Fig. 14.1, participants were overall satisfied with the quality and quantity of information the doctors provided them with in the pre-operative phase. However, half of the respondents perceived that information on the risks entailed in surgery and on the post-operative course was inadequate. Women also brought forward suggestions for enhancing the health service: 39.1% of them proposed relational and organizational improvements. As for their decisional styles, participants showed a high degree of NFC ($M=4.04$; $SD=0.7$). In particular they expressed high preference for order ($M=4.6$; $SD=0.7$) and intolerance to ambiguity ($M = 4.5$; $SD=0.8$). Moreover, some dimensions of NFC were related to the perceived adequacy of doctors' information, preference for social support during check-ups, and identification of illness-related negative consequences. Women who proposed improvements to the health service, who preferred going to check-ups being accompanied by meaningful others, and who reported negative consequences

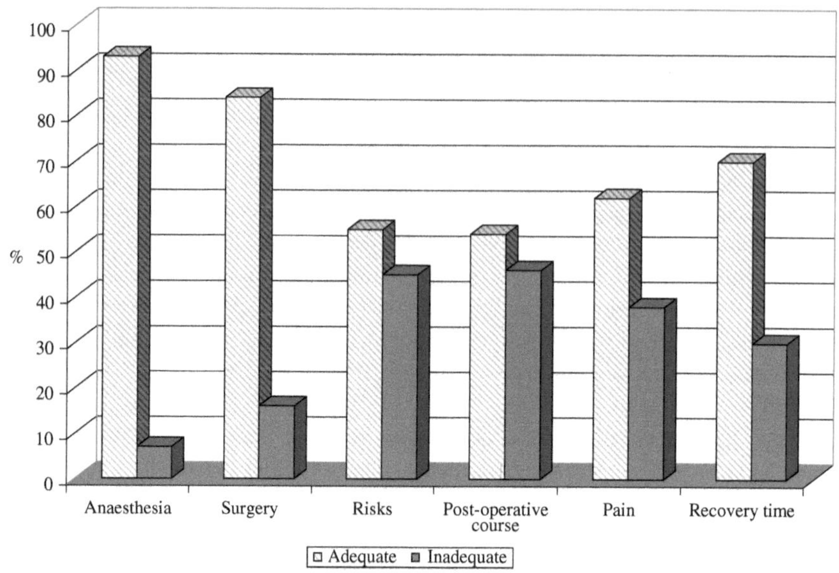

Fig. 14.1 Patients' evaluation of adequacy of the information received in the treatment stages. Values indicate the percentages of patients who provided evaluation ($N = 46$)

due to their disease, reported higher ratings of decisiveness than those who did not bring forward suggestions, preferred to see the doctor alone, or did not report negative disease consequences.

References

Affleck, G., & Tennen, H. (1996). Construing benefits from adversity: Adaptational significance and dispositional underpinnings. *Journal of Personality, 64*, 899–922.

Affleck, G., Tennen, H., Croog, S., & Levine, S. (1987). Causal attribution, perceived benefits and morbidity after a heart attack: An 8 year study. *Journal of Consulting and Clinical Psychology, 55*, 29–35.

Albrecht, G. L., & Devlieger, P. J. (1999). The disability paradox: High quality of life against all odds. *Social Science and Medicine, 48*, 977–988.

Antonovsky, A. (1987). *Unraveling the mystery of health: How people manage stress and stay well*. San Francisco: Jossey Bass.

Arnold, R., Ranchor, A., Koëter, G., De Jongste, M., & Sanderman, R. (2005). Consequences of chronic obstructive pulmonary disease and chronic heart failure: The relationship between objective and subjective health. *Social Science & Medicine, 61*, 2144–2154.

Atkinson, S., Rolim Medeiros, R. L., Lima Oliveira, P. H., & Dias de Almeida, R. (2000). Going down to the local: Incorporating social organization and political culture into assessments of decentralized health care. *Social Science and Medicine, 51*, 619–636.

Bandura, A. (1997). *Self-efficacy: The exercise of control*. New York: Freeman.

Bandura, A. (2004). Health promotion by social cognitive means. *Health Education and Behavior, 31*, 143–164.

Barge-Schaapveld, D. Q., Nicolson, N. A., van der Hoop, R. G., & deVries, M. W. (1995). Changes in daily life experience associated with clinical improvement in depression. *Journal of Affective Disorders, 34*, 139–154.

Bassi, M., & Delle Fave, A. (1999). Dreaming survival in Australian aboriginal populations. In A. Delle Fave & F. Meli (Eds.), *Modernization and cultural identity* (pp. 123–141). Milano: Casa Editrice Dell'Arco.
Bassi, M., & Delle Fave, A. (2007). L'esperienza della disabilità: selezione psicologica e promozione del benessere [the experience of disability: Psychological selection and well-being promotion]. *Psicologia della Salute, 1*, 31–46.
Bassi, M., Preziosa, A., & Pozzoli, S. (2007). Experience sampling method e lo studio dell'esperienza quotidiana: implicazioni per l'intervento [experience sampling method and the study of daily experience: Implications for intervention]. In A. Delle Fave (Ed.), *La condivisione del benessere. Il contributo della psicologia positiva* (pp. 169–189). Milano: Franco Angeli.
Bauer, J. J., McAdams, D. P., & Pals, J. L. (2008). Narrative identity and eudaimonic well-being. *Journal of Happiness Studies, 9*, 81–104.
Baumeister, R. F., & Vohs, K. D. (2002). The pursuit of meaningfulness in life. In C. R. Snyder & S. J. Lopez (Eds.), *Handbook of positive psychology* (1st ed., pp. 608–617). New York: Oxford University Press.
Beardsley, L., & Pedersen, P. (1997). Health and culture-centered intervention. In J. W. Berry, M. H. Segall, & C. Kacitçibasi (Eds.), *Handbook of cross-cultural psychology: Vol. 3. Social behavior and applications* (pp. 413–448). Needam Heights, MA: Allyn & Bacon.
Berry, J. W., & Sam, D. L. (1997). Acculturation and adaptation. In J. W. Berry, M. H. Segall, & C. Kagitçibasi (Eds.), *Handbook of cross-cultural psychology: Vol. 3. Social behavior and applications* (pp. 291–326). Needam Heights, MA: Allyn & Bacon.
Bickenbach, J. E., Chatterji, S., Badley, E. M., & Űstün, T. B. (1999). Models of disablement, universalism and the international classification of impairments, disabilities and handicaps. *Social Science and Medicine, 48*, 1173–1187.
Brady, M. (1995). Culture in treatment, culture as treatment. A critical appraisal of developments in addictions programs for indigenous North Americans and Australians. *Social Science and Medicine, 41*, 1487–1498.
Brickman, P., & Campbell, D. T. (1971). Hedonic relativism and planning the good society. In M. Appley (Ed.), *Adaptation-level theory* (pp. 287–305). New York: Academic Press.
Brown, A. S., Varma, V. K., Malhotra, S., Jiloha, R. C., Conover, S. A., & Susser, E. S. (1998). Course of acute affective disorders in a developing country setting. *Journal of Nervous and Mental Disease, 186*, 207–213.
Carver, C. S., & Gaines, J. G. (1987). Optimism, pessimism, and post-partum depression. *Cognitive Therapy and Research, 11*, 449–462.
Carver, C. S., Pozo, C., Harris, S. D., Noriega, V., Scheier, M. F., Robinson, D. S., et al. (1993). How coping mediates the effect of optimism on distress: a study of women with early stage breast cancer. *Journal of Personality and Social Psychology, 65*, 375–390.
Dasen, P. R., Berry, J. W., & Sartorius, N. (Eds.). (1988). *Health and cross-cultural psychology: Toward applications*. Newbury Park, CA: Sage.
Deci, E. L., & Ryan, R. M. (2000). The "what" and "why" of goal pursuits: human needs and the self-determination of behavior. *Psychological Inquiry, 11*, 227–268.
Delespaul, P. A. E. G., & deVries, M. W. (1992). The daily life of ambulatory chronic mental patients. In M. W. deVries (Ed.), *The experience of psychopathology: Investigating mental disorders in their natural settings* (pp. 110–122). New York: Cambridge.
Delle Fave, A. (1999). Individual development and bicultural identity: The Navajo way. In A. Delle Fave and F. Meli (Eds.), *Modernization and cultural identity* (pp. 49–68). Milano: Edizioni dell'Arco.
Delle Fave, A. (2005). Le dimensioni psicologiche e culturali della salute: esperienza ottimale e riabilitazione [the psychological and cultural dimensions of health: Optimal experience and rehabilitation]. *Psicologia della Salute, 8*, 29–40.
Delle Fave, A. (2006). The impact of subjective experience on the quality of life. A central issue for health professionals. In M. Csikszentmihalyi & I. Csikszentmihalyi (Eds.), *A life worth*

living. Contributions to positive psychology (pp. 165–181). New York: Oxford University Press.

Delle Fave, A. (2009). Optimal experience and meaning: Which relationship? *Psychological Topics, 18*, 285–302.

Delle Fave, A. (2010). Development through disability. The unfolding and sharing of psychological resources. In G. W. Burns (Ed.), *Happiness, healing, enhancement. Your casebook collection for applying positive psychology in the therapy* (pp. 88–99). Hoboken, NJ: Wiley & Sons.

Delle Fave, A., & Bassi, M. (2007). *Psicologia e salute. L'esperienza di utenti e operatori* [psychology and health. The experience of patients and professionals]. Torino: UTET Università.

Delle Fave, A., & Bassi, M. (2009). Sharing optimal experiences and promoting good community life in a multicultural society. *Journal of Positive Psychology, 4*, 280–289.

Delle Fave, A., Brdar, I., Freire, T., Vella-Brodrick, D. A., & Wissing, M. P. (2010). The eudaimonic and hedonic components of happiness: Qualitative and quantitative findings. *Journal of Happiness Studies*, published online, 4 May 2010.

Delle Fave, A., & Fava, G. A. (in press). Positive psychotherapy and social change. In R. Biswas-Diener (Ed.). *Positive psychology as social change*. Dordrecht, NL: Springer.

Delle Fave, A., Lombardi, M., & Massimini, F. (2003). Disability and development: Individual and cultural issues. In L. Loewenstein, D. Trent, R. Roth (Eds.), *Catching the future: Women and men in global psychology* (pp. 104–113). Lengerich: Pabst Science Publishers.

Delle Fave, A., & Maletto, C. (1992). Processi di attenzione e qualità dell'esperienza soggettiva nei non vedenti [attentional processes and quality of subjective experience in blind people]. In D. Galati (Ed.), *La psicologia dei non vedenti. Processi cognitivi, affettivi e strategie adattative* (pp. 321–353). Milano: Franco Angeli.

Delle Fave, A., & Massimini, F. (1992). The ESM and the measurement of clinical change: A case of anxiety disorder. In M. W. deVries (Ed.), *The experience of psychopathology: Investigating mental disorders in their natural settings* (pp. 280–289). New York: Cambridge.

Delle Fave, A., & Massimini, F. (2001). Promozione della salute e riabilitazione: alcune problematiche transculturali [health promotion and rehabilitation: Some cross-cultural issues]. In A. L. Comunian & A. Meneghini (Eds.), *Ri-abilitazione. Approccio multidisciplinare alla disabilità fisica* (pp. 74–86). Padova: Edizioni Progetto.

Delle Fave, A., & Massimini, F. (2003). Making disability into a resource. *The Psychologist, 16*, 9–10.

Delle Fave, A., & Massimini, F. (2004a). Bringing subjectivity into focus: Optimal experiences, life themes, and person-centered rehabilitation. In P. A. Linley & S. Joseph (Eds.), *Positive psychology in practice* (pp. 581–597). New York: Wiley.

Delle Fave, A., & Massimini, F. (2004b). The cross-cultural investigation of optimal experience. *Ricerche di Psicologia, 27*, 79–102.

Delle Fave, A., & Massimini, F. (2005). The relevance of subjective wellbeing to social policies: Optimal experience and tailored intervention. In F. Huppert, B. Keverne, & N. Baylis (Eds.), *The science of wellbeing* (pp. 379–404). Oxford: Oxford University Press.

deVries, M. W., Delespaul, P. A. E. G., & Dijkman-Caes, C. I. M. (1992). Consequences of depression for the experience of anxiety in daily life. In M. W. deVries (Ed.), *The experience of psychopathology: Investigating mental disorders in their natural settings* (pp. 141–147). New York: Cambridge.

Diener, E. (2009). *The science of well-being* (Vol. 37). Dordrecht: Springer.

Dijkman-Caes, C. I. M., & deVries, M. W. (1992). The social ecology of anxiety: Theoretical and quantitative perspectives. In M. W. deVries (Ed.), *The experience of psychopathology: Investigating mental disorders in their natural settings* (pp. 129–140). New York: Cambridge.

Elliott, T. R., Kurylo, M., & Rivera, P. (2002). Positive growth following acquired physical disability. In C. R. Snyder & S. J. Lopez (Eds.), *Handbook of positive psychology* (1st ed., pp. 687–699). New York: Oxford University Press.

Engel, G. L. (1977). The need for a new medical model: A challenge for biomedicine. *Science, 196*, 129–136.
Engel, G. L. (1982). The biopsychosocial model and medical education. *The New England Journal of Medicine, 306*, 802–805.
Fitzpatrick, R. (2000). Measurement issues in health-related quality of life: Challenges for health psychology. *Psychology and Health, 15*, 99–108.
Furnham, A., Akande, D., & Baguma, P. (1999). Beliefs about health and illness in three countries: Britain, South Africa and Uganda. *Psychology, Health & Medicine, 4*, 189–201.
Glick, I. D., Kamm, R., & Morse, E. (2009). The evolution of sport psychiatry. *Sports Medicine, 39*, 607–613.
Greenleaf, C. (2005). Self-objectification among physically active women. *Sex roles, 1/2*, 51–62.
Greer, S., Morris, T., Pettingale, K. W., & Haybittle, J. L. (1990). Psychological response to breast cancer and 15-year outcome. *Lancet, 335*, 49–50.
Helliwell, J. F., & Putnam, R. D. (2005). The social context of well-being. In F. Huppert, B. Keverne, & N. Baylis (Eds.), *The science of wellbeing* (pp. 435–460). Oxford: Oxford University Press.
Hernández-Quevedo, C., Jones, A., López-Nicolás, A., & Rice, N. (2006). Socioeconomic inequalities in health: A comparative longitudinal analysis using the European community household panel. *Social Science & Medicine, 63*, 1246–1261.
Hurley, C. C., & Shea, C. A. (1992). Self-efficacy: Strategy for enhancing diabetes self-care. *The Diabetes Educator, 18*, 146–150.
Ingstad, B. (1999). The myth of disability in developing nations. *The Lancet, 354*, 757–758.
Jackson, W. T., Taylor, R. E., Palmatier, A. D., Elliott, T. R., & Elliott, J. L. (1998). Negotiating the reality of visual impairment: Hope, coping and functional ability. *Journal of Clinical Psychology in Medical Settings, 5*, 173–185.
Jones, K. (2004). Schism ad heresy in the development of orthodox medicine: The threat to medical hegemony. *Social Science & Medicine, 58*, 703–712.
Kaplan, G., & Baron-Epel, O. (2003). What lies behind the subjective evaluation of health status? *Social Science & Medicine, 56*, 1669–1676.
Keyes, C. L. M. (2002). The mental health continuum: From languishing to flourishing in life. *Journal of Health and Social Research, 43*, 207–222.
Keyes, C. L. M. (2007). Promoting and protecting mental health as flourishing. A complementary strategy for improving national mental health. *American Psychologist, 62*, 95–108.
King, L., & Miner, K. (2000). Writing about the perceived benefits of traumatic life events: Implications for physical health. *Personality and Social Psychology Bulletin, 26*, 220–230.
Kruglanski, A. W. (1989). *Lay epistemics and human knowledge: Cognitive and motivational biases*. New York: Plenum Press.
Kuijer, R. G., & deRidder, D. T. D. (2003). Discrepancy in illness-related goals and quality of life in chronically ill patients: The role of self-efficacy. *Psychology and Health, 18*, 313–330.
Lanfranchi, F., Frecchiami, A., & Delle Fave, A. (under submission). Interventi riabilitativi ed esperienza ottimale nel contesto montano [Rehabilitation and optimal experience in the mountain context].
Leiter, M., Harvie, P., & Frizzell, C. (1998). The correspondence of patient satisfaction and nurse burnout. *Social Science and Medicine, 47*, 1611–1617.
Leshan, L. (1994). *Cancer as a turning point: A handbook for people with cancer, their families and health professionals*. Bath: Gateway Books.
Leventhal, H., Diefenbach, M., & Leventhal, E. (1992). Illness cognition: Using common sense to understand treatment adherence and effect cognition interactions. *Cognitive Therapy Research, 16*, 143–163.
Levin, B., & Browner, C. (2005). The social production of health: Critical contributions from evolutionary, biological, and cultural anthropology. *Social Science & Medicine, 61*, 745–750.

Mager, W., & Andrykowski, M. (2002). Communication in the cancer "bad news" consultation: Patient perceptions and psychological adjustment. *Psycho-oncology, 11*, 35–46.

Mahomed, N. N., Spellmann, M., & Goldberg, M. J. (1998). Functional health status of adults with achondroplasia. *American Journal of Medical Genetics, 78*, 30–35.

Massimini, F., & Delle Fave, A. (2000). Individual development in a bio-cultural perspective. *American Psychologist, 55*, 24–33.

Massimini, F., Inghilleri, P., & Delle Fave, A. (Eds.). (1996). *La selezione psicologica umana - teoria e metodo d'analisi* [human psychological selection – theory and method of analysis]. Milano: Coop. Libraria IULM.

Masten, A. S., & Reed, M. G. J. (2002). Resilience in development. In C. R. Snyder & S. J. Lopez (Eds.), *Handbook of positive psychology* (pp. 74–87). New York: Oxford University Press.

McLahan, M., Banda, D. M., & McAuliffe, E. (1995). Epidemic psychological disturbance in a Malawian secondary school: A case study in social change. *Psychology and Developing Societies, 7*, 79–90.

Merluzzi, T. V., & Sanchez, M. A. (1997). Assessment of self-efficacy and coping with cancer: Development and validation of the cancer behavior inventory. *Health Psychology, 16*, 163–170.

Merrick, W. A. (1992). Dysphoric moods in depressed and non-depressed adolescents. In M. W. deVries (Ed.), *The experience of psychopathology: Investigating mental disorders in their natural settings* (pp. 148–156). New York: Cambridge.

Michael, S. T. (2000). Hope conquers fear: Overcoming anxiety and panic attacks, in handbook of hope: Theory, measures and applications. In C. R. Snyder (Ed.), *Handbook of hope: Theory, measures, and applications* (pp. 301–319). San Diego, CA: Academic Press.

Moore, K. A. (2002). Positive psychology and health: Situational dependence and personal striving. In E. Frydenberg (Ed.), *Beyond coping: Meeting goals, visions, and challenges* (pp. 107–125). New York: Oxford University Press.

Myin-Germeys, I., Nicolson, N. A., & Delespaul, P. A. E. G. (2001). The context of delusional experience in the daily life of patients with schizophrenia. *Psychological Medicine, 31*, 489–498.

Nosenzo, M. A., Colombo, F., Corsi, F., Faini, I., Bossi, M., Sartani, A., et al. (2008). Neoplasia mammaria e mobilizzazione di risorse personali e relazionali [breast cancer and mobilization of personal and relational resources]. *Psicologia della Salute, I*, 9–22.

Peterson, C. (2000). The future of optimism. *American Psychologist, 55*, 44–55.

Peterson, C., & Park, C. (1998). Learned helplessness and explanatory style. In D. F. Barone, M. Hersen, & V. B. Van Hasselt (Eds.), *Advanced personality* (pp. 287–310). New York: Plenum.

Peterson, C., Seligman, M. E. P., & Vaillant, G. E. (1988). Pessimistic explanatory style is a risk for physical illness: A thirty-five year longitudinal study. *Journal of Personality and Social Psychology, 55*, 23–27.

Peterson, C., Seligman, M. E. P., Yurko, K. H., Martin, L. R., & Friedman, H. S. (1998). Catastrophizing and untimely death. *Psychological Science, 9*, 49–52.

Preziosa, A., Riva, G., & Delle Fave, A. (2008). L'esperienza soggettiva dell'obesità: implicazioni diagnostico-terapeutiche [the subjective experience of obesity: Therapeutical and diagnostical implications]. *Psicologia della Salute, I*, 39–55.

Rabkin, J. G., Wagner, G. J., & Del Bene, M. (2000). Resilience and distress among amyotrophic lateral sclerosis patients and caregivers. *Psychosomatic Medicine, 62*, 271–279.

Rohricht, F., Papadopoulos, N., Suzuki, I., & Priebe, S. (2009). Ego-pathology, body-experience, and body psychotherapy in cronic schizophrenia. *Psychology and Psychoterapy, 82*, 19–30.

Rolland, J. S. (2005). Cancer and the family: An integrative model. *Cancer, 104*(11 S), 2584–2595.

Rolland, J. S., & Walsh, F. (2005). Systemic training for healthcare professionals: The Chicago center for family health approach. *Family Process, 44*, 283–301.

Ryan, R. M., Patrick, H., Deci, E. L., & Williams, G. C. (2008). Facilitating health behavior change and its maintenance: Interventions based on self-determination theory. *The European Health Psychologist, 10*, 2–5.

Saraswathi, T. S. (1992). Child survival and health and their linkages with psycho-social factors in the home and community. *Psychology and Developing Societies*, *4*, 73–87.
Saravanan, B., Manigandam, C., Macaden, A., Tharion, G., & Bhattacharji, S. (2001). Re-examining the psychology of spinal cord injury: A meaning-centered approach from a cultural perspective. *Spinal Cord*, *39*, 323–326.
Scheier, M. F., & Carver, C. S. (2001). Adapting to cancer: The importance of hope and purpose. In A. Baum & B. L. Andersen (Eds.), *Psychosocial interventions for cancer* (pp. 15–36). Washington, DC: American Psychological Association.
Scheier, M. F., Matthews, K. A., Owens, G. F., Magovern, G. J., Lefebvre, R. C., Abbott, R. A., et al. (1989). Dispositional optimism and recovery from coronary artery bypass surgery: The beneficial effects on physical and psychological well-being. *Journal of Personality and Social Psychology*, *57*, 1024–1040.
Schulman, P., Keith, D., & Seligman, M. E. P. (1993). Is optimism heritable? A study of twins. *Behaviour Research & Therapy*, *31*, 569–574.
Schwarzer, R. (1994). Optimism, vulnerability, and self-beliefs as health-related cognitions: A systematic overview. *Psychology and Health*, *9*, 161–180.
Schwarzer, R. (1998). Optimism, goals, and threats: How to conceptualize self-regulatory processes in the adoption and maintenance of health behaviors. *Psychology and Health*, *13*, 759–766.
Schwarzer, R., & Fuchs, R. (1996). Self-efficacy and health behaviors, in predicting health behaviour: Research and practice with social cognition models. In M. Conner & P. Norman (Eds.), *Predicting health behaviour: Research and practice with social cognition models* (pp. 163–196). Maidenhead: Open University Press.
Seligman, M. E. P., & Csikszentmihalyi, M. (2000). Positive psychology. An introduction. *American Psychologist*, *1*, 5–14.
Sessa, D., Intini, S., Zagato, P., Cortinovis, I., Basso, P., Cavallo, M., et al (2006). Diversity as opportunity: Quality of life and psychological well-being of people with achondroplasia. Paper presented at the *3rd European Conference on Positive Psychology*. Book of Abstract, p. 62. Braga, Portugal, 3–6 July.
Sheldon, K., Williams, G., & Joiner, T. (2003). *Self-determination theory in the clinic: Motivating physical and mental health*. New Haven, CT: Yale University Press.
Shepperd, J. A., Maroto, J. L., & Pbert, L. A. (1996). Dispositional optimism as a predictor of health changes among cardiac patients. *Journal of Research in Personality*, *30*, 517–534.
Simeonsson, R. J., Lollar, D., Hollowell, J., & Adams, M. (2000). Revision of the international classification of impairments, disabilities, and handicaps. Developmental issues. *Journal of Clinical Epidemiology*, *53*, 113–124.
Snyder, C. R. (1994). Hope and optimism. In V. S. Ramachandren (Ed.), *Encyclopedia of human behavior* (pp. 535–542). San Diego, CA: Academic Press.
Snyder, C. R. (1998). A case for hope in pain, loss and suffering. In J. H. Harvey, J. Omarzu, & E. Miller (Eds.), *Perspectives on loss: A sourcebook* (pp. 63–79). Washington, DC: Taylor & Francis.
Snyder, C. R., & Pulvers, K. (2001). Dr. Seuss, the coping machine, and "oh, the places you will go", in coping with stress: Effective people and processes. In C. R. Snyder (Ed.), *Coping with stress: Effective people and processes* (pp. 3–29). New York: Oxford University Press.
Snyder, C. R., Rand, K. L., & Sigmon, D. R. (2002). Hope theory. In C. R. Snyder & S. J. Lopez (Eds.), *Handbook of positive psychology* (pp. 257–276). New York: Oxford University Press.
Snyder, C. R., Sympson, S. C., Ybasco, F. C., Borders, T. F., Babyak, M. A., & Higgins, R. L. (1996). Development and validation of the state hope scale. *Journal of Personality and Social Psychology*, *70*, 321–335.
Sodergren, S. C., & Hyland, M. E. (2000). What are the positive consequences of illness? *Psychology and Health*, *15*, 85–97.
Steele, J. P., & Fullagar, C. J. (2009). Facilitators and outcome of student engagement in a college setting. *Journal of Psychology*, *143*, 5–27.

Stewart, M. (1996). Effective physician-patient communication and health outcomes: A review. *Canadian Medical Association Journal, 152*, 1423–1433.

Tanaka-Matsumi, J., & Draguns, J. (1997). Culture and psychopathology. In J. W. Berry, M. H. Segall, & C. Kacitçibasi (Eds.), *Handbook of cross-cultural psychology: Vol. 3. Social behavior and applications* (pp. 449–492). Needam Heights, MA: Allyn and Bacon.

Tedeschi, R. G., & Calhoun, L. G. (1995). *Trauma and transformation: Growing in the aftermath of suffering*. Thousand Oaks, CA: Sage.

Tennen, H., & Affleck, G. (2002). Benefit-finding and benefit-reminding. In C. R. Snyder & S. J. Lopez (Eds.), *Handbook of positive psychology* (1st ed., pp. 584–597). New York: Oxford University Press.

Tiggemann, M., & Slater, A. (2001). A test of objectification theory in former dancers and nondancers. *Psychology of Women Quarterly, 25*, 57–64.

Tripathi, I., & Agarwal, A. (2000). Chronic illness, symptoms and efficacy in children as related to some psychological characteristics of mothers. *Psychology and Developing Societies, 12*, 31–42.

Tseng, W., & Hsu, J. (1980). Minor psychological disturbances of everyday life. In H. C. Triandis & J. G. Draguns (Eds.), *Handbook of cross-cultural psychology: Vol. 6. Psychopathology* (pp. 61–97). Boston, MA: Allyn and Bacon.

Ünalan, H., Gençosmanoğlu, B., Akgün, K., Karamehmetoğlu, Ş., Tuna, H., Önes, K., et al. (2001). Quality of life of primary caregivers of spinal cord injury survivors living in the community: Controlled study with short form-36 questionnaire. *Spinal Cord, 39*, 318–322.

Űstün, T. B., Chatterji, S., Bickenbach, J. E., Trotter II, R. T., Room, R., Rehm, J., Saxena, S. (Eds.). (2001). *Disability and culture. Universalism and diversity*. Göttingen: Hogrefe and Huber Publishers.

Walsh, F. (2003). Family resilience: A framework for clinical practice. *Family Process, 42*, 1–18.

Weinberg, N. (1988). Another perspective: Attitudes of people with disabilities. In H. E. Yuker (Ed.), *Attitudes toward persons with disabilities* (pp. 141–153). New York: Springer.

WHOQOL Group. (2006). A cross-cultural study of spirituality, religion, and personal beliefs as components of quality of life. *Social Science & Medicine, 62*, 1486–1497.

Williams, G., & Deci, E. (1998). The importance of supporting autonomy in medical education. *Annals of Internal Medicine, 129*, 303–308.

Williams, G., & Deci, E. (2001). Activating patients for smoking cessation through physician autonomy support. *Medical Care, 39*, 813–823.

Williams, G., Grow, V., Freedman, Z., Ryan, R., & Deci, E. (1996). Motivational predictors of weight loss and weight-loss maintenance. *Journal of Personality and Social Psychology, 70*, 115–126.

Williams, G., Rodin, G., Ryan, R., Grolnick, W., & Deci, E. (1998). Autonomous regulation and long-term medication adherence in adult patients. *Health Psychology, 17*, 269–276.

World Health Organization. (1946). Preamble to the Constitution of the World Health Organization. *Official records of the World Health Organization*, no. 2, p. 100.

World Health Organization. (2001). *International classification of functioning, disability and health (ICF)*. Geneva: WHO.

World Health Organization. (2004). *Promoting mental health: Concepts, emerging evidence, practice* (summary report). Geneva: WHO.

Chapter 15
Psychosocial Maladjustment and Mimetic Flow

15.1 Introduction

As discussed in the previous chapters, psychological selection is a ceaseless process that shapes an individual's life, and the quality of experience people associate with daily situations represents the key information for investigating this process and its moment-by-moment outcomes.

Optimal experience plays an important role in this process. Activities associated with it can be cultivated through the search for higher challenges, the refinement of personal abilities, and the achievement of increasing levels of order and complexity in behavior (Csikszentmihalyi, 1975/2000; Massimini & Delle Fave, 2000). However, most studies on optimal experience have been conducted among "normally" functioning populations, enjoying acceptable standards of living, decent housing and work conditions, a healthy network of relationships. What about people living under difficult circumstances?

This topic has been partially addressed in Chapter 13, through the discussion of findings gathered among first-generation immigrants moved to Europe from developing countries, and facing the challenge of acculturation. In this chapter, we will specifically focus on two categories of people suffering from severe psychosocial maladjustment: children and adolescents coming from dysfunctional families, and/or exposed to street life, and drug addicts. On the basis of information gathered through flow questionnaire, life theme questionnaire, and ESM, we will try to outline the features and role of optimal experiences in their lives, as well as their psychological selection pattern.

15.2 Cultural Change and Its Impact on Children

During the last few decades ecosystems, cultures and countries underwent dramatic changes. From a western, postmodern perspective we could maintain that these changes led to improvement in health, education, productivity, technology, cross-cultural relations, and communications. Democracy and citizens' participation have spread in several countries; decentralization of intervention and resources, the active

A. Delle Fave et al., *Psychological Selection and Optimal Experience Across Cultures*, Cross-Cultural Advancements in Positive Psychology 2,
DOI 10.1007/978-90-481-9876-4_15, © Springer Science+Business Media B.V. 2011

role of NGOs, and the private sector have created new opportunities for development in various areas. Such benefits are, however, counterbalanced by heavy costs: pollution, and severe damages to the natural environment; epidemics such as HIV/AIDS; an increase in drug abuse; a remarkable widening of the gap between the richest and the poorest in every country; a globalization process that is prominently resulting in world westernization; the unprecedented explosion of armed conflicts between cultures and ethnic groups within and between nations.

The transition from rural life to industrialization created severe unbalances in the life of people and cultures. At the individual level, complex and creative opportunities for optimal experience, such as traditional jobs, collective rituals and handicrafts, have been substituted by repetitive and mechanical tasks, passive leisure, and social isolation. The spreading of technology produced an increasing dependence on artifacts, more and more numerous and expensive, thus emphasizing socio-economic differences. In developing countries only élite groups benefit from modernization facilities, whereas the majority—especially in the outskirts of urban areas—is forced to abandon the traditional lifestyle, without finding meaningful opportunities for action—and survival—in the new context. Data collected in different cultural contexts have shown some of the negative effects of this phenomenon on the quality of experience (Delle Fave & Massimini, 1988).

The impact of these changes on children was effectively summarized by UNICEF (2001) by pointing out some paradoxical phenomena. The first one concerns resource distribution: despite global prosperity, the widening economic disparities have negatively affected the chances for improving children's conditions in most of the developing countries. The second one refers to health care: despite important achievements in this domain (medical treatments, disease prevention, and nutrition), millions of children have been exposed to the devastating consequences of HIV/AIDS; children still pay the largest tribute in terms of human lives to the association of poverty and poor hygienic conditions; wars, weapons, and mines have enormously increased the number of disabled children. The third paradox is related to legal provisions adopted for children's protection. While most nations ratified the 1989 Convention of Child Rights, and implemented laws and provisions in favor of minors, no decrease has been observed in work exploitation, violence, and sexual abuse involving children. Besides the persistent use of children as low-cost workers, the increase of armed conflicts has affected a huge number of children, either as victims or as soldiers. The diffusion of Internet has been used as vehicle for the spreading of pornography and prostitution involving minors, and the growing number of Westerners traveling abroad has incremented the sexual exploitation of boys and girls. A fourth paradox concerns the financial support provided to poor countries through international loans and reduction of debt. This support allowed for higher resource investments in children's health and education programs. On the other side, however, poor countries were also put under the pressure of reducing social expenditures and concentrating on productivity, in order to qualify for international lending assistance. As a consequence, in several cases both the dissemination and quality of primary education suffered at different levels: introduction of school fees, reduction of teachers' salaries, limited availability of learning materials. Moreover, governments often put other priorities and interests before education in budget plans.

The swelling number of children in developing countries has created a whole new set of issues that need to be addressed. Child abuse, illiteracy, malnutrition, disease, and delinquency are realities showing no signs of getting under control, in spite of prevention efforts undertaken by governmental and non-governmental bodies (Le Roux, 1996). They are, in fact, bouncing off into other areas, affecting families, societies, and countries.

15.2.1 Child Work: Resource or Exploitation?

In most developing countries a remarkable percentage of children is involved in some kind of work. The involvement of children in work shows great variations, according to the economic needs of the family, the features of the natural and cultural environment, the local opportunities for work, and the gender, age, and school attendance of the child. A survey conducted in 2000 on 49 developing countries showed that 19% of the children aged between 5 and 14 were involved in some form of work, with no significant differences between males and females (UNICEF, 2001). In rural areas working children accounted for a higher percentage (21%) than in towns (13%). Children most often contributed to family business (around 63%); they were less frequently involved in extra-family unpaid work (21%), paid jobs (14%), or domestic activities (14%).

The International Labor Organization (ILO, 2009) has recently estimated that over 215 millions of children aged between 5 and 14 work. However, not all work done by children should be classified as child labor, that is to be targeted for elimination. Children's participation in work that does not affect their health and personal development or interfere with their schooling is generally regarded as being something positive. This includes activities such as helping their parents around the home, assisting in a family business, or earning pocket money outside school hours and during school holidays. These kinds of activities contribute both to individual development and to family welfare; they provide children with skills and experience, and prepare them to be productive members of society during their adult life. The term "child labor," on the contrary, refers to work that deprives children of their potential and their dignity, that is harmful to physical and mental development, and that interferes with education, either preventing children to go to school or requiring excessively long and heavy engagement. In its most extreme forms, child labor involves children being enslaved, separated from their families, and exposed to serious hazards and illnesses. Whether or not particular forms of work can be called "child labor" depends on the child's age, the type and hours of work performed, the conditions under which it is performed, and the objectives pursued by individual countries. The answer varies from country to country, as well as among sectors within countries.

As previously reported, children's enrolment in formal education can be combined with their contribution to family income. The primary school net attendance ratio in 2000–2006 showed a growing trend compared with past reports, hitting 65% for children from the poorest fifth of households in developing countries (UNICEF, 2009). However, 115 millions of working children are still engaged in harmful and hazardous labor in homes, plantations, and factories. Moreover, 51 millions of children go unregistered at birth, do not get any form of education, and are often deprived of family care. Millions of children work in conditions that crush the right to normal physical and mental development. Working children are often deprived of their fundamental rights to survival and protection, but they are also exploited and discriminated in their everyday life. Moreover, in many places children are still being pushed into slavery.

Combating the exploitation of children in work activities and supporting their physical, mental, spiritual, moral, and social development (as stated by Article 32 of the Convention on the Rights of the Child) has been identified as one of the top priorities in the agenda of the major international organizations. In 1999 ILO adopted Convention no.182 that promotes the elimination of the worst forms of child labor. Article 3 quotes the activities comprised in this category: (a) all forms of slavery, such as sale and trafficking of children, debt bondage and serfdom, forced or compulsory labor including recruitment of children in armed conflicts; (b) the involvement of children in prostitution and pornography; (c) the involvement of children in illicit activities, in particular drug trafficking; (d) any hazardous work that is likely to harm the health, safety, or morals of children, by its nature or according to the circumstances in which it is carried out. This category includes activities such as mining, deep-sea fishing, fireworks and match production, work with dangerous chemicals, scavenging, informal sector work, commercial agriculture. The knowledge about the risks and negative consequences of these works is well documented in most countries.

At the beginning of the 1990s ILO launched the International Program on the Elimination of Child Labor (IPEC) in order to organize and support projects aimed at rescuing millions of children in the world from the burden of being the main family breadwinners, or victims of exploitation bound to a future of marginalization (ILO, 2001). IPEC established a wide network of governmental and social partners in many developing countries, with the priority aim of eliminating the worst forms of child labor in the short run, while progressively reducing children exploitation as income sources or producers. IPEC strategy is based on a broader perspective of people's empowerment through the promotion of education, decent work opportunities, and social protection for all citizens (Myrstad, 1999).

In spite of these efforts at the international level, millions of children around the world, and especially in the urbanized areas of developing countries, are still exposed to various forms of abuse and exploitation (Inciardi & Surratt, 1998; Jutkowitz, Spielmannm, Koeler, Lohani, & Pande, 1997; Le Roux, 1996; Sattaur, 1993). However, this phenomenon cannot be faced with ad hoc, circumscribed intervention programs (Rizzini, 1996). These children are the living consequences—and the victims—of the socio-economic inequality, the worldwide increasing gap between rich and poor people, the deep changes in urban and rural lifestyle and opportunities.

15.2.2 From Villages to Cities, from Home to the Streets

Rapid urbanization is among the most striking changes occurred in the second half of the twentieth century. Especially in developing countries, millions of families have moved to cities, mostly settling in peripheral slums and shantytowns under precarious living conditions (Harpham & Reichenheim, 1994). Recent studies estimated that in 2015 every fifth inhabitant of developing countries will live in towns (UNPD, 2002). Families' decision to migrate to cities is prominently related to widespread poverty and to expectations of better life and work conditions. However, such expectations are often frustrated, and urbanization turns into breakdown of family and social networks, unemployment, marginalization, and the involvement of children in income generating activities to support their families (Dallape, 1996; Gracey, 2002; Moazzam, Shahab, Ushijima, & de Muynck, 2004; Sen, 2009).

In particular, urbanization in developing countries has brought to the streets a ceaselessly increasing number of children. They are prominently boys, since girls are usually engaged in domestic work, and as street children they often get absorbed in the prostitution racket. There is a common misunderstanding concerning street children: they are globally perceived as minors with no place to live and without family ties. As a matter of fact, most of the children found in the streets all over the world do have parents daily interacting with them and caring for them to some extent. The United Nations defined street children as boys and girls who habitually stay and live in the street, without any kind of protection and supervision from responsible adults (International Catholic Children's Bureau, 1985). UNICEF (2005) distinguished among two broad categories of children that can be found in city streets. The first category comprises children *on the streets*, who work during the day, and join their family at night, often managing to combine job and school attendance. Some of these children live in the street together with their families, and help parents earn a living through occasional or structured jobs, mainly occurring in the street environment (Lusk, 1992). They are often enrolled in hazardous works, thus adding to their already harsh street condition the risk of labor-related accidents or diseases. Recent studies indicate that this group accounts for the vast majority of the children who work in the streets (Williams, 1993; Mathur 2009). The second category refers to children *of the streets*, who spend their life in the streets, far from their families or without relations with them. These children are very often workers, they do not attend school and find shelter, food, and a sense of family within a social network of peers sharing the street life. They can be involved in illegal actions such as theft, pickpocketing, and drug traffic. They primarily run away from their families because of neglect or abuse (Grundling & Grundling, 2005; MacAlpine, Henley, Mueller, & Vetter, 2010; Worthman & Panter-Brick, 2008), and in a lower percentage following solicitations from people depicting the city as a wonderland, rich in opportunities, and material attractions.

Several studies point out that the common view of street children as emotionally deprived and culturally impaired is a stereotype (Bar-On, 1998). According to

Aptekar and Abebe (1997), the ambiguity and vagueness characterizing the definition of street children depend on several reasons. The major reason is a political one: international agencies tend to inflate the number of street children, including categories that do not strictly fit the definition, in order to promote donations and financial investments (Aptekar, 1994). The living conditions and behavior of street children are often dramatized and exaggerated to draw the attention of the public. Second, street children are usually compared to "the children from a fictitious ideal middle-class family in the developed world" (Aptekar & Abebe, 1997, p. 478). Such an ethnocentric comparison is misleading in that, at least in the countries where street children are a widespread phenomenon, most of the other children (who should be the actual term of comparison) belong to low-income joint families. They are actively involved in solving the problems related to family daily survival, very differently from the middle-class children, and similarly to street children. Many of them can be actually included in the category of children "on the street."

Street children vary as their peers, and could become real resources for cultural change and development, instead of being regarded as problems (CWIN, 1995; De Oliveira, Baizerman, & Pellet, 1992). Living in socio-economic systems that are often both turbulent and insensitive, a street child develops varied strategies of survival (Panter-Brick, 2002). A study conducted among street children in Mumbai (Kombarakaran, 2004) showed that most of them were engaged in street work activities, such as scavenging, shoe-shining, and carrying loads at railways and bus stations, or employed by car workshop owners and shopkeepers. Their salary often exceeded their parents' earnings, they could get better food in the street restaurants than at home, and they used NGO's shelters and dispensaries for support and medical care. Some of the children "of the street" had established connections with families living in the city slums, and exchanged material and emotional support with peers sharing their street condition. They used friendship networks for finding job, and spent their earnings to buy clothes, to go to the movies, and to buy drugs. Only a small minority engaged in criminal activities and used maladaptive mechanisms to cope with street life stressors. Similar findings were obtained among street boys in Kenya (Davies, 2008; Kaime-Atterhoeg & Ahlberg, 2008) and in China (Lam & Cheng, 2008).

Street life leads to the development of social interactions patterns, belief systems, and behaviors that constitute an alternative cultural network. Well-defined rules and norms regulate social hierarchies, rights and duties, participation and information exchange, income production and distribution, material belongings, social support, and group decisions (Davies, 2008; Kudrati, Plummer, & Yousif, 2008; Turnbull, Hernandez, & Reyes, 2009; Unger et al., 1998). Street gangs develop their own individual and social values, though discrepant from those of the surrounding society. Street children, from this perspective, are living examples of the human tendency toward rule following highlighted by Harré and Secord (1972).

However, children who live in the street and/or are exploited as full-time workers are exposed to several risks at two different levels. At the individual level, their developmental potential is seriously hampered due to lack of socially meaningful opportunities for action and skill cultivation. At the social level, marginalization prevents them from becoming active members of the broader community.

Children of the street, who are deprived of emotional ties due to the lack of family connections, may suffer from various kind of psychological disorders (Schimmel, 2008). A recent study conducted on street youth in Ukraine detected higher levels of depression and emotional problems among children disconnected from their families (Kerfoot et al., 2007). Another study conducted in India highlighted the exposure of street children to various forms of abuse, such as work exploitation by employers, sexual abuse within and outside the street gang, physical harassment and maltreatment by policemen (Mathur, Rathore, & Mathur, 2009).

A major and worldwide problem among street children is drug abuse; most researchers have found a positive correlation between duration of street life, age of the children, and addiction levels (Morakinyo & Odejide, 2003; Praharaj, Verma, & Arora, 2008). Psychoactive substances widely vary: glue, typewriter correction fluid, and low-quality alcoholic beverages are relatively cheap and easy to find. Older children also use benzodiazepines or other kinds of medicaments that can be purchased at public dispensaries. Moreover, both boys and girls are exposed to sexual abuse (Towe, ul Hasan, Zafar, & Sherman, 2009).

Another serious problem underlined by Aptekar and Abebe (1997) concerns the public hostile attitude toward street children. The authors identify three kinds of hostility, each of them influencing the public perception of street children, and the strategies used to "rehabilitate" them. First, there is a penal-instructive hostility. The assumption that street children are criminals who have to be prosecuted results in violence, abuse, and severe punishments performed by educators and policemen in detention centers. Second, there is a collective frustrated hostility, deriving from the perception of failure in dealing with the huge social problems lying behind the phenomenon of street children. Citizens feel threatened by these children, who are seen as a public danger and, as a consequence, treat them harshly and aggressively. Third, there is a cultural hostility, identified with the dichotomy between the sedentary and the "peripatetic" way of life. Most cultures are basically sedentary, and attach a great value to the house as a private place where to hide inappropriate or shameful behaviors (Delle Fave, Massimini & Maletto, 1991). Street children lack this area of privacy, and they display all their good and bad aspects in the public space, including things that should be concealed.

15.2.3 Street Children in Western Countries

While the phenomenon of street children is most evident in developing countries, it represents a problem in affluent western societies as well. In the outskirts of big cities in North America and Europe many families live under difficult circumstances, suffering from unemployment, poor housing and hygienic conditions, and financial insecurity. Ethnic minorities and immigrants prominently face these difficulties, related to marginalization and discrimination problems. However, the growing tendency toward community and family disintegration in the peripheral areas of big cities, coupled with the widespread economic crisis, has recently contributed to the dramatic increase of the number of homeless children and youth, regardless of their ethnical background (Levy, 1996; Oles, 1991; Rew & Horner, 2003; Toro, 1999; van Wormer, 2003). Finally, with the breakdown of the Soviet Union most Eastern European countries had to cope with serious economic and political instability and their consequences, which include the dramatic phenomenon of street children (Alexandrescu, 1996; Kerfoot et al., 2007).

In addition, less extreme though socially alarming situations can be found among youth in North America and Europe. An increasing number of children and adolescents spend their days in the streets of the western towns. They usually live with their families, thus belonging to the typology "on the street." Their living conditions are substantially favorable: public medical and educational facilities are usually available to them, and they rarely need to contribute to family income. They are often organized in informal groups or gangs, exposed to drug abuse and to deviant and criminal behavior. Most of them officially attend school, but often irregularly or without commitment: dropout is quite common.

In spite of these substantial differences, these youth share some family and social problems with street children: a context lacking in social networks and community awareness (prominently decayed areas around big cities); family conflicts, abuses, and disruption; parents' unemployment and/or addiction; and lack of secure emotional ties. Intervention addressed to these children is substantially preventive in nature: its aim is to promote their development and socialization, to reintegrate them in the educational system, to provide them with a network of healthy relationships, and to help them define and pursue professional and personal goals (Regogliosi, 2000).

15.2.4 Successful Intervention: A Major Challenge

Although street children are among the most physically visible of all children, since they live and work in public areas, yet paradoxically they are also among the most invisible and, therefore, hardest children to reach with vital services, and the most difficult to protect (UNICEF, 2009). A wide variety of programs have been designed and developed to "rehabilitate" them; however, these programs face a considerable amount of dropouts all over the world. Many children go back to the streets, in spite of the genuine commitment and efforts of educators and social workers.

A major problem at the intervention level is children's refractoriness to institutionalization. Rehabilitation centers provide them with a safe environment, all material facilities, opportunities to learn and develop working skills, as well as a globally good quality of daily life. However, institutionalization implies forced observance of discipline, rules and obligations that represent major obstacles to successful intervention (Arieli, Beker, & Kashti, 1990). Several studies have pointed out this problem, that is recurrent across cultures, and that also entails an even more serious consequence: a great number of street children shun any contact with social workers, due to the fear to get secluded into centers (Kerfoot et al., 2007; Lam & Cheng, 2008; Mathiti, 2006).

Other intervention approaches are based on a greater flexibility, and they adopt a community-based perspective. The theoretical and empirical work of the Brazilian pedagogist Paulo Freire has given a major impulse to this approach. Freire stressed the importance of promoting adult education as a means toward emancipation from poverty and social participation (Freire, 1970, 1998). His model has been successfully applied in several countries, such as the Philippines (Too & Floresca-Cawagas, 1997) and African-American communities in the United States (Potts, 2003).

These projects are rooted in the local social system, and they include the active involvement of families and communities. Educators perform the most crucial part of their job in the streets to get a spontaneous and free contact with the children. Children are allowed to visit centers for spending the night and for getting food. They can attend Non-formal Education (NFE) courses that often take place directly in the streets (Rossi Doria 1999; Bhattarai & Delle Fave, 2002; Vithal, 2003). These courses provide basic notions in the domains of literacy, mathematics, history, and humanities, but they also foster children's awareness of social values and human rights. Children involved in them can subsequently decide to join residential communities, and at this point they are usually enrolled in public school curricula. Training programs are also offered, customized on individuals' interests; each child can freely choose among various activities, including traditional local skills, arts, and handicraft. Teaching strategies are used to promote children's autonomous discovery and awareness of their own learning potentials (Wilder, 2002).

Efforts are made to facilitate family reunion and the reintegration of the children in their original social context; however, this is not always possible, since in many cases children joined the street life to escape an abusing, conflictual and problematic family environment. At the community level, advocacy programs are run to raise awareness on child rights, and alphabetization courses for adults are organized as well. This approach is expected to affect society as a whole, because as selective transmitters of information, individuals influence the cultural evolution trend. Such a combined action of various individuals can foster social empowerment in the long run.

Several issues need to be addressed in this domain. The first one is program evaluation. The work done by governmental and non-governmental bodies is primarily programmatic, but there is little recorded research on its short-term and long-term impact on children's lives and quality of experience. Second, a wide range of laudable initiatives are largely unknown; there is lack of networking, communication, and dissemination of information. Therefore, action-based projects are needed in order to facilitate government and NGO work in strengthening existing programs through innovative strategies and sensitization of media. A third problem is the ethnocentric approach to intervention (Magazine, 2003). Local agencies should make the effort to customize intervention projects according to the cultural system in which children are expected to live, taking into account the failure potential of programs imported from other countries. Far too often international intervention in developing countries is unrelated to the local culture, being rather built on western standards. This tendency does not always depend on the intrusiveness of international donors, agencies, and volunteers. Very often local workers and educators rely on western models themselves, based on the education system they were offered at school, and on the still widespread stereotype assuming the superiority of western culture. Unfortunately, this still common practice introduces unrelated cultural information in a structured though dysfunctional social system, such as the street cultural network in which children are growing. Moreover, such strategy has few chances to be integrated into the local society, with its habits, beliefs, and traditions. It can even disrupt the local pattern of cultural evolution (Delle Fave & Massimini, 2005a).

15.2.5 Investigating Children's Experience and Expectations

A recent and very important acquisition in human development is the recognition of children as social agents, who can exert subjectivity and agency, can negotiate with adults from their own perspective, and can build articulated and structured social networks through peer relationships (Aubrey & Dahl, 2005; Mayall, 2002). Several authors have stressed that interventions should be based on an analysis of children's needs, as perceived by the children themselves (Veeran, 2005; Votta & Manion, 2003), in line with the UN convention of the rights of the child, which provides a legal basis for initiating activities aimed at promoting the well-being and growth of children in need.

In order to plan relevant and respectful interventions based on children's perception and situation, in-depth studies should be conducted on the quality of daily experience and perceived needs, from the perspective of both children and significant others in their lives (Davies, 2008). This, along with a monitoring of agencies and initiatives, will provide a better basis to chart out a course of action that is culturally relevant, acceptable, and feasible. The effectiveness of this strategy was assessed through the development and application of instruments, such as the Children's Perspective Protocol, used in surveys conducted in Bangladesh, Ethiopia, the Philippines, and Central America to get subjective reports of working and street life (Woodhead, 1999). Studies based on fieldwork have emphasized the central importance of children's active involvement in the research design in order to get authentic insights of their real life (Baker, Panter-Brick, & Todd, 1996; Kaime-Atterhoeg & Ahlberg, 2008; Turnbull et al., 2009; van Beers, 1996).

The investigation of children's experience still entails several problems and shows some research biases. First of all, it is necessary to gain children's trust, and this can require weeks of fieldwork, essential for sharing their daily life and challenges. Second, most children living in the streets or residing in centers since a short time never attended school, and they have difficulties in understanding questions often formulated in an academic, research style. Third, studies usually focus on the negative side of children's life, overlooking their strengths and resources, and ignoring the positive aspects of street life that could be one of the major reasons for children's dropout from the centers. Similarly, little attention is paid to the quality of experience children associate with intervention programs, a dimension that could shed further light on the opportunities for development and optimal experiences available to them.

In particular, the investigation of optimal experience and psychological selection trends could provide some hints for the development of projects centered on individual resources and subjective well-being. Presently, we can only offer some pilot findings from exploratory studies conducted in various countries. They show basic cross-cultural consistencies and highlight potentials and limitations shared by different intervention strategies. Most data have been gathered among children and adolescents "off the streets" (Merriman & Guerin, 2007), being in full-time care of NGOs or governmental institutions after a period of street life or severe family neglect. One study refers instead to Italian adolescents living "on the street."

15.2.5.1 Italy: Adolescents on the Street

A pilot investigation was conducted through flow questionnaire and life theme Questionnaire among ten boys and one girl, aged 14–16 and living in the periphery of a metropolitan area in North Italy. These teenagers had joined an intervention program developed by educationalists who regularly met them in the streets, and provided them with NFE courses (Delle Fave & Massimini, 2005a; Zanetti, 2002). All the participants had been raised in disrupted and/or harmful family environments. All had dropped out from school and spent most of their time in the street, going round in informal peer groups, listening to music, smoking, and fighting with other gangs. Seven of them were enrolled in a vocational training program. When asked about the occurrence of optimal experience in their life, only six (55%) identified this state, associating it with peer interactions, sexual activities, and sports. Their description of flow experience on Likert scales (Table 15.1) confirmed the theoretical assumptions: adolescents reported themselves highly excited, concentrated and relaxed, they perceived clear goals, high challenges and adequate skills.

Their description of the average experience associated with daily contexts offered a more complete overview of their resource investment. As illustrated in Table 15.1, being with peers was the most positive daily opportunity, and the associated experience closely overlapped flow. When invited to describe what did they mean by "being with friends," these adolescents referred to both structured and relaxed leisure activities such as "laughing, joking, having fun," "playing soccer," "going out, going to the park, talking, motorbiking." On the opposite, school was associated with dramatically low values for all the variables, including challenges and skills. A condition of apathy was clearly depicted (Delle Fave & Massimini, 2005b; Chapter 5), further confirmed in the answers to the open-ended question: "opening books, reading...dead bore!"; "a boring thing that also gave me anxiety"; "a loss of time." The experience perceived with family did not substantially differ from the descriptions provided by western adolescent participants in other studies (see Chapter 10), in spite of the fact that these participants lived in highly malfunctioning families. This ambivalence emerged when the participants described what did they mean by being with family: "eating, talking, quarrelling"; "being at home

Table 15.1 Italian adolescents on the street: the quality of experience during selected optimal activities and in daily contexts

Variables	Optimal activities (*N* = 6) *M (sd)*	Study (*N* = 11) *M (sd)*	Family (*N* = 11) *M (sd)*	Solitude (*N* = 11) *M (sd)*	Friends (*N* =) *M (sd)*
Involvement	5.3 (2.4)	1.1 (1.3)	5.0 (1.2)	2.4 (2.0)	6.4 (1.5)
Clear feedback	5.7 (2.3)	1.4 (1.8)	5.6 (1.7)	4.2 (2.1)	5.3 (2.1)
Intrinsic motivation	5.7 (2.9)	0.6 (1.4)	4.9 (2.9)	2.7 (2.6)	6.9 (1.4)
Excitement	7.0 (2.4)	1.1 (2.6)	6.2 (1.1)	3.8 (2.4)	7.1 (1.4)
Ease of concentration	4.7 (3.0)	0.6 (1.3)	5.6 (2.2)	4.7 (3.1)	6.7 (2.1)
Enjoyment	6.3 (1.5)	0.6 (0.9)	4.7 (1.8)	2.2 (1.7)	5.3 (2.1)
Concentration	7.6 (0.9)	0.6 (1.3)	4.7 (1.8)	3.6 (3.1)	5.3 (2.1)
Relaxation	7.3 (1.0)	4.6 (2.8)	6.6 (2.1)	6.0 (3.1)	7.6 (0.8)
Clear goals	7.0 (1.7)	2.7 (2.7)	5.5 (2.0)	4.7 (3.0)	6.2 (1.4)
Control of situation	4.3 (2.9)	1.3 (2.4)	4.2 (2.4)	4.0 (3.0)	5.1 (1.6)
Challenges	7.7 (0.8)	1.5 (1.5)	5.2 (2.7)	3.1 (3.2)	6.6 (2.5)
Skills	6.3 (1.6)	2.1 (2.0)	5.6 (2.6)	3.9 (3.4)	6.5 (2.5)

Note: N = Number of participants.

all together"; "just eating"; "a pleasant thing, talking." Being alone was prominently described as an experience of boredom, both in the scaled ratings and in the open descriptions: "being alone in the public park waiting for the friends," "getting bored," "sitting at home and watching TV."

When asked to report their wishes and desires (Table 15.2), these adolescents provided 21 answers, primarily referring to leisure. They quoted relatively unstructured activities such as traveling, going to the disco, driving the motorbike. Material goods followed in rank: adolescents wished to get plenty of money, a motorbike, a car. Three participants quoted professional aspirations: soccer player, racing car driver, selling fashion clothes. Only one boy was not able to express any desire.

The answers to the life theme questionnaire contributed to better define the psychological selection trend of these adolescents. Two participants could not identify any positive influence in their lives. Out of the 21 answers provided, 38.1% referred to family, and in particular to mother and siblings, and 28.6% to friends and love relationships. Two answers referred to the motorbike, as a status symbol and an expression of autonomy. As for negative life influences, again two adolescents did not report any. School accounted for 33.4% of the participants' answers, mostly including difficult relationships with teachers, considered too rigid, unfair, and biased against them. Social and family relationships followed, both with 17% of the answers. Parents' divorce, father's violence, and family conflicts were prominently quoted.

In spite of their drastically negative evaluation of the school, adolescents quoted education as their main present challenge in 38.5% of the 13 answers provided; they were well aware of the fact that in order to get a decent job they had to get at least

Table 15.2 Percentage distribution of wishes and goals reported by children under difficult circumstances across cultures

	Wishes				Goals			
Categories	Street Italy	Inst. Italy	Kenya	Brazil	Street Italy	Inst. Italy	Kenya	Brazil
Productive activities	14.3	9.6	21.4	22.6	50.0	25.8	50.0	51.7
Free time	38.1	16.9	21.4	–	8.2	12.9	–	6.9
Family	4.8	20.5	7.1	22.6	20.9	25.8	11.1	20.7
Social relations	–	18.1	7.1	–	–	9.7	5.6	–
Community, society issues	–	7.2	43.0	25.8	–	–	16.6	–
Personal growth	9.5	21.7	–	6.4	–	12.9	11.1	6.9
Material goods	33.3	6.0	–	22.6	20.9	12.9	5.6	13.8
N answers	21	83	14	31	24	31	18	29

the secondary school diploma. The relationship with the girlfriend and the identification of future projects were additional concerns. Two participants were not able to identify any challenge in their present life. Finally, and in line with the challenges, future goals (Table 15.2) prominently referred to work. Most participants seemed realistic as concerns their job opportunities, planning to become electricians, bakers, or shopkeepers, even though three of them indicated sports and music careers. Building a family and acquiring material goods (a car, a house, money) followed in rank, even though with a much lower percentage of answers.

From a general point of view, besides perceiving limited opportunities for engagement and skill development in daily life, these participants prominently associated optimal experience with free peer interaction. Previous cross-cultural studies on adolescents showed the two-sided effect of this activity on the quality of experience (Verma & Larson, 2003; Chapter 10). Spending free time with peers provides fun, positive affect and pleasure, it fosters the development of social roles, but it is often associated with low engagement and low mobilization of personal skills. As concerns street youth, it often means idling around without specific goals and aims. These findings suggest that street life, combined with a problematic family background, does not provide children with meaningful occasions for optimal experiences. The Italian adolescents examined, who rejected the pursuit of educational achievements through regular school attendance, lived in a low-challenging environment, prominently experiencing apathy, boredom, and disengaged fun with peers sharing their pathway. Their challenges and goals were adequate to promote their social integration, but the developmental relevance of their wishes and desires, centered on the acquisition of wealth and material goods, was alarmingly low.

15.2.5.2 Italy: Girls Living in Institution

To explore the impact of institutionalization on adolescents' quality of experience, we administered flow questionnaire and life theme questionnaire to 25 girls aged 14–21, entrusted to Institutions for Custody of Minors because of severe family problems and psychosocial maladjustment. The participants lived in small residential communities, whose programs aimed at building personal relationships between educators and adolescents, and at promoting girls' adjustment and integration in the social context. Contacts with the parents were frequent, and—if possible and advisable—the adolescents could join their families during weekends. Most of them (56%) attended high school, 36% had a full-time job, and two had a part-time occupation after school hours. In their family background different forms of deviant behavior were detected: parental alcoholism, drug addiction, sexual and/or physical violence, psychiatric syndromes, prostitution, and crime.

Most girls (80%) reported optimal experiences in their life, and associated it with various activities. Socialization and peer interactions were prominent (25.6% of the answers), followed by the use of media (23.1%), mostly comprising reading and watching TV. Both spending time with the boyfriend and practicing sports and hobbies accounted for 12.8% of the answers. In their ratings of the quality of

Table 15.3 The average quality of experience with family: comparison between girls living at home and girls living in institution

Variables	Home ($N = 25$) M (sd)	Institution ($N = 25$) M (sd)
Involvement	4.2 (2.1)	2.8 (2.8)
Clear feedback	6.4 (1.6)	5.1 (3.1)
Intrinsic motivation	4.7 (2.2)	3.8 (3.1)
Excitement	6.9 (2.1)	2.8 (2.5)
Ease of concentration	5.5 (2.2)	4.0 (3.0)
Unselfconsciousness	3.4 (2.2)	3.5 (3.0)
Enjoyment	4.7 (1.9)	2.8 (2.4)
Concentration	4.1 (2.1)	3.2 (2.6)
Relaxation	5.8 (1.9)	3.9 (3.0)
Clear goals	5.2 (2.2)	3.7 (2.7)
Control of situation	5.0 (2.3)	3.5 (2.8)
Challenges	5.0 (2.8)	2.5 (2.6)
Skills	6.0 (2.5)	3.6 (3.1)

Note: N = Number of participants.

experience associated with daily activities, these girls reported substantially low values for most variables in the family context. Compared with a group of 25 girls matched by age and education level, but living with their families (Table 15.3), institutionalized adolescents perceived significantly lower levels of involvement ($Z = 2.2$, $p < 0.05$), excitement ($Z = 4.0$, $p < 0.0001$), enjoyment ($Z = 2.7$, $p < 0.01$), clear goals ($Z = 2.0$, $p < 0.05$), challenges ($Z = 3.1$, $p < 0.01$) and skills ($Z = 2.7$, $p < 0.01$), as well as higher levels of anxiety ($Z = 2.2$, $p < 0.05$).

When asked "What do you mean with being with family?" most girls highlighted difficulties, such as "To talk about our problems, trying to understand why there are conflicts and to find compromises," "We don't live together the whole week, and the weekend goes by fast"; "I am very close to my family, even though I suffered because of them." The contrast between the ideal value and meaning of family relationships and the actually perceived situation clearly emerges from these descriptions.

When asked to report their wishes and desires (Table 15.2), these adolescents primarily referred to building relationships, within and outside the family context. However, they also expressed the desire to grow as individuals, and to become autonomous, mature, and satisfied persons. Free-time activities followed in rank, mostly comprising traveling and hobbies.

In the Life Theme Questionnaire only one girl was not able to identify any positive influence in her life. Most of the answers provided by the other participants referred to social relations (45%), followed by family (17.5%) and personal experiences (10%). All the girls described some negative influences, prominently quoting family (65.4% of the answers). Social relations came next, but in a much lower percentage (19.2%). Their main present challenge was personal growth (47.4%), followed by studying with a much lower percentage of answers (15.8%). Among goals (Table 15.2), building a family and study/work achievements accounted for over half of the answers; personal growth, material goods, and free-time goals followed with lower percentages of answers.

15.2.5.3 Kenya: The Children of Kivuli

The number of children living in the streets of Nairobi jumped from few hundreds in the 1970s to 60,000 in more recent times (Shorter & Onyancha, 1999). In 1992 a group of young Kenyan men from different professions and backgrounds, gathered around Fr. Kizito Sesana, a Comboni Priest, started a football team involving both street children and children from families living in the surrounding slum area. This initiative grew into a more structured program; street children were offered hot meals, medical care, school placement, and a temporary shelter. Few years later the Kivuli center was officially started (the word Kivuli means "refuge, shelter from the sun").

Today more than 50 children are provided with full care at Kivuli. Most of them attend local public schools or nonformal education courses, according to their age. Children are offered vocational trainings in tailoring, leather, and wood work. These activities allow them to develop skills and to sell their products through a net of fair trade. Children get psychological support through group meetings and individual counseling, and enjoy recreational activities such as sports and traditional dances. The boys are also allocated community responsibilities. Their families and guardians are regularly contacted, and in case of need they receive educational and material support. In addition, Kivuli offers various services to the local slum communities: animation, health care, financial contribution to children education, a well with drinkable water, a library, and a meeting room. The connection with families and the local community represents a crucial prerequisite to the reintegration of the children into their social network upon completion of the rehabilitation process.

The administration of flow questionnaire and life theme questionnaire to a group of boys at Kivuli provided some hints on their quality of experience and future expectations (Anselmo, 2000; Delle Fave & Massimini, 2005a). Moreover, as emphasized by Turnbull and colleagues (2009) and Kaime-Atterhoeg and Ahlberg (2008), the answers provided by the children and their pattern of task completion shed light on the strategies street children develop to cope with adults' inquiries about their life.

The questionnaires' administration was complex, and many boys repeatedly interrupted the task to go for other activities, retrieving it the following day and in several cases just leaving the questionnaires incomplete. The questionnaires were translated in Swahili, because most of the boys refused to speak and write in English. The translation was performed with the help of local volunteers and educators, who filled out the questionnaires themselves. Only 13 boys aged 11–16 completed the questionnaires, and among them only two reported the occurrence of optimal experience in their lives, and associated it with playing games (a 12-year-old child) and prayer (a 14-year-old teenager). Since adult volunteers and educators were also asked to complete the Swahili version of the questionnaires, and they did report flow in their life, the low rate of children's identification of the experience could be primarily related to their difficulty in achieving prolonged concentration and absorption in a task (basic components of flow), rather than to translation and comprehension problems. This issue will be addressed again in the final part of this section.

As concerns wishes (Table 15.2), children often referred to social issues, with answers such as "helping others," "to help here in Kivuli." Free time mostly comprised traveling and visiting new places, while productive activities included getting a good job and a high school diploma (participants' average level of education was 5th standard). The investigation of life influence highlighted the positive role of education, which accounted for 50% of the answers; family was never quoted instead. The most frequent negative influence was drug abuse (35% of the answers), followed by relational problems with family, policemen, and street gangs. Among present challenges children highlighted material needs, such as getting shoes and clothes, and learning (some children had difficulties with basic skills such as writing). Goals (Table 15.2) mostly comprised getting a job (becoming a sport professional, a judge, a pilot) and giving a contribution to society.

15.2.5.4 Brazil: Caminhos de Vida

Intervention addressed to street children in Brazil has been deeply influenced by the work of Paulo Freire, who highlighted that this problem is part of a more general and collective condition of discrimination and oppression. Only the emancipation from poverty, ignorance, and destitution of entire social classes can lead to the solution of children's exploitation, abuse, and neglect (De Roure, 1996; Freire, 1994, 1996). Street children are a dramatic reality in most Brazilian cities. Both the federal government and local authorities, in collaboration with national and international NGOs, have developed several projects to rescue children from the street life. In Goiania, the capital city of the state of Goias where the data presented here were gathered (Zanetti, 2002), an articulated network of institutions and associations is involved in this complex task. Children's social integration is promoted through a stepwise strategy, starting from informal contacts in the streets and ending in small residential centers, hosting a limited number of children, in order to foster the creation of a family atmosphere. Children are hosted in residential centers only upon their free acceptance of the proposal and its implications in terms of rights and duties. These centers offer them public school attendance, vocational trainings, psychological and emotional support, and the opportunity to rebuild or strengthen their contacts with the family of origin (Municipality of Goiania, 1999).

A visit to Casa Girassol (a center for boys) and to Casa Talithà-kum (a center for girls) led to the administration of flow questionnaire and life theme questionnaire to 11 participants, 5 girls and 6 boys, aged 15–22 (Zanetti, 2002). Only two participants had already completed primary school. Besides going to school, all the boys had a part-time job (as shoemakers, gardeners, and paperwork craftsman). The girls attended school and vocational courses in computer, tailoring, and weaving; four of them were mothers, and after school time they were supported in raising their children.

Time restrictions did not allow for an adequate translation of the first part of the flow questionnaire. Therefore, the occurrence of optimal experience in youth's lives was not explored. Other topics were, however, investigated. When participants were invited to report their wishes and desires (Table 15.2), their most frequent answers fell into the category "Community/society issues," referring to helping people in need, actively contributing to society, and seeing all people happy. Study and job achievements, financial and material improvements, and the well-being of parents, siblings, and children followed with the same percentage of answers.

When asked to quote the most positive influences in their lives, participants mostly referred to educators and street social workers (25% of the answers) and to the experience of motherhood (25%). Having left the street was quoted in 18.7% of the answers, and education in 12.5%. Among negative life influences, drug abuse was the prominent one (36.4% of the answers), followed by social relations (18.2%, mostly comprising treachery by friends, sexual abusers, and street gangs) and anti-social behaviors (stealing, 18.2%). Personal experiences accounted for 15.2% of the answers, and they referred to suffering caused by harsh conditions of street life. Only two participants quoted their family of origin.

For these youth, the prominent challenge in their present life was joining the productive society through work and study (33.4%), followed by personal growth (27.8%), which included answers expressing the difficulty to pursue long-term projects and to develop commitment to them through constant endurance and effort. The relationships with the other community members, and the rules to follow in daily life accounted for 15.2% of the answers. Three girls quoted raising their children as a prominent challenge. As for goals (Table 15.2), educational and work achievements accounted for over half of the answers, followed by building a family and getting material and financial security. Some participants reported ambitious work and learning goals: going to the University, becoming a lawyer or a physician.

15.2.6 Matching Opportunities with Expectations: A Crucial Issue

What can we learn from these findings, within the broader research literature on children under difficult circumstances, and from the perspective of psychological selection? The first consideration refers to optimal experience. Compared with the information gathered among adolescents from different cultures, described in Chapter 7 and in other parts of this book, a substantial limitation in the perceived opportunities for engagement and skill development emerged. Regardless of their country, children experiencing street or institutionalized life reported low exposure to optimal experience, and they mostly associated it with activities characterized by low challenge and complexity, as well as limited and short-term relevance. Peer relationships and unstructured leisure contexts were prominently reported, while learning and structured activities were almost absent. The optimal activities quoted by most of these participants neither fostered the cultivation of specific skills nor the youth's integration in the social context. They rather provided vicarious relations, and a way to escape a problematic life. Paradoxically, within a hostile and stressful environment, the risk of falling into disengagement states is persistent, due to the lack of structured situations. The daily experience of these children thus fluctuates between anxiety and thrill, on the one hand, and boredom and apathy, on the other hand. There is little room for optimal experiences in this setting.

Moreover, Italian and Brazilian youth stressed their difficulty in getting engaged in tasks requiring effort and prolonged concentration, such as learning and work activities. These combined findings suggest that street life, in spite of its appealing aspects of thrill, freedom and independence, does not help children develop emotional self-regulation and persistent attention focus. These abilities, which are essential tools for living in a structured human community, are substituted by more basic survival strategies such as circular attention, alertness and quick adaptive reactions to a continuously changing environment, more suited to the nomadic and peripatetic way of life typical of street children (Aptekar & Abebe, 1997). However, as studies on distress have widely shown, persistently high levels of activation lead to emotional exhaustion and reduced cognitive efficiency, especially in concomitance with the low levels of self-esteem and self-efficacy that often characterize children under difficult circumstances (Garmezy et al., 1984; Kanner, Coyne, Schaever, & Lazarus, 1981; Karademas & Kalantzi-Azizi, 2004). The widespread drug abuse among these children has to be partially related to stress-relief mechanisms (Morakinyo & Odejide, 2003; Stritzke, Lang, & Patrick, 1996). However, as discussed in detail in the following pages, addiction brings about a global deterioration in lifestyle, a gradual loss of interest in other challenges, a decrease in motivation to make plans and to develop competencies (Olievenstein, 2000). This is one of the major threats to these children's growth at the physical, social, and psychological levels.

Another problem emerged from all the interviews concerns the negative family context described by most children. Malfunction in family relationships can seriously affect children's behavior, as discussed in Chapter 10. Research studies showed that troubled communication within the family is a risk factor for adolescent deviant behavior (Cashwell & Vacc, 1996). Similar consequences derive from parental pathology, physical aggression, and alcoholism (Osuna, Alarcon, & Luna, 1992). Several intra-familial risk factors can be identified in dealing with children maladjustment, and their effect is additive: the more risk factors, the worse the outcomes (Sameroff, Seifer, & Bartko, 1997). Other studies highlighted the peculiar effect of psychological maltreatment, which turns to be one of the most predictive risk factors for maladjustment (McGee, Wolfe, & Wilson, 1997). The negative family experience shared by most adolescents in this chapter was counterbalanced by their prominent investment on peers, perceived as advisors and points of reference in the process of emotional, cognitive, and social development, with the evident dangers embedded in this solution. The reconstruction of attachment relationships represents both a major concern and a major challenge for social workers and educators dealing with street children (Schimmel, 2008). Nevertheless, across groups children reported family-related goals, mostly referring to getting their own family, but also including parents' care and support.

The comparison of goals and desires across groups partially shed light on the psychological selection pattern of these adolescents. Most participants were aware of the relevance of finding a job as a future life goal. They were also substantially realistic about their work opportunities, even though—in line with other studies (DiCarlo, Gibbons, Kaminsky, Wright, & Stiles, 2000; Merriman & Guerin, 2007)—popular and prestigious professions such as becoming a sport professional or a doctor were also quoted. As concerns desires, an interesting and partially unexpected difference between western and non-western teenagers was the prominence of material goods among the former and the emphasis on social contribution among the latter. This finding can be analyzed taking into account the cultural context these adolescents live in. Italian teenagers spending their days on the street do not face poverty, destitution, and lack of basic facilities. At the same time, they experience deprivation of meaningful challenges and relationships. Their aspiration to material achievements that would allow them to enjoy an easy and pleasant life without need for effort and commitment is consistent with the large resource availability in their environment. Moreover, they are typical representatives of a postindustrial individualistic culture, prominently oriented to materialism and individual success. On the opposite, Brazilian and Kenyan teenagers come from a first-hand experience of marginalization and forced exclusion. Their rehabilitation process made them aware of the importance of social action to promote more equity and a better life for disadvantaged populations. Friends and relatives of these teenagers still live in needy conditions; providing help to others is therefore not an abstract concept or a matter of wishful thinking; rather it is rooted in the direct experience of shared community hardship. Though we cannot exclude that this emphasis on social contribution was at least partially linked to social desirability biases, the fact that none of the western participants took it into consideration is a remarkable finding.

More generally, results offer some suggestions for intervention: street children should be provided with adequate training in the exercise of concentration and skill cultivation. Their specific abilities and competences are suited to the street environment, which does not support long-term planning and commitment to the intentional pursuit of complex and distal goals. These skills can be built through the promotion of optimal experience in complex and meaningful activities. Gradual challenge increase, support of self-determined goal-setting (Deci & Ryan, 2000), and the promotion of self-efficacy (Bandura, 1997), could be adequate strategies to pursue this aim. An optimistic explanatory style could be supported through internalization of children's locus of causality (Buchanan & Seligman, 1995). In line with this perspective, a study conducted in Tanzania among former street children living in a rehabilitative shelter (Nalkur, 2009) showed that, when solicited to generate narratives through the Thematic Apperception Test, these children emphasized the benefits derived from relationships and supportive achievement orientation. They also perceived the importance of exercising choices, thus highlighting the role of both self-determination and social support in setting and pursuing goals.

Finally, the promotion of children's agency should represent a central target in intervention. This construct has been variously conceptualized (for an overview see Bassi et al., 2010), but most important in the present context is the approach proposed by Sen (1987), who highlighted the connection between agency, intentionality, and responsibility. Through their sense of agency, individuals can commit themselves to relevant and meaningful actions in view of their impact on the person, the social context and other people's needs. This approach implies that people can actively and intentionally commit themselves to activities and goals that do not necessarily lead to immediate individual benefits and pleasure. They can invest psychic and material resources into activities which are relevant for the community, sometimes to the detriment of their own personal functionings (free time, relaxation, material goods, comforts). From this perspective, agency can promote children's active participation in their process of change, which includes lifestyle modifications, skill cultivation, active understanding, and re-interpretation of stressful events and of their psychological consequences. Individual and collective agency and responsibility can be mobilized in stressful situations (Quarantelli, 1985), and since one of the features of growth is its interpersonal aspect, growthful interactions should be offered to the children (Joseph & Linley, 2006). Such an approach moreover gives centrality to children's initiative and action, presently acknowledged as the core of any respectful and child-centered intervention (Magazine, 2003; Turnbull et al., 2009).

15.3 Can Flow Be Maladaptive?

Throughout this book, evidence is provided of the universality and relevance of optimal experience to individual functioning across cultures. However, optimal experience does not automatically bring about well-being and development. Several studies have highlighted that its outcomes vary according to the features of the associated activities and their role within the value system of the individuals and of their social environment, taking into account both cultural selection and psychological selection patterns. Some activities can be perceived as sources of optimal experience; they can be actively cultivated but eventually turn out to be inadequate means toward personal growth, self-actualization, and harmonious integration of the individual in the social context.

Evidence comes from studies conducted among recreational and pathological gamblers (Wanner, Ladouceur, Auclair, & Vitaro, 2006). Participants' description of flow during gambling was consistent with the theoretical assumptions and empirical evidence concerning optimal experience. However, pathological gamblers reported lower mean levels in most experiential variables and higher levels of self-consciousness than recreational gamblers.

Antisocial activities, such as stealing, were also sometimes quoted as sources of flow by homeless people and street youth (Delle Fave et al., 1991; Delle Fave & Massimini, 2005a). These activities are often articulated, they offer high challenge and opportunities for engagement, and for the mobilization of a considerable amount of knowledge and technical abilities. Some participants also reported enjoyment and intrinsic motivation in performing the activity, regardless of its outcomes. Similarly, flow-like absorption is often reported in combat situations, in which it contributes both to the subjective well-being and to the efficiency of soldiers (Harari, 2008).

The most detailed findings on the adverse consequences of optimal experiences have been obtained through the study of substance use and abuse. Therefore, the following pages will be specifically devoted to this topic.

15.3.1 Drug Intake and Mimetic Optimal Experiences

Several studies have highlighted the role of chemicals in promoting positive experiences, by lowering perceived stress in daily life and providing relaxation and recreation (Siqueira, Diab, Bodian, & Rolnitzky, 2001; Williams & Parker, 2001). In particular, research work based on experience sampling procedures shed light on the daily mechanisms underlying drug induced psychological positive effects. Tennen and colleagues (2000) showed the role of alcohol abuse as self-medication following experiences of anxiety or depression, within an emotion-centered coping strategy (Kessler et al., 1997). A study with ESM conducted by Larson and colleagues (1992) showed that alcohol intake among adolescents was recurrently associated with positive emotions, while during marijuana use participants reported average levels of mood, but they felt significantly more free and open than average.

Curiously enough, the diagnostic manual DSM-IV (American Psychiatric Association, 1994) does not give any emphasis to the positive experience associated with drug intake. Only generic cognitive and emotional changes are reported in the paragraph concerning "Intoxication," thus overlooking the core reason inducing people to take drugs. In fact, in our opinion the real problem of drug intake, which generates addiction, is the subjective experience associated with it (Nesse, 1994). From this perspective, the framework of positive psychology and, in particular, studies on optimal experience can help shed light on the psychological phenomenology of addiction as it is described by addicts themselves, and offer suggestions for treatment programs (Delle Fave & Massimini, 2003).

Besides substance-related variations, most drugs induce extremely positive experiences. A perception of complete absorption, deep involvement, isolation from the surrounding world, and psychophysical well-being are commonly described. This effect is grounded in a well-defined biological background, that is the activation of the dopaminergic reward circuits of the mesolimbic system, whose main anatomical structures are the nucleus accumbens and the ventral tegmental area (Palfai & Jankiewicz, 1997; Thombs, 1999; White, 1998). The mesolimbic structures are connected with the amygdala and the prefrontal cortex, and therefore they interact with the motivational and emotion regulation systems, and with learning and memory processes (Gardner & David, 1999; White, 1996).

However, differently from other reward mechanisms, the substance's positive effects decrease in frequency and intensity with time. This unfavorable evolution is related to two interdependent phenomena. The first one is represented by the control loss of psychoactive substance use in spite of its adverse consequences, and it includes the syndrome of biological dependence, and the psychological and behavioral addiction disorder (Maddux & Desmond, 2000; World Health Organization, 2005). The second phenomenon is tolerance, that is, the need to use increasingly larger amounts of substance to achieve the intended effect. Several biological and psychological mechanisms are involved in the development of dependence and tolerance. At the biological level, dependence is related to more or less stable changes occuring in the mesolimbic structures, as well as in the endocannabinoid system, in the endogenous opioid system (EOS), and in the brain-derived neurotrophic factor, which variously modulate the dopaminergic activity. Neuroanatomical modifications, such as reorganization of synapses and dendritic spine formation, take place in these areas, also involving the motivational and learning circuits connected with them (Hyman & Malenka, 2001). With time, a compensation mechanism involving EOS develops, in order to counterbalance the persistent increase of dopamine production and synaptic availability, thus opposing the drug effects on reward circuits (Trigo, Martin-Garcia, Berrendero, Robledo, & Maldonado, 2010) and inducing tolerance.

At the psychological level, addiction has been explained through conditioning and reinforcement mechanisms (McAuliffe & Gordon, 1980; Siegel, 1982). Cognitive models emphasized the role of self-efficacy, and of outcome expectancies in the various stages of addiction and recovery (Bandura, 1995). Kaplan (1992) explored with ESM the phenomenology of craving among heroin addicts, identifying two components of the syndrome: the first one is represented by the perceived need for the substance and the identification of a strategy to get it; the second one is the loss of control and the onset of abstinence symptoms, such as anxiety and restlessness. These findings confirmed previous hypotheses on the distinction between symbolic and physiological craving (Jellinek, 1960; Rankin, Hodgson, & Stockwell, 1979). Individual differences grounded in genetics (Harford, 1992; Li, Lumeng, McBride, & Murphy, 1994; Wall & Ehlers, 1995) and personality (Gunnarsdottir et al., 2000; Raylu & Oei, 2002) can also account for variations in vulnerability and reactivity to substance use and abuse.

Cultural and contextual attitudes toward substance use, in particular the influence of family (Ingram & Price, 2001; Ungar, 2004), peers, and significant others (Bake, Brandon, & Chassin, 2004; Leonard & Mudar, 2000), have been highlighted as major factors facilitating of preventing abuse (Khalily, 2001). As reported in the previous pages referring to street youth, poverty, marginalization, and a social environment lacking in challenges and opportunities for engagement can lead to drug abuse. Conversely, society and job pressures toward performance may induce substance use in order to be up to social requirements and expectations (Crowley, 1984). However, more often substance use and abuse are grounded in a multifactorial set of cultural, biological, individual, and situational components (Bailey & Rachal, 1993). The ultimate reason to indulge in these behavior is nevertheless the psychological reward derived from the attainment of a positive experience (Olievenstein, 2000).

The administration of flow questionnaire to drug addicts and ex-addicts highlighted the association of flow with drug intake (Delle Fave & Massimini, 2003). However, since participants were invited to rate the psychological features of flow on 0–8 scales, it was also possible to compare the variable ratings associated with drug intake with those related to the performance of other optimal activities. Differences were detected for some crucial dimensions of the experience: flow during drug intake was characterized by significantly lower levels of challenges, wish to do the activity, relaxation, control of the situation, and perceived goals (Delle Fave & Massimini, 2003).

These differences can be primarily related to the passive nature of the experience arising after drug intake. This experience is induced chemically. Individuals are neither solicited to mobilize specific skills in order to cope with challenges and to attain goals nor have they control on the quality and duration of the substance's effects. This lack of control prevents the person from perceiving high relaxation and intrinsic motivation. Moreover, once the chemically induced experience has extinguished, usually negative feelings arise, such as anxiety, depression, weariness, and difficult reinstatement into real life (American Psychiatric Association, 1994). In the long run, addicts become progressively disengaged from daily life and activities, physically weak, and marginalized from the social context. On the contrary optimal experience usually promotes personal growth, complexity in behavior, and social integration (Chapters 3 and 7). From this perspective, therefore, it is possible to maintain that the mimetic or pseudo-optimal experiences induced by substances deceive consciousness with an ephemeral perception of well-being, while entailing substantially maladaptive implications (Aarons, Brown, Stice, & Coe, 2001; Bogart, Collins, Ellickson, & Klein, 2007; Massimini & Delle Fave, 2000).

15.3.2 Detoxification Programs: The Role of Challenges and Meanings

In a recent editorial article, Miller and Miller (2009) claimed for the need of addressing addiction through a multifaceted approach. Drug abuse is usually just one of the problems addicts have to face, intertwined with other related ones involving all domains of life, from biological health to cultural norms and values. Moreover, only a minority of people with addiction problems seek help from specialists, and within this minority high rates of dropout have been recorded (McLellan, 2006). This alarming evidence suggests that, in order to be effective, intervention should be more tailored and person-centered, and it should address the multiplicity of problematic issues that addiction conveys.

Moreover, even though outcome evaluation is crucial to verify the effectiveness of a treatment, there is still lack of systematic investigation in this domain. In particular, the availability of optimal experience in the daily activities of ex-addicts undergoing treatment was only marginally explored. In the following pages we will provide some information on this topic, gathered in two different studies.

In the first study, flow questionnaire was administered to 61 participants aged 14–40 (46 men and 15 women), 52 involved in residential detoxification programs in three different communities, and 9 receiving outpatient pharmacological treatment with methadone from public health services (Delle Fave & Massimini, 2003).

Table 15.4 Detoxification and optimal activities. Percentage distribution of answers across activity categories

Optimal activities	Answers (%)
Work	19.7
Leisure	17.6
Media	16.2
Study	9.9
Drug intake	9.2
Religion	9.2
Family, partner	8.4
Social relations	4.9
Other	4.9
N. answers	142

The residential programs differed according to the approach followed in each of community: job training, Scientology, and religion-based treatment respectively. All the participants reported optimal experience in their present or past life. Table 15.4 shows the percentage distribution of the associated activities across categories. Work, leisure, and the use of media were prominent. However, differences in the activity distribution were detected according to the inspiring principles of each community, which oriented the treatment and channeled participants' investment of attention and psychological selection. Within the Scientology-based program, most participants (60%) quoted study, referring to the community founder's theories and their application to everyday life. Participants in the job-training center prominently quoted drug intake in the past (67%), and work in the present life (53%). Half of the participants in the religious community associated optimal experience with religious practices, followed by work (36%), while among the participants who received pharmacological treatment 44% quoted the use of media (mostly reading and watching TV), and 33% having sex. Differently from the other three groups, participants getting substitute pharmacological treatment were actually addicts. They had lost the exciting experiences derived from drug intake, but they were still dependent upon psychoactive substances. They associated optimal experiences with activities low in challenge, in individual and social meaning, and in opportunities for skill development.

Similar differences between community residents and outpatients were detected in a more recent study conducted with ESM among 29 Italian participants (3 women and 26 men) undergoing detoxification programs, ten of them as outpatients undergoing pharmacological treatment with methadone, and 19 of them living in a community following a psycho-educational approach (Bassi, Preziosa, & Pozzoli, 2007; Pozzoli, 2008). The community provided guests with a precise daily time structuration, comprising vocational trainings and work activities, self-help groups and counseling sessions, recreational and socialization initiatives.

ESM highlighted relevant differences in the time budget of the two groups: outpatients spent their time in maintenance activities (24% of the self-reports, comprising eating, resting, and personal care), reading and watching TV (19%), working (19%), socializing (13%), and leisure (15%). Community participants prominently reported work (29%) and interactions (23%), followed by maintenance (18%) and leisure (12%) as the prominent daily activities, while the use of media accounted only for 6% of their self-reports. This activity distribution resulted significantly different between the two groups ($\chi^2 = 90.4$, $p<0.0001$). Outpatients spent most of their time alone (61%), and in lower percentages with partner or family members (17%), while participants in residential treatment shared most part of their time with other community members (69%), being alone only in 24%. of the self-reports.

Group differences were also detected in the perceived relevance of the ongoing activity for future goals across life domains ($\chi^2 = 13.2$, $p<0.001$). Outpatients primarily quoted work (24%), followed by personal growth (17%) and material goods (15%). Among community members personal growth prevailed (37%), followed by future job opportunities outside the community (23%) and relations (21%).

As concerns the daily quality of experience, Table 15.5 shows the distribution of participants' self-reports across the channels of the Experience Fluctuation Model. Outpatients prominently reported low-challenge experiences (52.6%), and especially apathy, while among community participants high-challenge situations (45.3%), and especially anxiety, were most frequently quoted. The channel distribution significantly differed between groups ($\chi^2 = 22.4$, $p<0.001$). However, both outpatients and community members reported optimal experiences in similar percentages and in the same domains, namely, work and interactions.

These findings provide hints on some crucial aspects of treatment. The first one concerns the strategies used to promote participants' building of a new, non-addict identity (Biernacki, 1986). In particular, most communities aim at providing residents with challenges and opportunities for skill development in complex and culturally meaningful activities (such as work, study, and structured leisure), that can foster both their social integration and their personal growth. This training can transiently expose clients to experiences of anxiety, defined as a perceived imbalance between environmental demands and personal resources. However, as discussed in Chapter 3, this is the only pathway that promotes the development

Table 15.5 The percentage distribution of ESM self-reports across the EFM channels in participants attending detoxification in outpatient and residential community programs

Channels	Day care ($N = 10$)	Community ($N = 19$)
1. Activation	9.5	8.1
2. Optimal experience	19.6	16.9
3. Control	5.0	9.5
4. Relaxation	12.0	17.6
5. Boredom	14.6	13.5
6. Apathy	26.0	8.8
7. Worry	4.4	5.4
8. Anxiety	8.9	20.3
N self-reports	257	614

Note: N = Number of participants.

of any kind of competences and skills. The virtuous cycle through which individuals can attain optimal experience in the same activity throughout time is based on a gradual but ceaseless increase of challenges. This process necessarily implies periods in which these increasing challenges have to be faced with transiently inadequate skills. Constant practice and skill cultivation can re-establish the challenge/skill balance, thus urging the person to search for even higher challenges. From this perspective, the monitoring of guests' daily experience fluctuations in different activities can represent a useful tool for developing personalized residential treatments, and for evaluating treatment efficacy. Other studies based on sampling procedures showed the usefulness of monitoring emotions to evaluate transition processes among community residents (Ravenna, Hölzl, Costarelli, Kirchler, & Palmonari, 2001, 2002).

The second aspect concerns the different impact of treatment on participants' quality of experience, according to the features of the community. In particular, two of the communities examined in the study based on flow questionnaire provided their members with a whole set of behavioral instructions, inspired to Catholic religion and to Scientology, respectively. In these communities, guests were integrated within a cultural network that not only offered them opportunities for optimal experiences in structured and complex activities (such as work, study, and religious practice), but also a value system and opportunities for active contribution and participation (Cunningham, 1999; Downey, Rosengren, & Donovan, 2001). Even though there are substantial differences as concerns complexity and universality between the value system developed by a major human religion and the value system derived from a specific theory, elaborated and operationalized within a small subculture, in both communities guests were encouraged to harmonize their personal meaning-making process with the cultural meaning of the activities proposed to them (Delle Fave, 2009; McIntosh & McKeganey, 2000). A recent study conducted in a Brazilian religious community for detoxification provided similar evidence and outcomes (van der Meer Sanchez & Nappo, 2008). Great attention to identity building through a psycho-educational strategy was also paid in the community hosting the participants examined with ESM. Compared with outpatients, these people perceived their daily activities as prominently relevant for their personal and social growth.

Contrasting results were instead obtained through flow questionnaire among guests of the job training community. The participants frequently quoted drug intake as optimal activity, though referring to the past. This result can be related to the lack of a specific world outlook guiding the treatment. In this community individuals are free to build their own new identity according to self-selected beliefs and value system; however, they are not provided with specific support in this process, except for job skills and integration in the productive context. Due to the complex changes that ex-addicts have to face at every level, well-defined treatment contents and structure do not necessarily represent a constraint. Individuals have to rebuild their personal and social identity, often starting from basic grounds and values, and often coming from a condition of complete absence of reference points. Moreover, individuals who decide to undergo treatment can choose in advance among a variety of programs, thus having the opportunity to join the community whose approach most suits their cultural background and value system.

Finally, findings from both studies highlighted that pharmacological treatment alone does not represent an adequate solution to addiction. In particular, the ESM study shed light on the daily life of participants treated with methadone. Besides being physiologically dependent upon drug substitutes, they prominently spent their time in low-challenge contexts, engaging in scarcely relevant activities such as maintenance and TV watching. Their social network resulted dramatically restricted, due to their decision to undergo detoxification, that led them to interrupt most of the relationships developed and cultivated within the drug circle. Under these circumstances building a new, non-addict identity can be extremely difficult. Nevertheless, these participants reported optimal experience in almost one fifth of their self-reports, mostly associating it with work and interactions. They showed a good potential for engagement and skill development, but due to the lack of support in structuring time and attention they were exposed to frequent apathy experiences. As detected in several studies, and specifically described in Chapter 5, prolonged apathy predisposes to depressive symptoms, languishing, and drug abuse as compensation and self-medication (Delle Fave & Massimini, 1992; Larson, 2000), thus closing the vicious circle from which these participants were attempting to escape.

15.4 Building Positive Identities

The difficulties arising in treatment programs addressed to addicts and to youth under difficult circumstances can be at least partially related to the fact that drug intake and antisocial behaviors provide people with positive feelings and exciting experiences, even though transitory and substantially disruptive in the long run. Moving from these premises, from the perspective of psychological selection it is not surprising that addicts preferentially center their life upon drug, investing their resources in searching and using it as vehicle of rewarding and positive states. Similarly, street children who repeatedly run away from the rehabilitation centers look for the thrill, adventure, and independence that only a life free from discipline and constraints can offer.

An interpretation of human vulnerability to substance abuse, derived from the recent framework of evolutionary medicine, can help us better understand this mechanism (Nesse & Berridge, 1997; Smith, 1999). Our original Environment of Evolutionary Adaptation radically differed from the present one: it was a demanding context that challenged human survival through a permanent lack of resources, be they food or mating partners. These chronic resource limitation—and the consequent necessity to compete in order to get them—made emotions the most adaptive system available to humans for achieving an effective regulation of both approach and avoidance motivations and behavior. In today's environment, where resources are usually abundant, a higher flexibility in the regulation of emotions and of learning and evaluation patterns is essential for adaptation. However, wide variations can be detected between individuals in these fine-tuned regulation abilities, and not all individuals show the same level of behavioral, emotional, and learning flexibility, due to personal, social, and situational factors. Substance abuse can counterbalance this emotional and behavioral limitation through feelings of strengths, cognitive efficiency, and self-confidence that—though transiently—can enhance self-esteem, facilitate performance, and promote socialization through the relief of anxiety or depression symptoms. The same role could be played by the strong identification with a group, especially if characterized by assertive and aggressive behaviors, as often happens among street youth (Olley, 2006).

This approach, however, assumes that addicts, as well as street children and adolescents, do not possess some basic bio-psycho-social resources that prevent other people living under similarly difficult circumstances from "getting hooked" with addiction and/or street life thrills, especially when provided with the opportunity to change their life conditions. This lack of basic resources could partially explain the high rates of relapse among former addicts, and the frequent dropout of street children from rehabilitative centers. In fact, motivation to change alone does not exert a significant effect on substance abuse or treatment involvement (Carpenter, Miele, & Hasin, 2002), even though intrinsic reasons are more effective than extrinsic ones in promoting adherence to treatment (Downey et al., 2001; McBride et al., 1994).

Positive psychology has contributed to shed light on some of the resources that promote well-being and empowerment in the presence of unfavorable environmental conditions. They include resilience, optimism, hope, hardiness, self-efficacy, and self-determination. Since most of them can be learned and cultivated with time, they have a wide potential for application in intervention programs designed for these populations. In addition, the framework of psychological selection could provide hints about the developmental trend of each person, and about the domains that could be more easily cultivated by virtue of their association with optimal experiences, thus allowing for treatment personalization.

References

Aarons, G. A., Brown, S. A., Stice, E., & Coe, M. T. (2001). Psychometric evaluation of the marijuana and stimulant effect expectancy questionnaires for adolescents. *Addictive Behaviors, 26*, 219–236.

Alexandrescu, G. (1996). Street children in Bucharest. Programme note. *Childhood, 2*, 267–270.

American Psychiatric Association. (1994). *Diagnostic and statistical manual of mental disorders* (4th ed.). Washington, DC: American Psychiatric Association.

Anselmo, C. (2000). *Bambini di strada a Nairobi: il progetto Kivuli.* Unpublished Master dissertation, Università IULM Milano, Italy.

Aptekar, L. (1994). Street children in the developing world: A review of their conditions. *Cross-Cultural Research, 28*, 195–224.

Aptekar, L., & Abebe, B. (1997). Conflict in the neighborhood. Street and working children in the public space. *Childhood, 4*, 477–490.

Arieli, M., Beker, J., & Kashti, Y. (1990). Residential group care as a socializing environment: Toward a broader perspective. *Child and Youth Services, 13*, 45–58.

Aubrey, C., & Dahl, S. (2005). Children's voices: The view of vulnerable children in their service providers and relevance of services they receive. *British Journal of Social Work, 36*, 21–39.

Bailey, S. L., & Rachal, J. V. (1993). Dimensions of adolescent problem drinking. *Journal of Studies on Alcohol, 54*, 555–565.

Bake, T. B., Brandon, T. H., & Chassin, L. (2004). Motivational influences on cigarette smoking. *Annual Review of Psychology, 55*, 463–491.

Baker, R., Panter-Brick, C., & Todd, A. (1996). Methods used in research with street children in Nepal. *Childhood, 3*, 171–193.

Bandura, A. (Ed.). (1995). *Self-efficacy in a changing society*. New York: Cambridge University Press.

Bandura, A. (1997). *Self-efficacy: The exercise of control*. New York: Freeman.

Bar-On, A. (1998). So what's so wrong with being a street child? *Child & Youth Care Forum, 3*, 201–222.

Bassi, M., Preziosa, A., & Pozzoli, S. (2007). Experience sampling method e lo studio dell'esperienza quotidiana: implicazioni per l'intervento [Experience sampling method and the study of daily experience: implications for intervention]. In A. Delle Fave (Ed.), *La condivisione del benessere. Il contributo della psicologia positiva* (pp. 169–189). Milano: FrancoAngeli.

Bassi, M., Sartori, R. D. G., & Delle Fave, A. (2010). The monitoring of experience and agency in daily life: A study with Italian adolescents. In M. Balconi (Ed.), *The neuropsychology of agency* (pp. 81–106). Dordrecht: Springer Science.

Bhattarai, K., & Delle Fave, A. (2002). Children at work, children in the street: Present programs and future plans. In A. Delle Fave & M. B. Pun (Eds.), *In pursuit of a sustainable modernisation: Culture and policies in Nepal* (pp. 145–165). Milano: Arcipelago Edizioni.

Biernacki, P. (1986). *Pathways from heroin addiction: Recovery without treatment*. Philadelphia, PA: Temple University Press.

Bogart, L. M., Collins, R. L., Ellickson, P. L., & Klein, D. J. (2007). Are adolescent substance users less satisfied with life as young adults and if so, why? *Social Indicators Research, 81*, 149–169.

Buchanan, G. M., & Seligman M. (Eds.). (1995). *Explanatory style*. Hillsdale, NJ: Erlbaum.

Carpenter, K. M., Miele, G. M., & Hasin, D. S. (2002). Does motivation to change mediate the effect of DSM-IV substance use disorders on treatment utilization and substance use? *Addictive Behaviors, 27*, 207–225.

Cashwell, C. S., & Vacc, N. A. (1996). Family functioning and risk behaviors: Influences on adolescent delinquency. *School Counselor, 44*, 105–114.

Crowley, T. (1984). Contingency contracting treatment of drug-abusing physicians nurses and dentists: Behavioural intervention techniques in drug abuse treatments. *NIDA Research Monographs, 46*, 68–83.

Csikszentmihalyi, M. (1975/2000). *Beyond boredom and anxiety*. San Francisco: Jossey Bass.

Cunningham, J. (1999). Untreated remission from drug use: The predominant pathway. *Addictive Behaviors, 24*, 267–270.

CWIN. (1995). *Voice of child workers* (Special Issue No. 25). Kathmandu: Indreni Offset Press.

Dallape, F. (1996). Urban children: A challenge and an opportunity. *Childhood, 2*, 283–294.

Davies, M. (2008). A childish culture? Shared understandings, agency and intervention: An anthropological study of street children in northwest Kenya. *Childhood, 15*, 309–330.

De Oliveira, W., Baizerman, M., & Pellet, L. (1992). Street children in Brazil and their helpers: Comparative views on aspirations and the future. *International Social Work, 35*, 163–176.

De Roure, G. Q. (1996). *Vidas silenciadas. A violencia com crianças e adolescents na sociedade brasileira*. Campinas: Eda.

Deci, E. L., & Ryan, R. M. (2000). The "what" and "why" of goal pursuits: Human needs and the self-determination of behavior. *Psychological Inquiry, 11*, 227–268.

Delle Fave, A. (2009). Optimal experience and meaning: Which relationship? *Psychological Topics, Special issue on positive psychology, 18*, 285–302.

Delle Fave, A., & Massimini, F. (1988). Modernization and the changing contexts of flow in work and leisure. In M. Csikszentmihalyi & I. Csikszentmihalyi (Eds.), *Optimal experience. Psychological studies of flow in consciousness* (pp. 193–213). New York: Cambridge University Press.

Delle Fave, A., & Massimini, F. (1991). Modernization and the quality of daily experience in a southern Italy village. In N. Bleichrodt & P. J. D. Drenth (Eds.), *Contemporary issues in cross cultural psychology* (pp. 110–119). Amsterdam: Swets & Zeitlinger B.V.

Delle Fave, A., & Massimini, F. (1992). Experience sampling method and the measuring of clinical change: A case of anxiety syndrome. In M. W. deVries (Ed.), *The experience of psychopathology – investigating mental disorders in their natural settings* (pp. 280–298). Cambridge: Cambridge University Press.

Delle Fave, A., & Massimini, F. (2000). Living at home or in institution: Adolescents' optimal experience and life theme. *Paideia. Cadernos de Psicologia e Educaçao*, *19*, 55–66.

Delle Fave, A., & Massimini, F. (2003). Drug addiction: The paradox of mimetic optimal experience. In J. Henry (Ed.), *European positive psychology proceedings 2002* (pp. 31–38). Leicester: British Psychological Society.

Delle Fave, A., & Massimini, F. (2005a). The relevance of subjective wellbeing to social policies: Optimal experience and tailored intervention. In F. Huppert, B. Keverne, & N. Baylis (Eds.), *The science of wellbeing* (pp. 379–404). Oxford: Oxford University Press.

Delle Fave, A., & Massimini, F. (2005b). The investigation of optimal experience and apathy: Developmental and psychosocial implications. *European Psychologist*, *10*, 264–274.

Delle Fave, A., Massimini, F., & Maletto, C. (1991). Barboni [Homeless people]. *Psicologia Contemporanea*, *104*, 55–63.

DiCarlo, M. A., Gibbons, J. L., Kaminsky, D. C., Wright, J., & Stiles, D. (2000). Street children's drawings: Windows into their life circumstances and aspirations. *International Social Work*, *43*, 107–120.

Downey, L., Rosengren, D. B., & Donovan, D. M. (2001). Sources of motivation for abstinence. A replication analysis of the reasons for quitting questionnaire. *Addictive Behaviors*, *26*, 79–89.

Freire, P. (1970). *Pedagogy of the oppressed*. New York: Herder & Herder.

Freire, P. (1994). *Educaçao como pratica da liberdade*. Rio de Janeiro: Paz e Terra.

Freire, P. (1996). *Pedagogia da autonomia*. Rio de Janeiro: Paz e Terra.

Freire, P. (1998). Cultural action and conscientization. *Harvard Educational Review*, *68*, 499–521.

Gardner, E. L., & David, J. (1999). The neurobiology of chemical addiction. In J. Elster & O. J. Skog (Eds.), *Getting hooked. Rationality and addiction* (pp. 93–136). Cambridge: Cambridge University Press.

Garmezy, N., Masten, A. S., & Tellegen, A. (1984). The study of stress and competence in children: A building block for developmental psychopathology. *Child development*, *55*, 97–111.

Gracey, M. (2002). Child health in an urbanizing world. *Acta Paedeatrica*, *9*, 1–8.

Grundling, J., & Grundling, I. (2005). The concrete particulars of the everyday realities of street children. *Human Relations*, *58*, 173–190.

Gunnarsdottir, E. D., Pingitore, R. A., Spring, B. J., Konopka, L. M., Crayton, J. W., Milo, T., et al. (2000). Individual differences among cocaine users. *Addictive Behaviors*, *25*, 641–652.

Harari, Y. N. (2008). Combat flow: Military, political, and ethical dimensions of subjective well-being in war. *Review of General Psychology*, *12*, 253–264.

Harford, T. C. (1992). Family history of alcoholism in the United States: Prevalence and demographic characteristics. *British Journal of Addiction*, *87*, 931–935.

Harpham, T., & Reichenheim, M. (1994). *Health and disease in developing countries*. London: Macmillan.

Harré, R., & Secord, P. F. (1972). *The explanation of social behavior*. Totowa, NJ: Rowman and Littlefield.

Hyman, S. E., & Malenka, R. C. (2001). Addiction and the brain: The neurobiology of compulsion and its persistence. *Nature Reviews: Neuroscience*, *2*, 695–703.

ILO. (2001). *IPEC action against child labour 2000–2001: progress and future priorities*. http://www.ilo.org/public/english/standards/ipec

ILO. (2009). *Global Report*. http://www.ilo.org

Inciardi, J. A., & Surratt, H. L. (1998). Children in the streets of Brazil: Drug use, crime, violence and HIV risk. *Substance Use & Misuse*, *7*, 1461–1480.

Ingram, R. E., & Price, J. M. (2001). *Vulnerability to psychopathology. Risk across the lifespan.* New York: Guildford Press.
International Catholic Children's Bureau. (1985). *Forum on street children and youth.* Grand Bassam: International Catholic Children's Bureau.
Jellinek, E. M. (1960). *The disease concept of alcoholism.* New Haven, CT: Hillhouse Press.
Joseph, S., & Linley, A. (2006). Growth following adversity: Theoretical perspectives and implications for clinical practice. *Clinical Psychology Review, 26,* 1041–1053.
Jutkowitz, J. M., Spielmannm, H., Koeler, U., Lohani, J., & Pande, A. (1997). Drug use in Nepal: The view from street children. *Substance Use & Misuse, 7–8,* 987–1004.
Kaime-Atterhoeg, W., & Ahlberg, B. M. (2008). Are street children beyond rehabilitation? Understanding the life situation of street boys through ethnographic methods in Nakuru, Kenya. *Children and Youth Services Review, 30,* 1345–1354.
Kanner, A., Coyne, J., Schaever, C., & Lazarus, R. (1981). Comparison of two modes of stress measurement: Daily hassles and uplifts versus major life events. *Journal of Behavioral Medicine, 4,* 1–39.
Kaplan, C. D. (1992). Drug craving and drug use in the daily life of heroin addicts. In M. deVries (Ed.), *The experience of psychopathology* (pp. 193–218). New York: Cambridge University Press.
Karademas, E., & Kalantzi-Azizi, A. (2004). The stress process, self-efficacy expectations, and psychological health. *Personality and individual differences, 37,* 1033–1043.
Kerfoot, M., Koshyl, V., Roganov, O., Mikhailichenko, K., Gorbova, I., & Pottage, D. (2007). The health and well-being of neglected, abused and exploited children: The kyiv street children project. *Child Abuse and Neglect, 31,* 27–37.
Kessler, R. C., Crum, R., Warner, L. A., Nelson, C. B., Schulenberg, J., & Anthony, J. (1997). Lifetime co-occurrence of DSM-III-R alcohol abuse and dependence with other psychiatric disorders in the national co-morbidity survey. *Archives of General Psychiatry, 54,* 313–321.
Khalily, M. T. (2001). A comparison between the psycho-social characteristics of drug addicts and non-addicts. *Pakistan Journal of Psychological Research, 16,* 113–128.
Kombarakaran, F. A. (2004). Street children of Bombay: Their stresses and strategies of coping. *Children and Youth Services Review, 26,* 853–871.
Kudrati, M., Plummer, M. L., & Yousif, N. D. H. (2008). Children of the *sug*: A study of the daily lives of street children in Khartoum, sudan, with intervention recommendations. *Child Abuse and Neglect, 32,* 439–448.
Lam, D., & Cheng, F. (2008). Chinese policy reaction to the problem of street children: An analysis from the perspective of street children. *Children and Youth Services Review, 30,* 575–584.
Larson, R.W. (2000). Toward a psychology of positive youth development. *American Psychologist, 55,* 170–183.
Larson, R. W., Csikszentmihalyi, M., & Freeman, M. (1992). Alcohol and marijuana use in adolescents' daily life: A random sample of experiences. In M. deVries (Ed.), The experience of psychopathology (pp. 180–192). New York: Cambridge University Press.
Le Roux, J. (1996). The worldwide phenomenon of street children: Conceptual analysis. *Adolescence, 124,* 965–971.
Leonard, K. E., & Mudar, P. J. (2000). Alcohol use in the year before marriage: Alcohol expectancies and peer drinking as proximal influences on husband and wife alcohol involvement. *Alcoholism: Clinical and Experimental Research, 24,* 1666–1679.
Levy, Z. (1996). Conceptual foundations of developmentally oriented residential education: A holistic framework for group care that works. *Residential Treatment for Children and Youth, 13,* 69–83.
Li, Tk., Lumeng, L., McBride, W. J., & Murphy, J. M. (1994). Genetic and neurobiological basis of alcohol-seeking behaviour. *Alcohol & Alcoholism, 29,* 697–700.
Lusk, M. (1992). Street children of Rio de Janeiro. *International Social Work, 35,* 293–305.
MacAlpine, K., Henley, R., Mueller, M., & Vetter, S. (2010). A survey of street children in northern Tanzania: How abuse or support factors May influence migration to the street. *Community Mental Health, 46,* 26–32.

Maddux, J. F., & Desmond, D. P. (2000). Addiction or dependence? *Addiction, 95*, 661–665.
Magazine, R. (2003). Action, personhood and gift economy among so-called street children in Mexico City. *Social Anthropology, 11*, 303–318.
Massimini, F., & Delle Fave, A. (2000). Individual development in a bio-cultural perspective. *American Psychologist, 55*, 24–33.
Mathiti, V. (2006). The quality of life of "street children" accommodated at three shelters in Pretoria: An exploratory study. *Early Child Development and Care, 176*, 253–269.
Mathur, M. (2009). Socialization of street children in India: A socio-economic profile. *Psychology and Developing Societies, 21*, 299–325.
Mathur, M., Rathore, P., & Mathur, M. (2009). Incidence, type and intensity of abuse in street children in India. *Child Abuse and Neglect, 33*, 907–913.
Mayall, B. (2002). *Towards a sociology of childhood: Thinking from children's lives*. Buckingham: Open University Press.
McAuliffe, W. E., & Gordon, R. A. (1980). Reinforcement and the combination of effects: Summary of a theory of opiate addiction. In D. J. Lettieri, M. Sayers, & H. Wallestein Pearson (Eds.), *Theories on drug abuse. Research monograph (*30, pp. 137–141). Rockville, MD: NIDA.
McBride, C. M., Curry, S. J., Stephens, R. S., Wells, E. A., Roffman, R. A., & Hawkins, J. D. (1994). Intrinsic and extrinsic motivation for change in cigarette smokers, marijuana smokers, and cocaine users. *Psychology of Addictive Behaviors, 8*, 243–250.
McGee, R. A., Wolfe, D. A., & Wilson, S. K. (1997). Multiple maltreatment experiences and adolescents behavior problems: Adolescents' perspectives. *Development and Psychopathology, 9*, 131–149.
McIntosh, J., & McKeganey, N. (2000). Addicts' narratives of recovery from drug use: Constructing a non-addict identity. *Social Science and Medicine, 50*, 1501–1510.
McLellan, A. T. (2006). What we need is a system: Creating a responsive and effective substance use treatment. In W. R. Miller & K. M. Carroll (Eds.), *Rethinking substance abuse: What the science shows, and what we should do about it* (pp. 275–292). New York: The Guilford Press.
Merriman, B., & Guerin, S. (2007). Exploring the aspirations of Kolkatan (Calcutta) street children living on and off the streets using drawings. *International Journal of Psychology and Psychological Therapy, 7*, 269–283.
Miller, P. G., & Miller, W. R. (2009). What should web e aiming for in the treatment of addiction? *Addiction, 104*, 685–686.
Moazzam, A., Shahab, S., Ushijima, H., & de Muynck, A. (2004). Street children in Pakistan: A situational analysis of social conditions and nutritional status. *Social Science and Medicine, 59*, 1707–1717.
Morakinyo, J., & Odejide, A. O. (2003). A community based study of patterns of psychoactive substance use among street children in a local government area of Nigeria. *Drug and Alcohol Dependence, 71*, 109–116.
Municipality of Goiania. (1999). *Programa brasil criança cidada. Situaçao de rua*. Goiania: Fumdec.
Myrstad, G. (1999). What can trade unions do to combat child labour? *Childhood, 6*, 75–88.
Nalkur, P. (2009). Achievement orientations and strategies: A cultural comparison of Tanzanian street children, former street children, and school-going children. *Journal of Cross-Cultural Psychology, 40*, 1012–1027.
Nesse, R. M. (1994). An evolutionary perspective on substance abuse. *Ethology and Sociobiology, 15*, 339–348.
Nesse, R. M., & Berridge, K. C. (1997). Psychoactive drug use in evolutionary perspective. *Science, 278*, 63–66.
Oles, T. P. (1991). Resident's perceptions of change: A basis for after care. *Residential Treatment for Children & Youth, 9*, 29–37.
Olievenstein, C. (2000). *La drogue, 30 ans après*. Paris: Editions Odile Jacob.
Olley, B. (2006). Social and health behaviors in youth of the streets of Ibadan, Nigeria. *Child Abuse and Neglect, 30*, 271–282.

Osuna, E., Alarcon, C., & Luna, A. (1992). Family violence as a determinant factor in juvenile maladjustment. *Journal of Forensic Studies*, *37*, 1633–1639.
Palfai, T., & Jankiewicz, H. (1997). *Drugs and human behavior* (2nd ed.). Madison, WI: Brown & Benchmark.
Panter-Brick, C. (2002). Street children, human rights, and public health: A critique and future directions. *Annual Review of Anthropology*, *31*, 147–171.
Potts, R. G. (2003). Emancipatory education versus school-based prevention in African American communities. *American Journal of Community Psychology*, *31*, 173–183.
Pozzoli, S. (2008). *Tossicodipendenza e qualità dell'esperienza: confronto in un campione di soggetti ambulatoriali ed in comunità* [Drug addiction and experience: a comparison between outpatients and community residents]. Unpublished PhD Dissertation, University of Milano.
Praharaj, S. K., Verma, P., & Arora, M. (2008). Inhalant abuse (typewriter correction fluid) in street children. *Journal of Addiction Medicine*, *2*, 175–177.
Quarantelli, E. L. (1985). An assessment of conflicting views on mental health. The consequences of traumatic events. In C. R. Figley (Ed.), *Trauma and its wake* (pp. 173–215). New York: Brunner/Mazel.
Rankin, H., Hodgson, R., & Stockwell, T. (1979). The concept of craving and its measurement. *Behavioral Research and Therapy*, *17*, 389–396.
Ravenna, M., Hölzl, E., Costarelli, S., Kirchler, E., & Palmonari, A. (2001). Diary reports on emotion experience in the onset of a psychosocial transition: Becoming drug-free. *Journal of Community and Applied Social Psychology*, *11*, 19–35.
Ravenna, M., Hölzl, E., Kirchler, E., Palmonari, A., & Costarelli, S. (2002). Drug addicts in therapy—Changes in life space in the course of one year. *Journal of Community and Applied Social Psychology*, *12*, 353–368.
Raylu, N., & Oei, T. P. S. (2002). Pathological gambling: A comprehensive review. *Clinical Psychology Review*, *22*, 1009–1061.
Regogliosi, L. (2000). *La strada come luogo educativo. Orientamenti pedagogici sul lavoro di strada*. Milano: Unicopli.
Rew, L., & Horner, S. H. (2003). Personal strengths of homeless adolescents living in a high-risk environment. *Advances in Nursing Science*, *26*, 90–101.
Rizzini, I. (1996). Street children. An excluded generation in Latin America. *Childhood*, *3*, 215–233.
Rossi-Doria, M. (1999). *Di mestiere faccio il maestro* [My job is teaching]. Napoli: L'Ancora.
Sameroff, A. J., Seifer, R., & Bartko, W. T. (1997). Environmental perspectives on adaptation during childhood and adolescence. In S. S. Luthar, A. Burack, D. Cicchetti, & J. R. Weisz (Eds.), *Developmental psychopathology. Perspectives on adjustment risk, and disorder* (pp. 507–526). New York: Cambridge University Press.
Sattaur, O. (1993). *Child labour in Nepal*. Kathmandu: ASI-CWIN.
Schimmel, N. (2008). A humanistic approach to caring for street children: The importance of emotionally intimate and supportive relationships for the successful rehabilitation of street children. *Vulnerable Children and Youth Studies*, *3*, 214–220.
Sen, A. (1987). *On ethics and economics*. Oxford: Oxford University Press.
Sen, A. (2009). Street children in India: A non-government organization-based intervention model. *Journal of Developmental and Behavioral Pediatrics*, *30*, 552–559.
Shorter, A., & Onyancha, E. (1999). *Street children in Africa —A Nairobi case study*. Nairobi: Paulines Publications.
Siegel, S. (1982). Heroin "overdose" death: The contribution of drug-associated environmental cues. *Science*, *216*, 436–437.
Siqueira, L., Diab, M., Bodian, C., & Rolnitzky, L. (2001). The relationship of stress and coping methods to adolescents' marijuana use. *Substance Abuse*, *22*, 157–166.
Smith, E. O. (1999). Evolution, substance abuse, and addiction. In W. R. Trevatian, E. O. Smith, & J. J. McKenna (Eds.), *Evolutionary medicine* (pp. 375–405). New York: Oxford University Press.

Stritzke, W. G., Lang, A. R., & Patrick, C. J. (1996). Beyond stress and arousal: A reconceptualization of alcohol-emotion relations with reference to psychophysiological methods. *Psychological bulletin, 120*, 376–395.

Tennen, H., Affleck, G., Armeli, S., & Carney, M. A. (2000). A daily process approach to coping. *American Psychologist, 55*, 626–636.

Thombs, D. L. (1999). *Introduction to addictive behaviors*. New York: The Guilford Press.

Too, S. H., & Floresca-Cawagas, V. (1997). Towards a people-centred education: Possibilities and struggles in the Philippines. *International Review of Education, 43*, 527–545.

Toro, P. A. (1999). Advances in research on homelessness: An overview of the special issue. *Journal of Community Psychology, 27*, 115–117.

Towe, V. L., ul Hasan, S., Zafar, T., & Sherman, S. G. (2009). Street life and drug risk behaviors associated with exchanging sex among male street children in Lahore, Pakistan. *Journal of Adolescent Health, 44*, 222–228.

Trigo, J. M., Martin-Garcia, E., Berrendero, F., Robledo, P., & Maldonado, R. (2010). The endogenous opioid system: A common substrate in drug addiction. *Drug and Alcohol Dependence, 108*, 183–194.

Turnbull, B., Hernandez, R., & Reyes, M. (2009). Street children and their helpers: An actor-oriented approach. *Children and Youth Services Review, 31*, 1283–1288.

Ungar, M. U. (2004). The importance of parents and other caregivers to the resilience of high-risk adolescents. *Family Process, 43*, 23–41.

Unger, J., Kipke, M., Simon, T., Johnson, C., Montgomery, S., & Iversen, E. (1998). Stress and social support among homeless youth. *Journal of Adolescent Research, 13*, 134–157.

UNICEF. (2001). *Progress since the World Summit for Children*. http://www.childinfo.org

UNICEF. (2005). *The state of the world's children 2006*. New York: UNICEF.

UNICEF. (2009). *The state of the world's children. Special edition*. New York: UNICEF.

UNPD. (2002). *Human development report*. New York: Oxford University Press.

Van Beers, H. (1996). A plea for a child-centered approach in research with street children. *Childhood, 2*, 195–201.

van der Meer Sanchez, Z., & Nappo, S. A. (2008). Religious treatment for drug addiction: An exploratory study in Brazil. *Social Science and Medicine, 67*, 638–646.

Van Wormer, R. (2003). Homeless youth seeking assistance: A research-based study from Duluth, Minnesota. *Child & Youth Care Forum, 32*, 89–103.

Veeran, V. (2005). Working with street children: A child-centered approach. *Child Care in Practice, 10*, 359–366.

Verma, S., & Larson, R. W. (Eds.). (2003). *Examining adolescent leisure time across cultures: Developmental opportunities and risks. New directions in child and adolescent development*. San Francisco: Jossey-Bass.

Vithal, R. (2003). Teachers and 'street children': On becoming a teacher of mathematics. *Journal of Mathematics Teacher Education, 6*, 165–183.

Votta, E., & Manion, I. G. (2003). Factors in the psychological adjustment of homeless adolescent males: The role of coping style. *Journal of American Academy of Child and Adolescent Psychiatry, 42*, 778–785.

Wall, T. L., & Ehlers, C. L. (1995). Acute effects of alcohol on P300 in Asians with different ALDH2 genotypes. *Alcoholism: Clinical & Experimental Research, 19*, 617–622.

Wanner, B., Ladouceur, R., Auclair, A. V., & Vitaro, F. (2006). Flow and dissociation: Examination of mean levels, cross-links, and links to emotional well-being across sports and recreational and pathological gambling. *Journal of Gambling Studies, 22*, 289–304.

White, N. M. (1996). Addictive drugs as reinforces: Multiple partial actions on memory systems. *Addiction, 9*, 921–949.

White, F. J. (1998). Cocaine and the serotonin saga. *Nature, 393*, 118–119.

Wilder, L. K. (2002). The homeless are people, too: Including homeless students in educational programming. In F. E. Obiakor & P. A. Grant (Eds.), *Educating all learners: Refocusing the comprehensive support model* (pp. 68–83). Springfield, IL: Charles C. Thomas Publisher.

Williams, C. (1993). Who are the "street children"? A hierarchy of street use and appropriate responses. *Child Abuse and Neglect, 17*, 831–841.

Williams, L., & Parker, H. (2001). Alcohol, cannabis, ecstasy and cocaine: Drugs of reasoned choice amongst young adult recreational drug users in England. *International Journal of Drug Policy, 12*, 397–413.

Woodhead, M. (1999). Combating child labour. Listen to what the children say. *Childhood, 6*, 27–49.

World Health Organization. (2005). *Neuroscience of psychoactive substance use and dependence*. Geneva: WHO.

Worthman, C. M., & Panter-Brick, C. (2008). Homeless street children in Nepal: Use of allostatic load to assess the burden of childhood adversity. *Development and Psychopathology, 20*, 233–255.

Zanetti, E. (2002). *Educativa di strada: Brasile ed Italia a confronto*. Unpublished Master dissertation, Università Cattolica del Sacro Cuore di Milano, Italy.

Epilogue

...Time past and time future
Allow but a little consciousness.
To be conscious is not to be in time
But only in time can the moment on the rose-garden,
The moment in the arbour where the rain beat,
The moment in the draughty church at smokefall
Be remembered; involved with past and future.
Only through time time is conquered.
T.S. Eliot – Four Quartets: Burnt Norton, II

This book aimed at offering readers a journey into the labyrinthine realm of human consciousness, a journey dense of uncertainty and unsolved questions. A thin Ariadne's thread guided this journey: optimal experience, as an instrument to investigate the diverse pathways of development individuals follow and actively build during their lives.

Optimal experience is apparently a very fragile thread to walk across the mind labyrinth: it consists of moments—hours—arising and fading during daily life, providing enjoyment, engagement, and a feeling of mastery, but evading individual control. However, right because of this evasiveness and unpredictability, it is a precious resource supporting the laborious task of human growth and development, making it lighter and smoother.

Along the traces of optimal experience, our journey took us from the inner psychological processes to the external world, across the natural, social, and built environments in which individuals move, choose, and act. Framing optimal experience within the human biological and cultural inheritance systems allowed us to examine it from a time-space perspective, shedding light on its phenomenology as a transient event, on its origins and long-term implications for individuals and societies.

Along this journey, a powerful torch lit up our way: the enormous work of researchers and practitioners that in the last four decades have devoted their time and effort to understand optimal experience, its antecedents and consequences, its biological, cultural and psychological aspects, its potential as a tool for intervention. We tried to take into account all the contributions, and we apologize for having eventually overlooked some of them.

A. Delle Fave et al., *Psychological Selection and Optimal Experience Across Cultures*, Cross-Cultural Advancements in Positive Psychology 2,
DOI 10.1007/978-90-481-9876-4, © Springer Science+Business Media B.V. 2011

We hope that the readers can derive some useful information in accompanying us across the stories of men and women who had been generous enough to tell us about their optimal activities, their wishes and aspirations, their past and their future, thus allowing us to get some hints about the role of flow within the individual developmental path. We attempted to move from the individual level to the cultural one by comparing the experience of people coming from different countries, having different access to opportunities for flow in their life, experiencing hardship or affluence, living in metropolitan areas or in small villages, coping with extraordinary circumstances or with the little troubles of ordinary life. The collection of such a diversity of perspectives on the same issue allowed us to detect recurrences and discrepancies that could be partly related to culture, partly to the proximal social environment, and partly to idiosyncratic features.

We also found evidence of the fact that flow alone does not have the power to direct psychological selection. Activities providing flow in daily life, especially in the domain of leisure, are not included among individuals' present challenges and long-term goals. On the contrary, core pillars of individual well-being, such as family relations, are rarely quoted as opportunities for flow, and yet they predominate in the subjective lifelong perspective. Therefore, the study of flow has to be combined with the investigation of meaning and goal construction, at the individual level as well as at the social and cultural ones, in order to understand its role in the process of complexity development.

However, at the end of this journey we realize that there is a bulk of questions still to be answered, a great amount of topics still to be addressed from the biological, cultural, and psychological perspectives.

In spite of laudable efforts, little knowledge is available on the biological substrates of flow. As concerns its cultural dimensions, most studies were conducted among college students, teenagers, sport professionals and office or factory workers in industrialized countries. Our research group attempted to fill in this gap by visiting farmers, villagers, craftsmen, housewives, immigrants and members of ethnic minorities, people coping with physical and mental disease, drug addicts, street children, and religious people. We immodestly think that two decades of exploration allowed us to collect some evidence of both the universal- and culture-specific aspects of optimal experience. At the psychological level, still much research is needed to connect flow to basic psychological processes, and to other constructs in the research field of positive psychology and well-being promotion.

A major aspect is missing in this whole framework and in psychology in general. We ourselves have traveled the world assuming that flow would be a shared human feature, recurrent and stable across individuals and communities. This is actually what we found, or better, what we think we have found. Our studies led us to conclude that flow is the most positive state available to individuals within the daily fluctuations of experience. However, as some emotions are characteristic of specific cultures, or as self-construal patterns vary according to cultural features, we cannot rule out the possibility to identify positive states that have not yet been described by western psychologists. In Chapter 6 we offered only a limited example of the potential richness of studies adopting an emic perspective, and trying to understand flow from a different cultural and epistemological point of view. In order to do this, however, we need the contribution of non-western scholars willing to engage in this endeavor by taking a critical stance on the current pillars and certainties of scientific psychology.

We are still children...

Index

W

Y

Z